S0-AWV-398

Food and Cancer Prevention: Chemical and Biological Aspects

Food and Cancer Prevention: Chemical and Biological Aspects

Edited by

K.W. Waldron, I.T. Johnson, and G.R. Fenwick
AFRC Institute of Food Research, Norwich

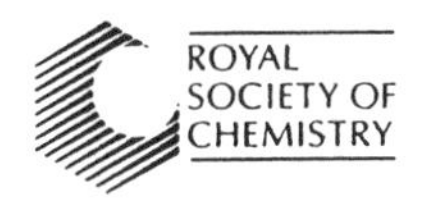

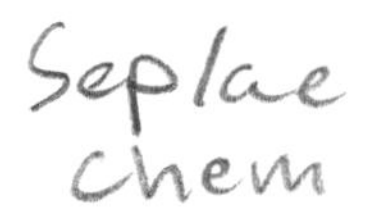

The Proceedings of an International Conference sponsored by the Food Chemistry Group of the Royal Society of Chemistry, held at Norwich, UK September 13–16, 1992.

Special Publication No. 123

ISBN 0-85186-455-4

A catalogue record for this book is available from the British Library

Published by The Royal Society of Chemistry,
Thomas Graham House, Science Park, Cambridge CB4 4WF

Printed by Bookcraft (Bath) Ltd.

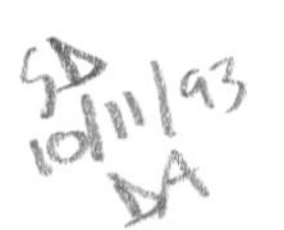

Preface

From the somewhat narrow perspective of the industrialised Western world we often think of cancer primarily as a disease of old age and affluence. In fact the environmental influences upon cancer are extremely complex. The geographical distribution of many cancers spans cultures and age groups and there is compelling statistical evidence to suggest that diet is amongst the most important determinants of cancers such as carcinoma of the oesophagus and stomach, which are common in the Middle East and Asia. In the West, carcinoma of the breast and colon are major causes of morbidity and death which often begin in middle age and also seem strongly linked to diet. Even lung cancer, for which the causal connection with cigarette smoking is beyond dispute, shows evidence of other environmental influences which may include a protective effect of diet.

Epidemiological evidence makes it clear that diet can protect against the development of cancer, and in some circumstances promote it. Developments in molecular and cell biology have recently led to significantly increased understanding of cell proliferation and differentiation, but there remains much to learn about the impact of diet on these basic biological mechanisms. Food and Cancer Prevention '92 was designed to explore these issues and to promote, and facilitate, constructive interdisciplinary interactions.

The meeting, held on the campus of the University of East Anglia, represented the third in a series of biennial conferences exploring the diet/health interface. The first meeting (Bioavailability 88), examined the area of nutrient availability, whilst Fibre 90 focused on dietary fibre. As befits a series of meetings organised and underwritten by the Food Chemistry Group of the Royal Society of Chemistry all three meetings emphasised the central role of chemistry and chemists, and also served to educate members of the profession in the challenges and opportunities inherent in these exciting areas.

The concept of Food and Cancer 92 originated from a workshop organised by RIKILT (State Institute for Quality Control) and the Wageningen Agricultural University in 1990, and it is appropriate, therefore, that at the time of writing a follow up meeting is being arranged for 1995. The field is rapidly moving and it is clear that over the next few years there will be many advances in techniques and understanding. It is to be hoped that the ideas presented, and discussed, in Norwich will have stimulated research, and encouraged progress.

The organisation of any meeting is a team effort. We are very grateful to the Scientific and Organising Committees for their hard work, to the numerous staff of the AFRC Institute of Food Research for their unflagging enthusiasm and efficiency, and to the Food Chemistry Group for its financial support. In the end, of course, the success of a meeting depends upon the participants and we would finally like to thank all those who attended the meeting.

K.W. Waldron
I.T. Johnson
G.R. Fenwick
January 1993

Contents

Part 5 Suppressing Tumour Development: The Role of Diet in the Modulation of Cell Proliferation

Part 6 Immune Mechanism: The Role of Food Components as Immunoregulators

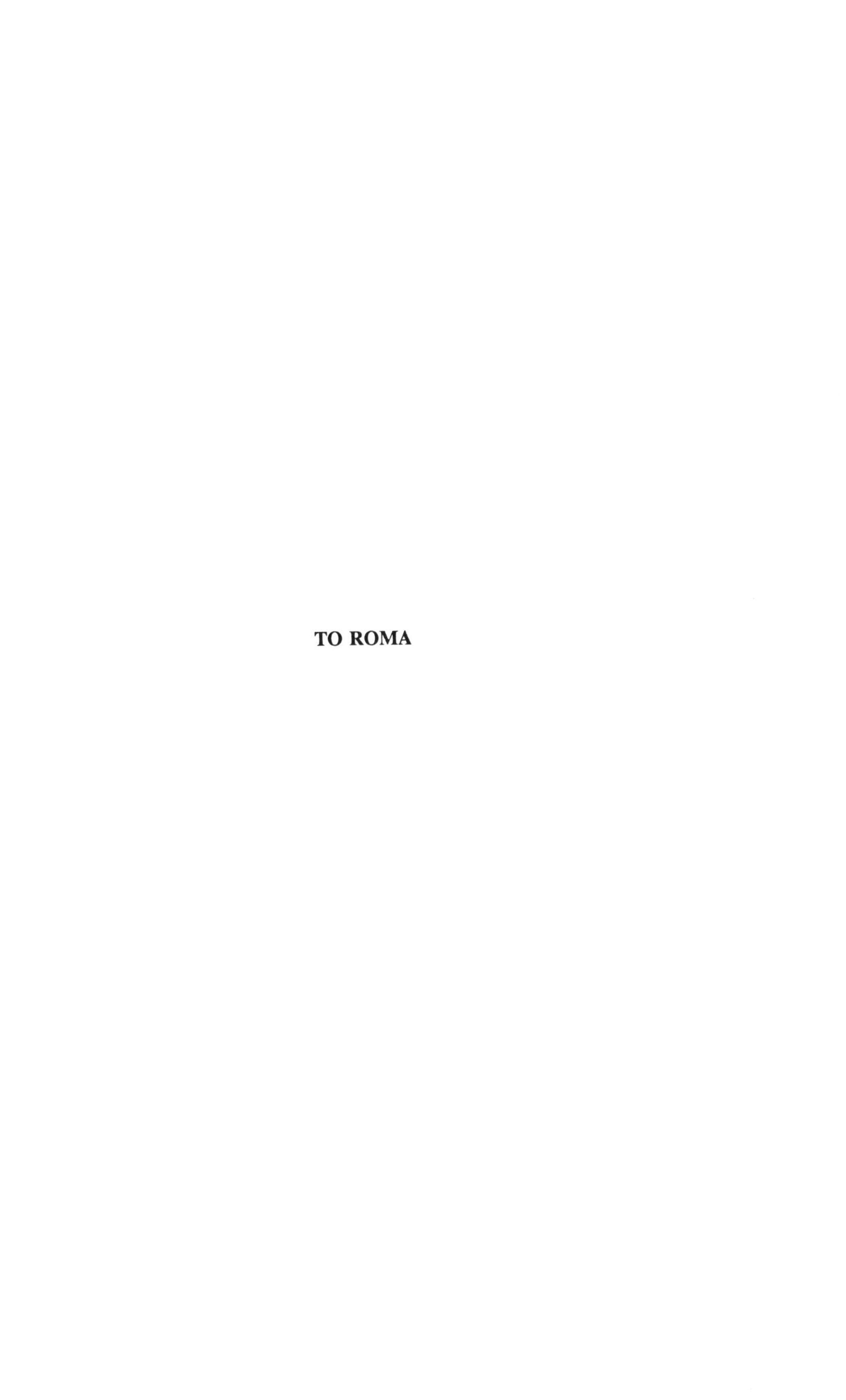

TO ROMA

PART 1 THE RELATIONSHIPS BETWEEN DIET AND CANCER IN HUMAN POPULATIONS

FOOD: ITS ROLE IN THE ETIOLOGY OF CANCER

Gary M. Williams, M.D.

American Health Foundation
Valhalla, NY 10595

1 INTRODUCTION

Apart from the necessity of food for the support of life, many healthful or harmful components of food have been known for centuries. The impact of nutrition on chronic diseases, however, began to emerge only in the early part of the century when cancer and cardiovascular diseases began to replace infectious diseases as the most important causes of early mortality. By 1908 in a major treatise on cancer, W. R. Williams concluded that "the incidence of cancer is largely conditioned by nutrition".[1] Knowledge of the role of diet has continued to accrue,[2,3] such that analysis of mortalities from cancers in the United States with respect to the prevalence of associated risk factors reveals that about 40% of cancer may be due to diet (Table 1).

Food contains both naturally occurring and synthetic components that either inhibit or facilitate the carcinogenic process.[4,5] The protective properties of food are described by Wattenberg (these proceedings) and hence, this paper focuses on causative elements. It must be kept in mind, however, that some protective elements act to a large extent by displacing causative elements. For example, a high fiber diet is usually a low fat diet.

Table 1 Estimated Causes of Cancer Mortality in the United States, 1992

TYPE	% OF TOTAL
Lifestyle cancers	
Tobacco-related: lung, pancreas, bladder, kidneys	30-35
Diet-related:	
High fat, low fiber, broiled or fried foods? - large bowel, breast, pancreas, prostate, ovary endometrium	30-35
Nitrate-nitrite, low vitamin C - stomach	2-3
Alcohol, mycotoxins - liver	3-4
Tobacco and alcohol related: oral cavity, esophagus	3-4
Viruses: human papilloma - cervix, penis, anus; hepatitis B - liver; HTLV-1 - adult T-cell leukemia; Epstein-Barr - B-cell lymphoma	1-5
Sunlight - skin (melanoma)	1-2
Occupational cancers: various carcinogens - bladder and other organs	1-2
Lifestyle and occupational exposures: tobacco and asbestos; tobacco and mining; tobacco and uranium and radium - lung, respiratory tract	3-4
Iatrogenic: radiation, drugs - diverse organs, leukemia	1-2
Genetic: retinoblastoma, ?soft tissue sarcomas	0-1

Based on 2 and 15

2 MECHANISMS OF CARCINOGENESIS

In the evolution of a neoplasm, there are two necessary and distinct sequences, the generation of a neoplastic cell and the growth and development of the neoplastic cell into a tumor.[5] Generally, agents that effect neoplastic conversion do so by causing genetic alterations whereas those that facilitate neoplastic development act through epigenetic effects. Both sequences are caused and modulated by a variety of factors, including components of diet.[6] Cancer is a multi-factorial disease and for each type of cancer it is necessary to identify the factors that initiate the process, presumably genotoxic agents, and those that enhance the process, co-carcinogenic or promoting agents.

3 NUTRITION AND CANCER

One of the major ways in which diet contributes to cancer etiology is through imbalances in nutrients, either inadequacies or excesses (Table 2).

Table 2 Dietary Impacts on Cancer in 1992

FACTOR	ESTIMATED IMPORTANCE	
	Western Communities	Asian/African Communities
Nutritional excesses	+++	+
Nutritional inadequacies	++	++
Carcinogens formed in food	?+	+
Food contaminants and additives	0	++

Nutritional Inadequacies

Deficiencies in micronutrients have been associated with cancer under specific circumstances, for example riboflavin and iron deficiencies and cancer of the esophagus[7]. The most significant inadequacy in the Western diet is low fiber intake (less than 25g per day). A protective effect of dietary fiber against colon cancer[7] was suggested by Burkitt.[8] The support from epidemiologic studies has not been consistent[9], due to some extent to the difficulty in defining fiber. Nevertheless, there have been sufficient negative associations[10] to conclude that fiber is important. Moreover, animal studies have revealed a protective effect of fiber on colon cancer[3] and also on breast cancer.[11] The mechanism for the protective effect of fiber against colon cancer involves complexing of bile acids, which are promoters of colon cancer, as well as other possible effects.[3,12]

Another inadequacy that has been identified epidemiologically to be linked to cancer risk is low intake of fruits and vegetables and stomach cancer.[13,14] This may relate to inadequate levels of micronutrients or antioxidants.[15]

Nutritional Excesses. Excess fat consumption (greater than 20% of calories or 40 g per day) is strongly associated with an increased prevalence of colon and breast cancer and possibly prostate and pancreas cancer.[3] Animal models generally reveal that dietary fat influences cancer development in the breast,[16] colon,[17] pancreas and prostate, although specific exceptions have been observed. Some experiments have been interpreted to show that the effect of high fat diets is entirely attributable to increased caloric intake, but analysis of the collective literature reveals a specific enhancing effect of dietary fat, as well as a general enhancing effect of calories.[18] Nevertheless, caloric intake and possibly nutrient density are of importance. It is noteworthy that in animal models, the only modulation of diet that consistently maintains maximal longevity is caloric restriction.[19]

An important aspect of fat is the content of fatty acids.[20] Generally, diets high in n-6 polyunsaturated fatty acids (linoleic acid) enhance tumor development, whereas those high in n-3 polyunsaturated fatty acids (linolenic acid) diminish tumor development.[17,21]

Excess salting of foods has been associated with increased risk of stomach cancer[22] and animal studies provide support.[23]

Overall, nutritional excesses have greatest impact on cancers in the Western world (Table 2).

4 FOOD COMPONENTS AND CANCER

Specific carcinogenic substances can occur in food through several sources (Table 3).

Highly sensitive techniques are available for the detection of these and generally they have been held to very low levels. In the past, however, nitrate was used at high levels for food preservation and likely contributed to the formation of carcinogens suspected to be involved in the high incidence of stomach cancer prevalent in the early 1900's.[24] Also, aflatoxins, which were not discovered until 1960, were likely at significant levels in some crops prior to this time.[25] It is tempting to speculate that the decline in liver cancer in the U.S. may relate to reduced mycotoxin exposure. Obviously, the large number of rodent hepatocarcinogens such as organochlorine pesticides that have been present in food have not led to an increase in human liver cancer.

During the cooking of food, a variety of heterocyclic amines are formed in the browning reaction.[26] These genotoxic agents are potent multispecies and multiorgan carcinogens. It has been postulated that they may be the initiating agents for breast and colon cancer in the Western world.[15]

Nitrosamines are formed from common precursors in the diet and are postulated to be the initiating agents for esophageal cancer.[27] Certain nitrosamines induce esophageal cancer in rodents.[28]

Table 3 Sources of Carcinogens in Food

SOURCE	EXAMPLE
Naturally Occurring	
Plant	cycasin
Microbial	mycotoxins
Contaminant	
Introduced before processing	DDT
Introduced during processing	trichloroethylene methylene chloride
Additive	butylated hydroxytoluene saccharin
Formed from food components	
Formed during processing	nitrosamines phenol diazonium compounds
Formed during preparation	benzo(a)pyrene heterocyclic amines
Formed in the body	nitrosamides/nitrosamines

No synthetic food additive has been associated with cancer in humans.[29] This is as would be expected since carcinogens are not allowed as food additives. Thus, the conclusion of Shubik[30] in 1980 that the contribution of then used intentional food additives, processing agents, pesticides and packaging materials to the total cancer incidence appears to be nil is still valid. Nevertheless, one food "additive", salt, appears to play a role in stomach cancer.[22,23]

5 CONCLUSIONS

It is well established that patterns of food consumption are associated with incidences of certain cancers and that food contains specific carcinogens. The information reviewed here supports the conclusion that food-borne elements contribute to the prevalence of the main cancers (Table 4).

Table 4 Food-Borne Etiologic Agents for Human Cancers

CANCER	GENOTOXIC CARCINOGEN	ENHANCING OR PROMOTING FACTOR
Colon	?heterocyclic amines	high fat diet low fiber diet
Breast	?heterocyclic amines	high fat diet low fiber diet
Stomach	?phenol diazonium compound	low intake of fruits and vegetables high intake of salted food
Liver	aflatoxins	alcohol
Esophagus	?nitrosamines	alcohol
Prostate		high fat diet
Pancreas		high fat diet

Thus, a major focus for cancer prevention must be on assessment of the role of nutrition and food components. The potential for dietary modification to affect cancer rates is illustrated by the decline of stomach cancer in the Western world. Rates in the United States have decreased from 38 deaths per 100,000 white males in 1930 to 7 per 100,000 in 1985 and from 28 deaths per 100,000 white females to 4 per 100,000.[24] The most likely explanation for this decline is changes in methods of food preservation. The use of salting and nitrates has diminished[31] in favor of canning, freezing and refrigeration. Salt and nitrates provide substrates for the formation of carcinogens and salt is a promoter of stomach cancer in animal models. Thus, reduction of these elements could lessen carcinogenic effects in the stomach.

Another cancer that has declined in the United States in both males and females is liver cancer. This is in spite of increased exposure to food-borne animal liver carcinogens such as DDT and BHT. One liver carcinogen that has been carefully controlled over the past 25 years is aflatoxins. Since mutations in the p53 gene in hepato cellular cancer show a specific pattern similar to that induced by aflatoxin in rodents,[32,33] it may be possible to retrieve material from before 1960 to assess the contribution of aflatoxin.

Regardless of the basis for the decline of these cancers, their reduction clearly demonstrates that cancer can be prevented. The current knowledge of the role of nutrition in the etiology of major cancers such as colon and breast offers a compelling opportunity for cancer reduction.

REFERENCES

1. W. R. Williams, The Natural History of Cancer, William Wood & Co., New York, 1908, p. 350.
2. J.H. Weisburger and G.M. Williams, 'Cancer Medicine, 2nd Edition', Lea and Febiger, Philadelphia, 1982, Chapter I-4, p. 42.
3. B.S. Reddy and L.A. Cohen (eds), 'Diet, Nutrition and Cancer: A Critical Evaluation', CRC Press, Boca Raton, FL, 1986.
4. B.N. Ames, Science, 1983, 221, 1256.
5. G.M. Williams and J.H. Weisburger, Casarett and Doull's Toxicology The Basic Sciences of Poisons, 4th Ed., Pergamon Press, New York, 1991, Chapter 5, p. 127.
6. G.M. Williams, J.H. Weisburger and E.L. Wynder, 'Carcinogens and Mutagens in the Environment, Volume 1: Food Products', CRC Press, Boca Raton, FL, 1982, p. 53.
7. E.L. Wynder and J.H. Fryer, Ann Int Med. 1956, 49, 1106.
8. D. Burkitt, Cancer, 1971, 28, 3.
10. G.E. McKeown-Eyssen, Prev Med, 1987, 16, 532.
11. J.L. Freudenheim, S. Graham, P.J. Horvath, J.R. Marshall, B.P. Haughey and G. Wilkinson, Cancer Res, 1990, 50, 3295.
11. D.P. Rose, Nutr. Cancer, 1990, 13, 1.
12. D.M. Klurfeld, Cancer Res (Suppl), 1992, 52, 2055s.
13. D. Trichopoulos, G. Ouranos, N.E. Day, A. Tzanou, O. Mansusos, Ch. Papadimitriou and A. Trichopoulos, Int. J. Cancer, 1985, 36, 291.
14. P.H. Chyou, A.M.Y. Nomura, J.H. Hankin and G.N. Stemmerman, Cancer Res., 1990, 50, 7501.
15. J.H. Weisburger, 'Macronutrients. Investigating Their Role in Cancer', Marcel Dekker, Inc., New York, 1992.
16. C.W. Welsch, Cancer Res., 1992, 52, 2040s.
17. B.S. Reddy, C. Burill and J. Rigotty, Cancer Res., 1991, 51, 487.
18. L.S. Freedman, C. Clifford and M. Messina, Cancer Res., 1990, 50, 5710.
19. E.J. Masoro, 'The Potential for Nutritional Modulation of Aging Processes', Food & Nutrition Press, Inc. Trumbull, CN, Chapter 8, p. 123.
20. W. T. Cave, Jr. FASEB J. 1991, 5, 2160.
21. K.K. Caroll and L.M. Braden, Nutr. Cancer, 1984, 6, 254.
22. R.W. Kneller, W.D. Guo, A.W. Hsing, J.S. Chen, W.J. Blot, J.Y. Li, D. Forman and J.F. Fraumeni, Jr., Cancer Epidem. Biomarkers and Prev., 1992, 1, 113.
23. M. Takahashi, T. Kokubo, F. Furukawa, Y. Kurokawa, M. Tatematsu and Y. Hayashi, Gann, 1983, 74, 28.
24. C.C. Boring, T.S. Squires and T. Tong, 'Cancer Statistics', American Cancer Society, Atlanta, GA, 1992.
25. V. Betina, Mycotoxins. Chemical, Biological and Environmental Aspects,

Elsevier Science Publ. Co., New York, 1989.
26. K. Wakabayashi, M. Nagao, H. Esumi and T. Sugimura, Cancer Res., 1992, 52, 2092s.
27. V.M. Craddock, Eur. J. Cancer Prev., 1992, 1, 89.
28. V.M. Craddock and H.E. Driver, Carcinogenesis, 1987, 8, 1129.
29. International Agency for Research on Cancer, IARC Monographs on the Evaluation of Carcinogenic Risks to Humans. Overall Evaluations of Carcinogenicity: An Updating of IARC Monographs Volumes 1 to 42, Suppl. 7, Lyon, 1987.
30. P. Shubik, Prev. Med., 1980 9, 197.
31. P.E. Hartman, Environ. Mut., 1983, 5, 111.
32. I.C. Hsu, R.A. Metcalf, T. Sun, J.A. Welsch, N.J. Wang and C.C. Harris Nature (Lond), 1991, 350, 427.
33. B. Bressar, M. Kew, J. Wands and M. Ozturk, Nature (Lond), 1991, 350, 429.

INHIBITION OF CARCINOGENESIS BY NONNUTRIENT CONSTITUENTS OF THE DIET

Lee W. Wattenberg, M.D.

Department of Laboratory Medicine & Pathology
University of Minnesota
Minneapolis, MN 55455, USA

INTRODUCTION

The occurrence of cancer can be prevented by a surprisingly large number of chemical compounds. This type of prevention is referred to as "chemoprevention."[1] Two forms exist. One, designated "general population chemoprevention," entails efforts at providing measures that are applicable to large population groups; the other, "targeted chemoprevention," is directed toward individuals at increased risk of cancer in specific tissues. The two differ in terms of allowable toxicity and specificity of agent targeting. A driving force for general population chemoprevention has been both epidemiological and experimental data indicating protective effects of dietary constituents against the occurrence of cancer.

Epidemiological studies have shown that diets containing large quantities of vegetables and, to a lesser extent, fruits are associated with relatively low risks of cancer.[2] The assignment of which constituents of these foods of plant origin are responsible for protection has been indecisive. In the search for inhibitory compounds, a group currently under investigation is that of the minor nonnutrient constituents of the diet.[3,4] This presentation provides an overview of experimental studies in which members of this very diverse group of compounds have been shown to inhibit carcinogenesis. The implications of these data could be quite profound. Ultimately, they could be relevant to decisions on food selection and composition for the purpose of providing increased protection against cancer, as well as for possible use of individual compounds as specific dietary adjuncts.

Foods contain both major and minor constituents. The major ones are protein, fat, carbohydrate and fiber. Foods also contain many minor dietary constituents. Some of these are nutrients, such as vitamins and minerals. In addition, there are a large number of nonnutrients, i.e. compounds that have no nutritional value. It is this latter group that will be the principle focus of this paper. Many of the nonnutrient compounds are unfamiliar to individuals in the biomedical sciences and even to those whose specialty is nutrition. They have been ignored because they seem to be biologically quite inert. However, it is becoming apparent that some of these compounds can have rather profound effects in preventing the occurrence of cancer.

The role of nonnutrients in the diet in preventing cancer comes from three levels of data, each of which is successively more defined.[4] The first level consists of data derived from studies in which comparisons of carcinogenic responses were made between animals fed crude diets composed of natural constituents containing both nutrients and nonnutrients and semi-purified diets composed almost entirely of purified materials and almost completely lacking nonnutrients. In several of these experiments, the comparisons show a lower tumor response in animals fed the crude diets.[5-8] The results of these studies are of particular importance because they suggest a protective role of nonnutrients in some carcinogenic processes, and in addition that the concentration of the nonnutrients in conventional diets is adequate to bring about this preventive effect. The second level of information consists of studies in which a single crude dietary constituent, such as a vegetable or fruit or a crude product derived from these foods of plant origin, have been investigated. Some examples are cruciferous vegetables, citrus fruit oils, garlic oil and tea, all of which have been shown to inhibit carcinogenesis in experimental animals.[3,4]

Inhibition of carcinogenesis by specific nonnutrient constituents of the diet

The finding of specific compounds of plant origin that have inhibitory effects on carcinogenesis has been the result of two lines of investigation. One of these has been the identification of a constituent from crude plant materials. The plant material employed had carcinogen inhibitory effects or was shown to produce a biological response, such as enhancement of detoxification systems, likely to result in cancer prevention. Thus, d-limonene, a major constituent of citrus fruit oils that inhibit carcinogenesis, was found to be a preventive agent.[1,9] In the case of cruciferous vegetables that inhibit carcinogenesis, several groups of inhibitors have been identified. These include indoles, aromatic isothiocyanates, dithiolethiones, and phenols.[1,3,4] Studies in progress aimed at identifying the active constituents of garlic and onion oils that result in inhibition of carcinogenesis have shown that a number of organosulfur compounds present in these oils have inhibitory properties.[4,10]

The second type of investigation that has resulted in identification of nonnutrient dietary inhibitors has focused initially on synthetic compounds. Subsequently, the presence of the compound itself or a structurally related compound was found in natural products. Thus initial studies of a series of synthetic chemicals resulted in identification of flavone as an inhibitor. Flavone, itself is a synthetic compound. However, in subsequent work, a large number of naturally-occurring flavone derivatives were found to be inhibitors of carcinogenesis.[1]

The mechanisms of action of many of the minor nonnutrient inhibitors of carcinogenesis are poorly understood making it difficult to organize them into a precise pattern. One way of providing an organizational framework is to classify inhibitors according to the time in the carcinogenic process at which they are effective.[1] Utilizing this framework, inhibitors of carcinogenesis can be divided into three categories. The first consists of compounds that prevent the formation of carcinogenesis from precursor substances. The second are compounds that inhibit carcinogenesis by preventing carcinogenic agents from reaching or reacting with critical target sites in the tissues. These inhibitors are called "blocking agents", which is descriptive of their mechanism of action. They exert a barrier function. The third category of inhibitors acts subsequent to exposures to carcinogenic agents. These inhibitors are termed "suppressing agents", since they act by suppressing the expression of neoplasia in cells previously exposed to doses of carcinogen that otherwise would cause cancer. During the course of studies of various inhibitors it became apparent that some inhibitors act at more than one time point in the carcinogenic process.[1,4]

Blocking agents

Blocking agents can prevent genotoxic compounds from reaching or reacting with critical target sites. Characteristically they are effective when administered prior to or simultaneously with carcinogenic agents. The genotoxic consequences such as reduced adduct formation can be found. A large literature exists describing the mechanisms of action of blocking agents. There are three known means by which blocking agents act. One is to inhibit activation reactions of genotoxic compounds requiring metabolic activation. A second entails induction of increases in the activity of enzyme systems that can detoxify these compounds. A third mechanism is the trapping of reactive genotoxic species. The work on inhibition of genotoxic compounds has been extensively reviewed.[1] Table 1 contains a list of nonnutrient blocking agents that inhibit genotoxic compounds.

Table 1. Some nonnutrient blocking agents effective against genotoxic compounds

Terpenes[1,9,11]	Curcumin[24,25]
Organosulfides[12,13,14]	Coumarins[1]
Aromatic isothiocyanates[4,15,16]	Conjugated dienoic linoleic acids[26,27]
Indoles[1]	Nucleophiles[1,28]
Dithiolethiones[1,17]	18-β-Glycyrrhetinic acid and related triterpenoids[29,30]
Phenols[1]	Glucarates[3,31]
Flavones[1]	Rosemary extract[32]
Tannins[18-20]	
Ellagic acid[21-23]	

In addition to effect on genotoxic compounds, some blocking agents are effective against neoplastic responses to nongenotoxic compounds. The most extensive studies of this nature are of inhibition of tumor promoters. Table 2 contains a list of major groups of blocking agents that inhibit the actions of tumor promoters.

Table 2. Some nonnutrient blocking agents effective against tumor promoters

Inhibitors of arachidonic acid metabolism[1]	Chalcones[36]
Phenols[1]	Organosulfides[37]
Modulators of polyamine metabolism[1]	Tannins[33]
Protease inhibitors[1]	Curcumin[38]
Glycyrrhetinic acid and related tri-terpenoid compounds[39]	Flavonoids[34,35]

One of the most common characteristics of inhibitors of tumor promotion is the capacity to inhibit the arachidonic acid cascade.[1,40] A second feature that frequently is found in blocking agents inhibiting tumor promotion is the capacity to prevent attack by oxygen radicals. This can be brought about by the inhibitor acting as an antioxidant or by the compound preventing formation of oxygen radicals.[41-43] For example, an antioxidant function is a common attribute of phenolic or polyphenolic compounds. In contrast, protease inhibitors and inhibitors of the arachidonic acid cascade can inhibit tumor promotion by preventing formation of oxygen radicals.[40,43] It will be noted that some chemopreventive agents appear in both Table 1 and Table 2. This can be the result of the compound being multifunctional. For example, a phenolic compound such as butylated hydroxyanisole, is an antioxidant and, in addition, it is capable of induction of detoxification systems.[1] The appearance in both tables also may be due to the capacity of a compound, such as a thiol, to block the actions of different categories of attacking molecules, some genotoxic and other non-genotoxic.

Suppressing agents

Suppressing agents prevent the evolution of the neoplastic process in cells previously exposed to doses of carcinogenic agents that otherwise would cause cancer.[1] Characteristically these inhibitors are effective when given subsequent to all administrations of carcinogenic agents i.e. full carcinogens, tumor promoters and progressing (converting) agents. With these time relationships they can be distinguished from blocking agents. Table 3 contains a list of minor nonnutrient constituents of the diet that can act as suppressing agents in animal models.

Table 3. Some nonnutrient suppressing agents

- Protease inhibitors[43-46]
- (-)-Epigallocatechin gallate[33]
- Inhibitors of the arachidonic acid cascade[1,47-49]
- Terpenes[50]
- Aromatic isothiocyanates[1]
- Inositol hexaphosphate[51,52]
- Nerolidol[53]
- 4-hydroxy-2(or 5)-ethyl-5(or 2)-methyl-3(2H)-furanone[54]

The number of suppressing agents that have been identified is considerably less than that for blocking agents. As described previously, the concept of the mechanisms by which blocking agents act is relatively simple, although the systems themselves can be very complex. Both in vitro and in vivo test systems for identifying potential blocking agents are available and a substantial number of these compounds have been found. In the case of suppressing agents, the mechanisms of their action often are not well defined. This might be expected since the events that they must counteract are those basic to cancer, which itself is incompletely understood. Four mechanisms by which suppressing agents may act are listed in Table 4. Others almost certainly exist. Some suppressing agents act by more than one mechanism.

Table 4. Some mechanisms of action of suppressing agents

1. Prevent endogenous formation of "attacking" molecules or inactivate those that are formed.
2. Directly counteract consequences of genotoxic events.
3. Produce differentiation.
4. Selectively inhibit cellular proliferation of potentially neoplastic cells.

In Table 4, the first mechanism listed by which suppressing agents may act is "prevention of endogenous formation of attacking molecules or inactivation of those that are formed." The first three groups of suppressing agents discussed below would have the capacity to inhibit by this mechanism. However all three are multifunctional so that other mechanisms may be involved as well.

The first group of suppressing agents listed in Table 3 are the protease inhibitors. In vitro studies showing suppressive effects by protease inhibitors on cellular transformation are well documented[55,56] In addition, these compounds have been found to inhibit carcinogenesis in experimental animals.[45,46] Protease inhibitors have been shown to prevent formation of oxygen radicals.[44,45,55,56] Thus one component of their suppressing mechanism may reside in the capacity to prevent formation of attacking molecules, in this instance oxygen radicals. Protease inhibitors have biological effects other than preventing oxygen radical formation as has been described in several reviews of this interesting group of compounds.[44,45] At present it is not clear which of the attributes of these compounds is critical for the chemopreventive capacities that they exhibit.

The second group of suppressing agents listed in Table 3 are the arachidonic acid cascade inhibitors. These are a very important group of suppressing agents. After the retinoids, there are more studies showing inhibition of carcinogenesis with arachidonic acid cascade inhibitors than any other group of chemopreventive agents. Most of the animal studies with the arachidonic acid cascade inhibitors have been done with two synthetic compounds, indomethacin and piroxicam.[1,47-49] They inhibit carcinogenesis of the large bowel and breast. In some instances inhibition has been obtained in experiments in which the compounds were administered starting several months after the last dose of a carcinogenic agent. In humans, piroxicam has been reported to cause regression of adenomatous polyps of the large bowel.[57] Epidemiology studies in the human suggest that aspirin, a less potent arachidonic acid cascade inhibitor, may reduce the occurrence of large bowel cancer in humans.[58] The overall background of efficacy of the arachidonic acid cascade inhibitors is impressive. Its importance to the area of diet and cancer resides in the fact that a relatively large number of naturally occurring nonnutrient constituents of food have inhibitory effects on the arachidonic acid cascade in vitro. These include monophenols, polyphenols, flavonoids, and curcumin.[1,40,70,71] Some, but not all of the in vitro inhibitors prevent carcinogenesis in vivo.

The third inhibitor listed in Table 3 is (-)-epigallocatechin gallate.[20,33] This compound is an antioxidant but has other functional attributes.[20] Evidence as to which of these is critical to its suppressive effects is lacking. There are compounds such as synthetic derivations of ascorbic acid that have strong scavenging capacities for active oxygen species and do not have other apparent attributes that could account for their inhibiting effects.[42] Under these conditions chemoprevention appears due to the radical trapping function.

Protease inhibitors, arachidonic acid cascade inhibitors and (-)-epigallocatechin gallate have been shown to inhibit the effects of tumor promoters when administered prior to or simultaneously with the promoting agent and to suppress carcinogenesis in experiments in which they were given days or weeks subsequent to all administrations of promoters or other carcinogenic agents. The data on inhibition of tumor promotion suggests that the mechanism of action entails prevention of oxygen or peroxy radical formation due to exposure to the exogenous promoting agent or to scavenging the radicals that are formed. It is possible that a similar mechanism may be involved in the capacity of these compounds to act as suppressing agents at least in some instances. Under these conditions, the suppressing agents would be acting against, radical formation due to endogenous stimuli. Endogenous formation of mutagenic compounds, in particular oxygen radicals has been discussed in detail by Ames and his colleagues.[59,60] The protease inhibitors, arachidonic acid cascade inhibitors and (-)-epigallocatechin gallate have a variety of biological effects other than those related to oxygen radicals so that the mechanism(s) of inhibition of carcinogenesis by these compounds remains to be firmly established.

Although trapping mechanisms have generic implications, considerable specificity may be present in vivo. This may be due to the nature of the attacking species as well as pharmacological properties such as those due to tissue and species differences. It should be emphasized that a compound showing trapping capacities in vitro may not act by this mechanism in vivo. Many compounds are multifunctional. This caveat is particularly relevant to considerations of the mechanisms of inhibition by the protease inhibitors, the arachidonic acid cascade inhibitors and

(-)-epigallocatechin gallate, all of which are multifunctional.

A second mechanism by which suppressing agents may act is by directly counteracting mechanistic consequences of genotoxic events, Table 4. Conceptually, this is a very attractive mechanism of inhibition since it relates a specific defect to a specific remedy. As increasing information is obtained about the carcinogenic process, the data show sequences of mutational events occurring during the carcinogenic process. Studies by Vogelstein and his colleagues highlight such sequences and accumulations.[61] For each mutational event, the possibility of counteracting its manifestations by some chemopreventive agent exists. Several investigators have focused on this strategy. Of particular interest in this regard has been work on mutated ras oncogenes, a common early event in the carcinogenic process. The ras oncogene product is a protein designated $p21^{ras}$ which becomes isoprenylated. The mevalonic acid pathway results in the synthesis of farnesyl pyrophosphate which becomes bound to the $p21^{ras}$ protein by the enzyme farnesyl:protein transferase.[62-64] Inhibition of isoprenylation can reduce the amount of the active mutated gene product.

One line of investigation pertinent to nonnutrient constituents of the diet that can inhibit activated oncogene activity has been directed at inhibiting isoprenylation of the ras protein. Monoterpenes can act in this manner. In early studies (±)-menthol and 1,8-cineole were reported to be inhibitors of HMG-CoA reductase activity in vivo.[65] This enzyme is pivotal for the synthesis of farnesol. However, the most detailed work on inhibition of isoprenylation has focused on d-limonene. This compound has been shown to inhibit $p21^{ras}$ isoprenylation in mammalian cells cultured in vitro and also in mammary tissue in vivo.[66] In related in vivo studies, d-limonene had a suppressive effect against N-methyl-N-nitrosourea induced mammary tumor formation in rats. Many of the mammary tumors produced in this experimental model contain an activated ras oncogene.[50] Orange oil, which contains over 95% limonene, also has been found to suppress mammary tumor formation in this experimental model.[4,50] Nerolidol, a naturally occurring compound structurally related to farnesol, and a putative analogue, has been reported to inhibit azoxymethane induced large bowel neoplasia.[53] The above data indicate that nonnutrient food constituents may impact on the consequences of oncogene activation.

In Table 4, the third mechanism of action listed for suppressing agents entails induction of differentiation. Differentiating agents have been studied in terms of their impact on both chemoprevention and also chemotherapy. The most extensively investigated differentiating agents are the retinoids, which are synthetic analogues of vitamin A. These compounds are very potent differentiating agents. Vitamin A itself has this attribute. However, it is relatively toxic at the high dose levels generally required to produce suppressing activity in vivo. Nevertheless, in a careful study, supplementation of the diet with vitamin A has been shown to inhibit carcinogen induced neoplasia of the breast in the rat.[67] β-Carotene has been studied extensively for its suppressing activity in animal models. Most of these studies have been negative. A few positive studies have been published, but most of these have not been confirmed. The one exception is inhibition of ultraviolet carcinogenesis of the skin, which is a special situation.[29] β-Carotene also has been reported to be effective against leukoplakia in the human.[68]

A fourth mechanism of action listed for suppressing agents in Table 4 consists of direct inhibition of cell proliferation. Hormone antagonists come under this heading. Inhibitors of ornithine decarboxylase inhibit cell proliferation. Difluoromethylornithine has been extensively studied in this regard. This compound, which is synthetic, appears to preferentially inhibit cell proliferation of preneoplastic cells as compared to normal cells. With difluoromethylornithine, it is possible to achieve a dose level that suppresses carcinogenesis by inhibiting cell proliferation of potentially neoplastic cells without producing significant toxicity in the host.

In Table 3, aromatic isothiocyanates are listed as suppressing agents. Only minimal data as to their suppressive effects are available. These compounds are multifunctional and their mechanism of inhibition is not known. Inositol hexaphosphate has been shown to inhibit large bowel carcinogenesis in the rat and the mouse. Inhibition occurs at relatively high dose levels, and solid data as to the mechanism of inhibition is lacking. As noted previously, nerolidol is a putative analogue of farnesol. However, its mechanism of action has not been established experimentally. Recently, 4-hydroxy-2(or 5)-ethyl-5(or 2)-methyl-3(2H)-furanone, a constituent of soy sauce has been reported to be a suppressing agent. This compound is an antioxidant but a full investigation of its mechanism of action has not been carried out. An additional nonnutrient, glycyrrhizin, has been reported to suppress spontaneous liver tumor formation in C3H/He male mice.[39] In summary, a variety of suppressing agents have been identified in foods. There is some knowledge as to their mechanisms of inhibition, but in most instances the information is incomplete.

CONCLUSIONS

Experimental studies have shown that foods contain a wide variety of nonnutrient compounds that can inhibit carcinogenesis. Most are of plant origin. These data are in accord with epidemiological observations of protective effects of vegetables and fruits against the occurrence of cancer. Many of the inhibitors are blocking agents, i.e. they prevent carcinogenic agents from reaching or reacting with critical target sites. Some are suppressing agents, i.e. compounds that prevent the evolution of the neoplastic process in cells that otherwise would become malignant. The precise role that the nonnutrient inhibitors of carcinogenesis play under various conditions of dietary selection that exist currently, or could play under optimal conditions, remains to be established. Ultimately some of the compounds may be useful as chemopreventive agents to be taken as dietary supplements.

REFERENCES

1. L.W. Wattenberg, Cancer Res., 1985, 45, 1.

2. Anonymous, Diet, Nutrition and Cancer, National Acad Press, Washington, D.C., 1982, pp 358.

3. L.W. Wattenberg, Cancer Res., 1983, 43, 2448s.

4. L.W. Wattenberg, Cancer Res., 1992, 52, 2085s.

5. H. Silverstone, R.D. Solomon, and A. Tannenbaum, Cancer Res., 1952, 12, 750.

6. S.S. Hecht, M.A. Morse, A. Shantu, G.D. Stoner, K.G. Jordan, C.-I. Choi, and F.-L, Chung, Carcinogenesis, 1989, 10, 1901.

7. L.W. Wattenberg, P. Borchert, C.M. Destafney, and J.B. Coccia, Cancer Res., 1983, 43, 4747.

8. D.S. Longnecker, B.D. Roebuck, J.D. Yager, H.S. Lilja, and B. Siegmund, Cancer, 1981, 47, 1562.

9. C.E. Elson, J.L. Maltzman, J.L. Boston, and M.A. Tabber, Carcinogenesis, 1988, 9, 331.

10. H. Sumiyoshi, and M.J. Wargovich, Cancer Res., 1990, 50, 5084.

11. L.W. Wattenberg, V.L. Sparnins, and G. Barany, Cancer Res., 1989, 49, 2689.

12. M.J. Wargovich, C. Woods, V.W.S. Eng, L.C. Stephens, and K. Gray, Cancer Res., 1988, 48, 6872.

13. V.L. Sparnins, G. Barany, and L.W, Wattenberg, Carcinogenesis (Lond.), 1988, 9, 131.

14. V.L. Sparnins, A.W. Mott, G. Barany, and L.W. Wattenberg, Nutr. Cancer, 1986, 8, 211.

15. F.L. Chung, in: Cancer Chemoprevention, 1992, CRC Press, Boca Raton, Fla (in Press).

16. M.A. Morse, C.X. Wang, G.D. Stoner, S. Mandal, P.B. Conran, G.A. Shantu, S. Hecht, and F.L. Chung, Cancer Res., 1989, 49, 549.

17. T.W. Kensler, J.D. Groopman, and B.D. Roebuck, in: Cancer Chemoprevention, 1992, CRC Press, Boca Raton, Fla (in press).

18. H. Mukhtar, M. Das, W.A. Khan, Z.Y. Wang, D.P. Bik, and D.R. Bickers, Cancer Res., 1988, 48, 2361.

19. M. Athar, W.A. Khan, and H. Mukhtar, Cancer Res., 1989, 49, 5784.

20. H. Fujiki, M. Suganuma, H. Suguri, K. Takagi, S. Yoshizawa, A. Ootsuyama, H. Tanooka, T. Okuda, M. Kobayashi, and T. Sugimura, Antimutagens and Anticarcinogenesis Mechanisms II, 1990, pp. 205.

21. S. Mandel and G.D. Stoner, Carcinogenesis, 1990, 11, 55.

22. R.L. Chang, M.-T. Huang, A.W. Wood, C.Q. Wong, H.L. Newmark, H. Yagi, J.M, Sayer, D.M. Jerind, and A.H. Conney, Carcinogenesis, 1985, 6, 1127.

23. T. Tanaka, H. Iwata, K. Niwa, Y. Mori, and H. Mori, Jpn. J. Cancer Res., 1988, 79, 1297.

24. M.-T. Huang, T. Lysz, T. Ferraro and A.H. Conney, in: Cancer Prevention, 1992, CRC Press, Boca Raton, Fla, (in press).

25. M.-T. Huang, R.C. Smart, and A.D. Conney, Proc. Am. Assoc. Cancer Res., 1987, 28, 173.

26. M.W, Pariza in: Cancer Prevention, 1992, CRC Press, Boca Raton, Fla (in press).

27. Y.L. Ita, J. Storkson, and M.L. Pariza, Cancer Res., 1990, 50, 1097.

28. R. Kato, T. Hakadate, S. Yamamoto, and T. Sugimura, Carcinogenesis, 1983, 4, 1301.

29. H. Nishino, K. Kitagawa, and A. Iwashima, Carcinogenesis, 1984, 5, 1529.

30. H. Tokuda, H. Ohigashi, K. Koshimizu and Y. Ito, Cancer Lett., 1986, 33, 279.

31. Z. Walaszek, M. Hanavsek-Walaszek, and T.E. Webb, Cancer Lett., 1986, 33, 25.

32. K.W. Singletary and J.M. Helshopper, Cancer Lett., 1991, 60, 175.

33. Y. Fujita, T. Yamane, M. Tanaka, K. Kuwato, J. Okuzumi, T. Takashi, H. Fujiki, and T. Okuda, Jap. J. Cancer Res., 1989, 80, 503.

34. R. Kato, T. Nakadate, S. Yamamoto, and T. Sugimura, Carcinogenesis, 1983, 4, 1301.

35. H. Wei, L. Tye, E. Bresnick and D.F. Birt, Cancer Res., 1990, 40, 499.

36. S. Yamamoto, E. Aizu, H. Jiang, T. Hakadate, I Kiuoto, J.C. Wang, and R. Kato, Carcinogenesis, 1991, 12, 317.

37. S. Belman, J. Solomon, H. Segal, E. Block, and G. Barany, J. Biochem Toxicol, 1989, 4, 151.

38. M.-T. Huang, T. Lysz, T. Ferraro, and A.H. Conney, in: Cancer Chemoprevention, 1992, CRC Press, Boca Raton, Fla (in press).

39. H. Hishino,in: Cancer Chemoprevention, 1992, CRC Press, Boca Raton, Fla (in press).

40. S. Yamamoto and R. Kato, in: Cancer Chemoprevention, 1992, CRC Press, Boca Raton, Fla (in press).

41. R.C. Smart, M.-T. Huang, Z.T. Han, M.C. Kaplan, A. Focella, and A.H. Conney, Cancer Research, 1987, 47, 6633.

42. H. Kushida, K. Wakabayashi, M. Suzuki, S. Takahashi, K. Imaida, T. Sugimura, and M. Hagao, Carcinogenesis, 1992, 13, 913.

43. W. Troll, J.S. Lim, and S. Belman, in: Cancer Chemoprevention, 1992, CRC Press, Boca Raton, Fla (in press).

44. W. Troll, R. Wiesner, and K. Frankel, Advances in Cancer Research, 1987, 49, 265

45. A.R. Kennedy and P.C. Billings, in: Proc. of 2nd International Conf. on "Anticarcinogenesis and Radiation Protection", P.A. Cerotti, O.F. Nygaard and M.S. Simic (eds), 1987, Plenum Press, N.Y. pp. 285.

46. P.E. Billings, P.M. Newberne, and A.R. Kennedy, Carcinogenesis, 1990, 11, 1083.

47. B.S. Reddy, K. Tokumo, N. Kulkarni, C. Aligia and G. Kelloff, Carcinogenesis, 1992, 13, 1019.

48. B.S. Reddy, H. Maruyama, and G. Kelloff, Cancer Research, 1987, 47, 5340.

49. T. Narisawa, M. Sato, M. Tani, T. Kudo, T. Takahashi, and A. Goto, Cancer Research, 1981, 41, 1954.

50. T.H. Maltzman, L.H. Hort, C.E. Elson, M.A. Tanner, and M.N. Gould, Carcinogenesis, 1989, 10, 771.

51. A. Shamsuddin, P M Elsayed, and A. Ullah, Carcinogenesis, 1988, 9, 577.

52. A. Shamsuddin and A. Ullah, Carcinogenesis, 1989, 10, 625.

53. L.W. Wattenberg, Carcinogenesis, 1991, 12, 151.

54. A. Nagahara, H. Benjamin, J. Stockson, J. Krewson, K. Sheng, W Liv and M.W Pariza, Cancer Res., 1992, 52, 19g2.

55. J. Yavelow, M. Collngs, Y. Birck, W. Troll, and A.R. Kennedy, Proc. Natl. Acad. Sci. USA, 1985, 82, 5395-5399.

56. A.R. Kennedy and J.B. Little, Cancer Research, 1981, 41, 2103.

57. D.L. Earnest, L.J. Hixson, P.R. Finley, G.G. Blackwell, J. Einspahr, S.S. Emerson, and D.S. Alberts, in: Cancer Chemoprevention, 1992, CRC Press, Boca Raton, Fla, (in press).

58. M.J. Thun, M.M. Namboodri, and C.W. Hath, Jr., New Engl. J. Med., 1991, 325, 1593-1596.

59. B N Ames and L.S. Gold, Mutation Res., 1991, 250, 3.

60. J.R. Wagner, C.C Hu and B.N. Ames, Proc Nat. Acad. Sci. USA, 1992, 89, 3380.

61. E.R. Fearson, and B Vogelstein, Cell, 1990, 61, 759.

62. J L Goldstein and Brown, Nature, 1990, 343, 425.

63. Y. Reiss, J.L. Goldstein, M.C. Seabra, P.J. Casey, and Brown, Cell, 1990, 62, 81.

64. W.A. Maltese, FASEB, 1990, 15, 3319.

65. R.J. Clegg, B. Middleton, C.D. Bell, and D.A. White, J Biol Chem, 1982, 257, 2294.

66. P.L. Crowell, R.R. Chang, Z. Ren, C.E. Elson, and M.N. Gould, J. Biol. Chem, 1991, 266, 176-79.

67. M.H. Zile, M.E. Cullum, I.A. Roltsch, J.V. DeHoog, and C.W. Welsch, Cancer Res., 1986, 46, 3503.

68. H. Garewol, F.L. Meyskens, D. Killen, D. Reeves, T.A. Kiersch, H. Elletson, A. Strosberg, D. King, and K. Steinbronn, J. Clin Oncol, 1990, 8, 1715.

69. F.L. Meyskens, D. Pelot, H. Meshkinpour, P. Plezia, E. Gerner, and S. Emerson, Cancer Chemoprevention, 1992, CRC Press, Boca Raton, Fla, (in press).

70. F.E. Dewhirst, Prostaglandins, 1980, 20, 209.

71. C. Kemal, P. Louis-Flamberg, R. Knopinsli-Olsen, and A.L. Shorter, Biochemistry, 1987, 26, 7064.

CONTRIBUTION OF EPIDEMIOLOGY IN ELUCIDATING THE ROLE OF FOODS IN CANCER PREVENTION

D. Kromhout, H.B. Bueno de Mesquita and M.G.L. Hertog

Division of Public Health Research
National Institute of Public Health
and Environmental Protection
P.O. Box 1
3720 BA Bilthoven
The Netherlands

1 ABSTRACT

Epidemiologic research suggests an important role for dietary factors in the occurrence of cancer. There is however much uncertainty about the strength of this association due to limitations of observational epidemiologic research and of dietary assessment methods. In cancer research mainly retrospective case-control studies are carried out. The most consistent finding of these studies is the inverse association between vegetable and fruit consumption and the occurrence of epithelial cancers. Whether this protective effect is due to nutrients e.g. carotenoids or non-nutritive substances e.g. flavonoids is not known. An example is given of a multidisciplinary project in which analytical chemists and epidemiologists work together to elucidate the importance of flavonoids as anticarcinogenic agents.

2 INTRODUCTION

Epidemiology has played a major role in identifying risk factors for cancer. Already in the nineteen fifties it became clear that smoking is an important risk factor for lung cancer. Later on it was shown that smoking was not only a risk factor for lung cancer but also for cancer of the mouth, pharynx, larynx, oesophagus, pancreas, kidney and bladder. Results from cross-cultural studies carried out in the nineteen sixties and seventies suggested that dietary factors could also play a role in the etiology of different types of cancer. In their landmark report on the causes of cancer Doll and Peto estimated that 30% of the occurrence of cancer is due to tobacco consumption and 35% may be related to dietary factors (1). However there is a large difference in the reliability of the estimates for smoking and diet. In 1981 the confidence limits for smoking were 25-40% and for diet 10-70%. The evidence for the important role of smoking not only for the occurrence of cancer but also for vascular diseases and chronic non-specific lung diseases was stressed in a recent article by Peto and co-workers (2). There is no doubt that smoking is a major risk factor for cancer. Although evidence is accumulating that certain dietary factors may be involved in cancer etiology it is still uncertain how important the dietary factors are. In the ILSI conference on "Nutrition and cancer" held April 1991 in Atlanta, Georgia, Doll gave as his current best estimate for the importance of diet in cancer causation 20-60%. The reason for this large range is that only limited evidence is available from (non)-experimental prospective studies. Most evidence is from cross-cultural and case-control studies.

In this paper strengths and weaknesses of observational epidemiologic studies in elucidating the role of food constituents in cancer etiology will be discussed. Special attention will be paid to the limitations of different epidemiologic designs and dietary survey methods. The possible protective effect of vegetables and fruits in relation to cancer occurrence will be taken as an illustration of the difficulties in elucidating the role of dietary factors in cancer prevention.

3 EPIDEMIOLOGIC STUDIES

Time plays an important role in classifying epidemiologic studies. If information on a dietary factor is collected before the occurrence of a disease the design of the study is called prospective. In retrospective studies information on diet is collected after disease occurrence. Retrospective studies are always observational in nature but prospective studies can have either an observational or an experimental design. The difference between these two is the manipulation of the dietary factor. In observational studies the investigator does not manipulate the dietary factor in contrast to experimental studies. This means that generally the contribution of experimental studies to the evidence on diet-cancer relations is larger than that from observational studies. However a well designed observational study in which besides information on the dietary factor also information is collected on important confounders, can be very informative.

Besides time it is also important to know whether the epidemiologic information was collected at the group or at the individual level. Cross-cultural studies use information at the group level e.g. dietary data describing the food consumption patterns of countries are related to cancer mortality patterns in these countries. In this type of study generally information on important confounding factors is lacking. Another important drawback of these studies is that the so-called ecologic fallacy may occur. Relations observed at the group level are not necessarily present at the individual level. This may be due to the fact that by averaging the dietary factors in a population artificial relations between diet and cancer may be described. It may also be possible that the determinants of a disease may be different at the population level compared with the individual level (3).

In judging the evidence for relations between dietary factors and cancer occurrence the most important factors to take into account are:
* time (prospective * retrospective)
* design (observational * experimental)
* person (individual * group)
Taking these factors into account it will be possible to make a reliable judgement on the relation between a dietary factor and cancer based on the available evidence. Generally speaking the informativeness of epidemiologic studies increases from cross-cultural-, case-control- and cohort studies to experimental studies.

4 DIETARY SURVEY METHODS

Different dietary survey methods can be used in epidemiologic studies. These methods can be characterized by the way food intake data are collected. This can be done either by record, interview or food frequency method (4). The record method is used if an investigator wants accurate information about current food intake during a limited period e.g. 1-7 days. If the usual food intake is of primary importance to an investigator repeatedly collected food records during a certain time period can be used. The dietary information collected by this method can either be obtained by weighing all foods or by recording in household measures. Record methods are laborious and can only be used when a small number of persons is examined.

The interview methods can be divided into recall and dietary history methods. The most commonly used method is the 24-hour recall, which attempts to obtain a complete description of all foods eaten during the 24 hours preceding the interview. An important drawback is that no picture is obtained about the usual food intake of an individual, but only a snapshot of the food intake during the previous day, although repeatedly collected 24-recalls can be used as an estimate of the usual food intake. Another approach is to ask the respondent to estimate his/her usual intake, as applied in the dietary history methods. These methods provide information about the usual food intake of an individual during a considerable period of time between two weeks and one year. The most extensive method in this category is the so-called cross-check dietary history method originally developed by Burke (1947). Besides information about the usual food consumption pattern during and between meals the consumption of specific foods is checked either in combination with a three-day record or by information on the quantities of various foods purchased per week for the whole family (5). This method is therefore time consuming and can only be carried out in epidemiologic studies of not more than a couple of thousands participants.

In nutritional epidemiology there is a need for simple methods that can be applied to large populations. Food frequency methods are very well suited for this purpose; they are characterized by the collection of information about the frequency with which certain foods are eaten during a specified period (6). Self-administered structured questionnaires with a limited number of foods are most popular. The number of foods in the questionnaire is generally derived from large data bases or pilot studies in which complete information about food intake is collected. Only those foods that contribute substantially to the nutrients of interest are selected so that the number of foods can be limited to as few as 60 foods. In the more advanced food fequency methods photographs are used to obtain information about portion sizes of the foods consumed. Food frequency methods do not provide information on all foods consumed and are therefore time and population dependent.

5 VALIDITY AND REPRODUCIBILITY OF DIETARY SURVEY METHODS

In studying diet-cancer relations information about the accuracy of dietary survey methods is needed. Accuracy has to do with the difference between the estimate and the true value of the parameter (the total error in the estimate);high accuracy meaning small total error. Generally, accuracy is divided into two components: validity and reproducibility.

The validity of a method is assessed by comparing it with an independent method of unquestionable accuracy. Dietary survey methods of unquestionable validity do not exist. Information about the relative validity of dietary survey methods may be obtained by evaluating the method of interest with another generally accepted method, designed to measure the same concept e.g. comparing the 24-hour recall with the one-day record method. Dietary survey methods can also be validated by comparing energy and nutrient intakes with a biochemical indicator of these intakes e.g. 24-hour nitrogen in urine as an indicator of protein intake and total energy expenditure estimated by the doubly labelled water technique as an indicator of total energy intake (7,8). Besides the validity also the reproducibility of a dietary survey method is of importance. A method is reproducible if two independent measurements give the same result in the same situation. Reproducibility studies using dietary survey methods estimating the current food intake, e.g. the 24-hour recall, are mainly influenced by the intra-individual variation in the intake of foods. The dietary history method however, is based on the concept that the participant has to recall the food consumption and to integrate this information to an usual food consumption pattern during at least the two weeks preceding the interview. Reproducibility studies using dietary history methods provide therefore information about the ability of the participant to give reproducible information on the usual intake of foods.

The cross-check dietary history method is frequently used in case-control studies. It is essential in this type of study to estimate what the food intake of the cases was before the occurrence of the disease. It is therefore of interest to investigate the validity of the dietary assessment in both cases and controls with respect to their dietary habits in the past. Within the context of the Zutphen Study such a study has been carried out(9). Of 43 myocardial infarction patients and 86 healthy controls information was available on their food intake collected in 1970 when all participants were free of disease. In 1985 information was collected on the current food intake of those subjects and they were also asked to estimate their food intake 15 years ago. The retrospectively assessed food intake was compared with the actual food intake in 1970. Retrospectively the energy intake was overestimated by approximately 300 kcal/day. The data collected in 1970 showed a significantly lower energy intake in myocardial infarction cases compared with controls. However, the retrospectively assessed energy intake data did not show a significant difference between cases and controls. The results of this study suggest that the power to detect a significant difference in energy intake between cases and controls was considerably reduced when dietary data were assessed retrospectively.

In reproducibility studies using the dietary history method the time interval between the measurements is crucial: it should not be too short to avoid recollection of the first interview but should also not be too long to prevent changes in food habits. Within the Zutphen Study it was shown that the differences in reproducibility estimations of different nutrients in elderly men were small when repeated surveys were carried out three and 12 months after the initial survey (10). For most nutrients the attenuation factor was 0.8. This implies that the observed relation between a nutrient and a disease is only slightly attenuated due to lack of reproducibility of the measurement of the nutrient. Consequently repeated application of the cross-check dietary history method in the case of low-order correlations, is of little help.

The Zutphen Study showed that the reproducibility differed for different foods (10). Alcoholic beverages, bread, sugar products and milk products reproduced well. Potatoes, fruit, cheese, edible fats and pastry were moderately well reproduced. Vegetables and meat were least reproducible. This has consequences for the design of future studies on diet-cancer relations. Poorly reproduced foods should either be better estimated during the interview or another method should be used for their estimation.

The validity and reproducibility of a semi-quantitative food frequency questionnaire has been described by Willett and co-workers (11). A 61-item questionnaire was administered twice at an interval of approximately one-year. During the same period four one-week dietary records were collected of the same 173 nurses. Overall 48% of the subjects in the lowest and 49% of the subjects in the highest quintile of the caloric adjusted intake computed from the dietary records were also in the lowest and the highest quintile of the questionnaire. The intra-class correlations were similar for the questionnaire and one-week record (range 0.41-0.79) indicating a similar reproducibility of both methods. The authors conclude that a simple self-administered questionnaire can provide useful information about individual intakes during a one-year period. This conclusion may be over-optimistic because a substantial number of subjects are misclassified in the distribution of the different nutrients.

It can be concluded that validation and reproducibility studies should always be a part of an epidemiologic study investigating diet-cancer relations. Semi-quantitative food frequency questionnaires can be validated against a large number of 24-hour recalls or records preferably taken over a period of a year. The reproducibility of the questionnaire should be tested by repeating the questionnaire after one year.

Objective measures of energy and protein intake obtained by the doubly labelled water technique and measurement of nitrogen in 24-hour urine collections respectively should be obtained. Blood samples could be collected for the validation of the intake of certain micronutrients e.g. beta-carotene. Only if these types of validation and reproducibility studies are carried out will a good picture of the accuracy of semi-quantitative food frequency questionnaires be obtained. This strategy is already being put in practice in the international study on diet, cancer and health being carried out in seven european countries and coordinated by the International Agency for Research on Cancer in Lyon (12).

6 VEGETABLES AND FRUITS IN RELATION TO CANCER

In reviews on diet and cancer three dietary factors are generally mentioned as the most important e.g. fat, mutagenic products formed during food preparation and vegetables and fruits.Dietary fat may be important in relation to commonly occurring types of cancer e.g. breast and colon cancer(13). The evidence for a promoting effect of fat for these types of cancer derives mainly from cross-cultural studies. The evidence from case-control and cohort studies is conflicting. There is a need for properly designed cohort studies with an accurate measurement of fat intake in order to establish the importance of fat intake in the etiology of breast and colon cancer.

There is evidence from epidemiologic studies that cooked meat and fish are associated with the occurrence of colon and pancreatic cancer (14,15). During the cooking process mutagenic heterocyclic amines may be formed (16). These pyrolytic products can be metabolically activated by humans both through N-oxidation and O-oxidation to produce highly reactive metabolites that form DNA-adducts (17). In rats these compounds readily develop tumors. Turesky and co-workers concluded that these genotoxins should be regarded as potential human colo-rectal carcinogens.

Burkitt suggested 20 years ago that dietary fiber may be important for the prevention of colo-rectal cancer (18). Peto and co-workers suggested in 1981 that the inverse association between vegetable and fruit consumption and the occurrence of epithelial cancers may be due to the protective effect of the provitamin A, beta-carotene, by scavenging free radicals (19). These articles generated a lot of interest in the role of vegetable and fruit consumption in cancer prevention. A large number of epidemiologic studies, mainly case-control studies, have been carried out to investigate this association.

A systematic review of 115 case-control studies was performed by Steinmetz and Potter (20). This review revealed several interesting results. Lung cancer was strongly related with carrots and green leafy vegetables, both rich sources of beta-carotene. Colon cancer was primarily associated with cruciferous vegetables and carrots suggesting a role of (non)- nutritive anticarcinogenic substances e.g. indoles and beta-carotene, beyond that potentially conferred by dietary fiber. For rectal cancer a specific pattern of vegetable and fruit comsumption was not found.

Fruit consumption was consistently inversely associated with esophageal-, laryngeal-, oral- and pharyngeal cancer suggesting an influence of vitamin C or another substance in fruits. Stomach cancer was consistently inversely associated with both fruits and vegetables. The consumption of potatoes was often positively related with stomach cancer. Vegetables and fruits were consistently inversely related with both pancreatic and bladder cancer.

The hormone-dependent cancers appeared to be less affected by fruits and vegetables. There was some evidence for an inverse relation between fruit and vegetable consumption and cancer of the breast, ovary and endometrium. No association was found between fruit and vegetable consumption and prostatic cancer.

A summary of the case-control studies to type of vegetables and fruits showed also some interesting results. In more than 80% of the studies inverse associations were found for raw and fresh vegetables and lettuce. In 60-80% of the studies inverse associations were observed for leafy green-, cruciferous-, and allium vegetables, carrots, broccoli, cabbage, raw or fresh fruit and citrus fruit. The evidence for potatoes was equivocal with about 50% of the studies showing either an inverse or positive association. A consistent positive association was found for legumes.

The consistency in the associations between vegetable and fruit consumption in relation to cancer is striking. In most case-control studies the odds ratios were in the order of 0.5. These moderate odds ratios may be due to attenuation because of the imprecision of dietary assessment. We showed in the Zutphen Study that of all foodgroups vegetables were least reproducible (10). From that point of view the consistency in the results is remarkable.

The effect of attenuation may be illustrated with the following example. In a case-control study carried out in our institute a protective effect was found for vegetable consumption in relation to pancreatic cancer (15). The odds ratio of the highest quintile of vegetable consumption compared with the lowest quintile was 0.34 (95% CL:0.18-0.64). In the context of that case-control study also the reproducibility of the different foodgroups and nutrients was estimated (21). Therefore the attenuation factor could be calculated. Adjustment for attenuation resulted in an odds ratio of 0.11.This example suggests that the associations between vegetable and fruit consumption and cancer are probably much stronger than observed in studies in which random misclassification is not taken into account.

7 WHAT ARE THE CAUSAL AGENTS IN VEGETABLES AND FRUITS?

Vegetables and fruits are rich sources of nutrients and non-nutritive substances. Carotenoids are present in green-yellow vegetables, vitamin C in citrus fruits, polyphenols are found in most vegetables and fruits. Glucosinolates are present in cruciferous vegetables e.g. Brussels sprouts, broccoli etc. Due to the diversity of substances present in vegetables and fruits it is difficult to say what constituent is causally related to cancer.

Specific information on vegetables and fruits may help in elucidating what constituent(s) are causally related to cancer. The evidence available so far suggests that especially cruciferous vegetables and carrots are associated with colon cancer. This suggests that non-nutritive anticarcinogenic agents present in cruciferous vegetables, e.g. glucosinolates, indoles, isothyocyanates and dithiolthiones,and carotenoids present in carrots may be the important agents. These substances may be more important than dietary fiber. In addition these substances showed anticarcinogenic effects in experimental studies (22).

A problem in elucidating the role of non-nutritive substances in the prevention of cancer is the lack of quantitative data on their content in foods. If we like to study the effect of non-nutritive substances in foods chemical analyses of these constituents in foods are needed. Due to the large number of non-nutritive substances in vegetables and fruits it is necessary to make a priority listing for the different classes of these constituents. In 1990 we organized a international workshop in Wageningen, The Netherlands in order to prepare such a list. At that workshop it was concluded that polyphenolic flavonoids are an important group of substances to be studied.

After this workshop we started a project to determine the content of flavonoids in foods. We developed and validated a High Performance Liquid Chromatographic (HPLC) method for the determination of five major flavonoids e.g. quercetin, kaempferol, myricetin, apigenin and luteolin in foods (23). This method was used for the determination of the flavonoid content of vegetables, fruits and beverages commonly consumed in the Netherlands (24). This study showed that quercetin was the most common flavonoid in foods and the highest concentrations were found in tea, onions and apples. The results of these analyses will be used to study the associations between quercetin and cancer in the Zutphen Study. In this study detailed information on the intake of vegetables, fruits and drinks was collected in 1985. These data can be related to five year cancer incidence.

The above described example shows how analytical chemists and epidemiologists can work together in identifying the importance of dietary constituents in the prevention of cancer. This multidisciplinary approach is needed because currently used food tables do not provide epidemiologists with the information they need. It is however unlikely that in this way the constituent may be identified that could prevent cancer. It is more likely that the total anticarcinogenic potential of vegetables and fruits e.g. the sum of nutritive and (non)-nutritive anticarcinogens is responsible for the preventive effect. Multidisciplinary research may help in identifying what substances are more or less important.

8 ACKNOWLEDGEMENT

The comments of G. Elzinga on an earlier version of this manuscript are gratefully acknowledged.

REFERENCES

1. Doll R, Peto R. The causes of cancer. J Nat Cancer Inst 1981; 66: 1195-1308.

2. Peto R, Lopez AD, Boreham J, Thun M, Heath C. Jr. Mortality from tobacco in developed countries: indirect estimation from national vital statistics. Lancet 1992; 339: 1268-1278.

3. Rose G. Sick individuals and sick populations. Int J Epidemiol 1985; 14: 32-38.

4. Bingham S. The dietary assessment of individuals; methods, accuracy, new techniques and recommendations. Nutr Abstr Rev (Series A) 1987; 57: 705-742.

5. Burke BS. The dietary history as a tool in research. J Am Diet Ass 1947; 23: 1041-1046.

6. Willett WC. Nutritional epidemiology, Oxford University Press. New York Oxford 1990.

7. Isaksson B. Urinary nitrogen output as a validity test in dietary surveys. Am J Clin Nutr 1980; 33: 4-5.

8. Livingstone MBE, Prentice AM, Strain JJ, Coward WA, Black AE, Barker ME, Mc Kenna PG, Whitehead RG. Accuracy of weighed dietary records in studies of diet and health. Brit Med J 1990; 300: 708-712.

9. Bloemberg BPM, Kromhout D, Obermann-de Boer GL. The relative validity of retrospectively assessed energy intake data in cases with myocardial infarction and controls (The Zutphen Study). J Clin Epidemiol 1989; 42: 1075-82.

10. Bloemberg BPM, Kromhout D, Obermann-de Boer GL, Van Kampen-Donker M. The reproducibility of dietary intake data, assessed with the cross-check dietary history method. Am J Epidemiol 1989; 130: 1047-1056.

11. Willett WC, Sampson L, Stampfer MJ, Rosner B, Bain C, Witschi J, Hennekens CH, Speizer FE. Reproducibility and validity of a semi- quantitative food frequency questionnaire. Am J Epidemiol 1985; 122: 51-65.

12. Riboli E. The IARC program of prospective studies on nutrition and cancer. Recent progress in research on nutrition and cancer. Wiley-Liss, New York, 1990: 189-204.

13. Willett WC. The search for the causes of breast and colon cancer. Nature 1989; 338: 389-394.

14. Willett WC, Stampfer MJ, Colditz GA, Rosner BA, Speizer FE. Relation of meat, fat, and fiber intake to the risk of colon cancer in a prospective study among women. N Engl J Med 1990; 323: 1664-1672.

15. Bueno de Mesquita HB, Maisonneuve P, Moerman CJ, Runia S. Intake of foods and nutrients and cancer of the exocrine pancreas: a population-based case-control study in the Netherlands. Int J Cancer 1991; 48: 540-549.

16. Sugimura T, Wakabayashi K. Mutagens and carcinogens in food. In: Pariza MW, Felton JS, Aeschbacher HU, Sato S (eds). Mutagens and carcinogens in the diet. Wiley-Liss, New York, 1990: 1-18.

17. Turesky RJ, Lang NP, Butler MA, Tutel CH, Kadlubar FF. Metabolic activation of carcinogenic heterocyclic aromatic amines by human liver and colon. Carcinogenesis 1991; 12: 1839-1845.

18. Burkett DP. Epidemiology of cancer of the colon and rectum. Cancer 1971; 28: 3-13.

19. Peto R, Doll R, Buckley JD, Sporn MB. Can dietary beta-carotene materially reduce human cancer rates? Nature 1981; 290: 201-208.

20. Steinmetz KA, Potter JD. Vegetables, fruit, and cancer. I Epidemiology. Cancer Causes Control 1991; 2: 325-357.

21. Bueno de Mesquita HB, Smeets FWM, Runia S, Hulshof KFAM. The reproducibility of a food frequency questionnaire among controls participating in a case-control study on cancer. Nutr Cancer 1992; 18: 143-156.

22. Steinmetz KA, Potter JD. Vegetables, fruit, and cancer. II Mechanisms.Cancer Causes Control 1991; 2: 227-242.

23. Hertog MGL, Hollman PCH, Venema DP. Optimization of a quantitative HPLC determination of potentially anticarcinogenic flavonoids in vegetables and fruits. J Agric Food Chem. In press.

24. Hertog MGL, Hollman PCH, Katan MB. The content of potentially anticarcinogenic flavonoids in 28 vegetables and 9 fruits commonly consumed in the Netherlands. Submitted.

DIET AND MAMMOGRAPHIC PATTERNS: WORK IN PROGRESS

Timothy Key, David Forman, Louise Cotton, Ann Lewis, Gwyneth Davey, John Moore, Graham Clark, Christine Mlynek, Joyce Tarrant, Philip Savage, Ruth English and Basil Shepstone

Imperial Cancer Research Fund Cancer Epidemiology Unit and Research Assay Laboratory, Radcliffe Infirmary, Oxford; Stoke Mandeville Hospital, Aylesbury; and Department of Radiology, University of Oxford

1 INTRODUCTION

Wolfe[1] classified the mammographic appearance of breast parenchyma into four patterns: N1 = normal, mainly fat; P1 = prominent duct pattern, mild; P2 = prominent duct pattern, moderate to severe; DY = extremely dense parenchyma, "dysplasia". He claimed that these patterns predict the risk for developing breast cancer. Subsequent epidemiological studies have confirmed that risk is increased in women with P2 or DY patterns in comparison with women having N1 or P1 patterns. In 28 studies reviewed by Goodwin and Boyd,[2] there was a median relative risk of 2.0 for DY versus N1 patterns.

The proportion of women with P2 or DY patterns increases with age in premenopausal women and decreases with age in postmenopausal women. The proportion of women with P2 or DY patterns also decreases with increasing weight and with increasing parity.[3,4]

Two recent studies have reported associations of mammographic patterns with nutritional factors. Brisson and colleagues[5] found that high risk mammographic patterns were associated with a high intake of saturated fat and with low intakes of carotenoids and fibre. Boyd and colleagues[6] found that high risk mammographic patterns were associated with a high intake of alcohol and with a high serum concentration of HDL cholesterol.

The purpose of the study described here was to test the hypotheses generated by these two studies.

2 METHODS

Subjects

Women attending for breast cancer screening in the Aylesbury Vale Health District were invited to participate in the study. Participating women answered a general questionnaire, gave a blood sample, and had their weight measured. They then completed a dietary questionnaire at home and returned it by post. The women included in the analyses reported here were the first 242 premenopausal and 247 postmenopausal women for whom mammograms, blood samples and dietary questionnaires were obtained.

Mammographic patterns

Mammographic patterns were classified according to Wolfe's criteria. Due to the small number of mammograms classified as N1, the N1 and P1 categories have been combined for presentation of the results.

Dietary questionnaire

This was a semi-quantitative food frequency questionnaire of 127 items, modified from that of Rimm and colleagues for use in Britain.[7] Nutrient intakes were calculated using standard portion sizes, mostly from the compilation by Crawley.[8] Nutrient values were mostly from Paul and Southgate.[9]

A validation study of our food frequency questionnaire among 163 middle aged women in Cambridge showed the following Spearman correlation coefficients with nutrient intakes calculated from 16 days of weighed food intake: energy, 0.53; total fat, 0.55; alcohol, 0.90; non-starch polysaccharides, 0.58; fibre, 0.33; carotene, 0.47; vitamin C, 0.56 (Bingham and colleagues, in preparation).

Blood samples and biochemical measurements

After venepuncture, the blood samples were kept in the dark at approximately 4°C for up to seven hours, before centrifugation and storage of aliquots of serum at -80°C.

Serum concentrations of retinol, carotenoids and α-tocopherol were measured by HPLC.[10] Serum concentrations of total cholesterol and HDL cholesterol were measured with an automatic analyser.

The results for fat soluble vitamins are for the first 168 premenopausal women for whom assays have been completed. The results for lipids are for the 109 premenopausal and 113 postmenopausal women selected for measurement of serum sex hormones (the hormone measurements are not reported here).

Statistical analysis

Mean values were calculated and adjustments made using analysis of covariance. Variables with skewed distributions were logarithmically transformed, and the mean values presented for these variables are geometric means. Means were adjusted for age, weight and parity, and for menopausal status where appropriate. Two sided tests of significance were used.

3 RESULTS

Age, menopausal status, parity, weight

In comparison with women with N1 or P1 patterns, women with P2 or DY patterns were significantly younger, more likely to be premenopausal, and lighter (Table 1). The proportion of women who were nulliparous was small in all three groups.

Nutrient intake

Differences between groups in the adjusted geometric mean intakes of energy, fat, saturated fat, fibre and alcohol were small and not statistically significant (Table 1). Adjusted geometric mean intakes of carotene and of vitamin C were lower in women with DY patterns than in women with N1 or P1 patterns, and the difference between groups was statistically significant.

Serum nutrients and lipids

There were no significant differences between groups in serum concentrations of retinol or carotenoids, although adjusted geometric mean retinol was 8% lower in women with DY than with N1 or P1 patterns, and adjusted geometric mean carotenoid concentrations were between 2% and 20% lower in women with DY patterns than in women with N1 or P1 patterns (Table 2). Mean concentrations of α-tocopherol were 10% and 11% lower in women with P2 and DY patterns respectively than in women with N1 or P1 patterns, and the difference between groups was statistically significant. Serum cholesterol measurements were available for 101 of the 168 subjects for whom α-tocopherol was measured; among these women, geometric mean α-tocopherol was 15% lower in women with DY than with N1 or P1 patterns ($p=0.02$), and this difference was unchanged after adjusting for serum cholesterol.

Adjusted mean serum HDL cholesterol concentration was 18% higher among postmenopausal women with DY than in those with N1 or P1 patterns, but otherwise there were no significant differences between groups in cholesterol concentrations.

4 DISCUSSION

As reported in previous studies, women with high risk mammographic patterns were younger, lighter and more often premenopausal than women with low risk patterns.

Our results did not support the hypotheses that high risk mammographic patterns are associated with high intakes of saturated fat and alcohol or with low intakes of fibre. They did support the hypothesis that high risk patterns are associated with a low intake of carotene, and suggested that high risk patterns might also be related to a low intake of vitamin C.

Table 1 Patient characteristics and nutrient intakes

Variable	N1+P1	P2	DY	P[1]
Number	207	144	138	
Age, years	53.8	52.2	49.3	<0.001
Premenopausal, percent	36.7	45.1	73.2	<0.001
Nulliparous, percent	7.7	9.7	9.4	0.77
Weight, kg	69.0	65.0	63.7	<0.001
Energy, kcal	1918	1947	1905	0.80
Fat, g	77.9	79.8	78.9	0.84
Fat, percent energy	37.0	37.2	37.6	0.63
Saturated fat, g	28.4	29.3	29.0	0.78
Fibre, g	24.7	24.6	23.5	0.45
Alcohol, g	2.9	2.9	3.0	0.98
Carotene, μg	4320	4201	3659	0.02
Vitamin C, mg	111	116	102	0.04

[1] Test for heterogeneity between means.
Nutrient values are geometric means (except for percentage energy from fat, arithmetic means), adjusted for age, weight, parity and menopausal status.

Table 2 Serum nutrient and lipid concentrations

Variable	N1+P1	P2	DY	P[1]
Premenopausal nutrients				
Number	49	46	73	
Retinol, μmol/l	1.83	1.73	1.69	0.11
α-carotene, μmol/l	0.10[2]	0.09[3]	0.08	0.59
ß-carotene, μmol/l	0.47	0.40	0.40	0.41
Lycopene, μmol/l	0.40	0.39	0.39	0.93
Total carotenoids, μmol/l	3.87	3.80	3.67	0.78
α-tocopherol, μmol/l	32.7	29.4	29.0	0.01
Premenopausal lipids				
Number	29	32	48	
Total cholesterol, mmol/l	5.9	5.8	5.7	0.74
HDL cholesterol, mmol/l	1.4	1.3	1.3[4]	0.43
Postmenopausal lipids				
Number	65	33	15	
Total cholesterol, mmol/l	5.9	6.0	5.9	0.93
HDL cholesterol, mmol/l	1.1	1.1[5]	1.3	0.04

[1] Test for heterogeneity between means. [2] N=47. [3] N=45. [4] N=47. [5] N=32.
Values are geometric means for vitamins and arithmetic means for lipids, adjusted for age, weight and parity.

The measurements of serum concentrations of carotenoids in premenopausal women were only very weakly supportive of the hypothesis that women with high risk mammographic patterns have relatively low carotenoid concentrations. The finding of an association between high risk patterns and relatively low serum α-tocopherol requires confirmation. Our results were supportive of the hypothesis that high risk mammographic patterns are associated with high concentrations of HDL cholesterol, but this effect was confined to postmenopausal women.

In a subsequent publication we will report dietary intakes of individual carotenoids and of α-tocopherol, and serum concentrations of carotenoids and α-tocopherol in postmenopausal women.

5 ACKNOWLEDGEMENTS

We thank the staff of the Aylesbury Vale Breast Screening Unit for recruiting the subjects, Dr David Yeates for providing the computer programme to calculate nutrient intakes, and Suzanne Shortland for preparing the manuscript.

6 REFERENCES

1. J.N. Wolfe, Cancer, 1976, 37, 2486.
2. P.J. Goodwin and N.F. Boyd, Am. J. Epidemiol., 1988, 127, 1097.
3. A.F. Saftlas and M. Szklo, Epidemiol. Rev., 1987, 9, 146.
4. B.L. de Stavola, I.H. Gravelle, D.Y. Wang, D.S. Allen, R.D. Bulbrook, I.S. Fentiman, J.L. Hayward and M.C. Chaudary, Int. J. Epidemiol., 1990, 19, 247.
5. J. Brisson, R. Verreault, A.S. Morrison, S. Tennina and F. Meyer, Am. J. Epidemiol., 1989, 130, 14.
6. N.F. Boyd, V. McGuire, E. Fishell, V. Kuriov, G. Lockwood and D. Tritchler, Br. J. Cancer, 1989, 59, 766.
7. E.B. Rimm, E.L. Giovannucci, M.J. Stampfer, G.A. Colditz, L.B. Litin and W.C. Willett, Am. J. Epidemiol., 1992, 135, 1114.
8. H. Crawley, 'Food Portion Sizes', Her Majesty's Stationery Office, London, 1988.
9. A.A. Paul and D.A.T. Southgate, 'McCance and Widdowson's The Composition of Foods', Her Majesty's Stationery Office, London, 1978.
10. D.I. Thurnham, E. Smith and P.S. Flora, Clin. Chem., 1988, 34, 377.

WORKSHOP REPORT: NEW DEVELOPMENTS IN EPIDEMIOLOGY

W.P.T. James

Rowett Research Institute
Greenburn Road
Bucksburn
Aberdeen

Epidemiology is a crucial component of any analysis of the role of diet in cancer but it suffers three problems. First the need to encompass a whole range of potential dietary factors which makes the specificity of the epidemiological analysis very difficult. Secondly the lack of a coherent mechanistic understanding of the role of diet in carcinogenesis. Studies are handicapped by the paucity of tests or indices of processes which can be applied to epidemiology studies. Finally although these population studies have the great advantage of providing immediate relevance to practical issues this very relevance makes the epidemiologist vulnerable to immediate misinterpretation by the media who want to translate the significance of a single study, with all its drawbacks, into practical advice for the public.

On a design basis epidemiological progress has been made with the use of nested studies within prospective monitoring and with analyses of familial dietary patterns to overcome the disadvantages of assessing diets in case control studies. The new approach of combining studies by performing meta-analyses is an important new development which needs to be taken further. Indeed in Europe we are guilty of neglecting the importance of integrating information by allocating funds to the collective analysis and sifting of pre-existing studies.

A conflict in future needs is evident. There is much to be said for concentrating on a well thought out major study in Europe where a number of centres combine their expertise to ensure a rigorously assessed and logical programme. This has the advantage of allowing the total funds in this area to be spent more effectively but this approach also implied a large and probably long study. However, given the rapidity of research in mechanistic terms there was a move to only fund studies which are completed in 3-5 years despite the protracted period needed for the development of cancer.

Nutritional epidemiology is beset by the problem of monitoring the diet. In the last decade a huge effort has gone into numerous case control, retrospective studies with dietary monitoring by such inexact methods that most nutritionists would consider the results unlikely to be helpful. Despite these drawbacks considerable progress has been made on the three themes emerging as of importance viz. fat intakes, meat consumption and fruit and vegetable intakes. Whilst these potential modulators of risk were not new we are now faced with developing a more refined view of which components are responsible and developing tools which can give greater specificity to particular dietary components.

One of the fundamental problems is how best to cope with the myriad changes in food production and the evident variation in food composition depending on the variety of the plant or food product. These are two conflicting issues. First it is now impossible to keep up with maintaining an up to date European, let alone a world, database on foods set out in a consistent manner. This means that dietary surveys will always be imperfect. On the other hand new approaches e.g. of the quercetin content of foods still provides new insights into the total intake of a bioactive molecule of interest provided there is already available at least a reasonable set of dietary data with sufficient specificity of foods to allow approximate estimation of the varied intake of such newly recognised compounds within the population. We have to accept that too much emphasis has been given to nutrients and not enough to the activity of other bioactive dietary compounds.

The complexity of foods means that greater benefit may accrue by concentrating on biomarkers of intake e.g. from blood and urine samples which are already being stored in prospective studies in the hope that they can be used for subsequent reappraisals using new analyses of compounds of interest. Clearly, however, what is really needed is the development of biomarkers of risk which can be applied to a population. This will allow the newly emerging approach in epidemiology to be developed more rigorously, ie. the testing by dietary monitoring of intervention of those at high risk. We have only a few high risk groups currently identified although within the next year or two we confidently expect gene probes to be developed for those prone to breast cancer (perhaps associated with differences in chromosome 17) and colon cancer. At present epidemiological analyses show a familial trait in defined groups e.g. of breast cancer but the prevalence of this trait seems low when based only on familial disease monitoring. More specific monitoring of blood groups or the use of gene probes will help but this will probably be needed to be specified on an organ specific basis so that host responsiveness can be monitored.

Given the array of initiators, metabolic promoters, inhibitors and metabolic blockers it would be argued that we should either develop generic tests of the net effect of an array of processes which can then be applied to epidemiology to concentrate on a reasonable hypothesis e.g. free radical damage and develop markers of host reactivity. The link between free radical damage and ageing was important and we now have a number of tests emerging which are worth exploiting.

The public response to epidemiological studies depends in the short terms on their presentation by the media but the real significance of dietary studies conducted in an epidemiological setting is that they allow practical advice to be given. If the studies are conducted responsibly and rigorously they will lead to effective prevention policies for envisaging the eventual decline in the incidence of cancer.

PART 2 THE OCCURRENCE AND SIGNIFICANCE OF CARCINOGENS IN FOODS

GENOTOXIC EFFECTS OF NITROSAMINES AND COOKED FOOD MUTAGENS IN VARIOUS ORGANS OF MICE AND THEIR MODIFICATION BY DIETARY FACTORS

S. Knasmüller, W. Parzefall, W. Huber, H. Kienzl and R. Schulte-Hermann

Institute of Tumor Biology and Cancer Research, University of Vienna, Borschkegasse 8a, A-1090 Vienna, AUSTRIA

1. INTRODUCTION

In recent years evidence has accumulated that certain dietary constituents might be able to reduce the genotoxic effects of mutagens. However, for the majority of compounds proof for antigenotoxic properties is hitherto restricted to results obtained under *in vitro* conditions and it is not known whether they also maintain their efficiency in the living animal[1].

In particular constituents of *Brassica* vegetables have been found in long term carcinogenicity studies [2,3] to protect against the carcinogenic effects of certain representatives of food genotoxins, but it is not known at general if the observed anticarcinogenic properties are paralleled by antigenotoxic effects *in vivo* and it is also unclear if there might be protection in combination with other genotoxins as well.

Aim of our experiments was to clarify some of these questions by studying the effect of putative antigenotoxins in combination with nitrosamines and cooked food mutagens in animal mediated differential DNA repair assays with *E. coli* K-12.

In initial experiments we found that this test system is, in contrast to other *in vivo* assays, very sensitive towards the genotoxic effects of representative compounds of these two classes of carcinogens which might play an important role in the etiology of human cancer.

2. METHODS

DNA repair assays with *E. coli* K-12 strains

Detection of DNA damage is based on the determination of the differential survival of two streptomycine resistent *E. coli* K-12 strains which differ in DNA repair capacity (# 343/753 is *uvr*B/*rec*A, # 343/765 is uvr^+/rec^+)[4]. Both strains are streptomycine resistant to prevent contaminations of the agar medium.

Mixtures of the two strains were exposed either *in vitro* (liquid holding assays) or *in vivo*. Following appropriate dilution, the survival of each strain was determined by plating on selective agar which contained the antibiotic and neutralred as pH indicator. The repair deficient strain is lac^+ and forms red colonies on this agar medium, the wildtype strain is repair proficient and forms white colonies. Media were composed as described[4].

In vitro assays. Genotoxins were incubated with a mixture of the strains (1-2 x 10^7cells of each strain/ml), various concentrations of the putative modifiers and liver S-9 mix prepared from untreated male mice. Following incubation for 120 min at 37°C under shaking, the mixtures were diluted (10^{-4}) with PBS and plated. Two days later, the individual strain survival was determined by counting.

In vivo assays. Mixtures of the strains (2-4x10^8 cells of each strain in 0.2 ml PBS) were injected *i.v.* into male Swiss Albino mice (ca. 25 g) which had been pretreated with a putative modifier or had remained untreated. Immediately thereafter the mice received the genotoxins either i.p. or orally. After 120min the animals were killed, the organs transferred into PBS, homogenized, and appropriate dilutions plated on NRS-agar plates for determination of the individuals strain survival as described[4,5].

Experiments with rat hepatocytes

Hepatocyte suspensions were prepared from perfused livers of untreated male Fisher 344 rats as described[6]. The cells were transferred into histidine-free MEM-medium. Incubation mixtures contained 1x10^6 hepatocytes (0.9 ml), 0.1 ml of a stationary phase overnight culture of *Salmonella typhimurium* TA 98,10 μl of the test compound dissolved in DMSO and 1-10 μl of the putative antimutagen. Following incubation for 60 min in the dark at 37°C, the suspensions were plated with two fold concentrated top agar.

3. RESULTS

Genotoxic effects of nitrosamines and cooked food mutagens

Table 1 summarizes repairable DNA damage measured in *E. coli* cells exposed in animal hosts which had been treated orally with nitrosamines or cooked food mutagens.

Nitrosodiethanolamine (NDELA) was the strongest genotoxin of all compounds tested; N-nitrosopyrrolidine (NPYR) and the structurally related, tobacco specific N-nitrosonornicotine (NNN) had a similar genotoxic potency and were less effective as the dimethyl-analogue. 4-(N-methyl-N-nitrosamino)-1-(3-pyridil)-1-butanone (NNK) gave a clear cut positive result at a dose of 360 mg/kg.N-diethanolnitrosamine (NDELA) caused only marginal effects at extremely high concentrations.

Most cooked food mutagens induced clear effects at a dose of 40 mg/kg, with PhIP a higher dose (200 mg/kg) was required. The general ranking order of genotoxic potency in the *in vivo* assays was MeIQ ⩾ IQ > MeIQx ⩾ Trp-P-2 > PhIP. In contrast to the pronounced differences of genotoxic activity measured in earlier *in vitro* assays, the effects of the various compounds measured *in vivo* were much the same.

With NDELA, NNN and NPYR, the order of acitivity was liver ⩾ lungs ⩾ kidneys > testes ⩾ spleen. NNK induced, in contrast, pronounced effects only in the livers, with NDELA no clear differences in the organspecificity could be measured.

Also the heterocyclic amines caused the strongest effects in the livers and lungs, also in the spleens pronounced effects occurred and the activity in the kidneys was only moderate (ranking order liver > lungs > spleen > testes). The effects measured in bacteria recovered from the blood varied strongly. In general, the effects were similar to those measured in the livers and lungs, but a precise determination of genotoxic activity was not possible.

The results presented in Table 1 were all gained under comparable experimental conditions (exposure time 120 min, oral administration of the test compounds). In other experimental series, in which the test compounds were given i.p., essentially the same ranking order of genotoxic potency and the same pattern of organ distribution of genotoxicity were measured, but the doses required to cause clear effects were consistently lower (data not shown).

Modifying effects of dietary constituents on the genotoxicty of NDMA and NPYR

The inhibitory effects of unsaturated fatty acids on the mutagenicity of nitrosamines in microbial *in vitro* assays have been reported repeatedly by Japanese groups[1], but it is not known so far if they are also effective in the living animal. This is also the case with vitamin A, which reduced the mutagenic effects of NDMA and NDEA in Ames tests and inhibited

Table 1

Induction of genotoxic effects in *E. coli* cells recovered from various organs of mice treated orally with nitrosamines or heterocyclic amines. [a)]

Compound	Dose (mg/kg bw.)	Number of animals	Relative differential survival (#343/753 *uvr*B/*rec*A vs. #343/765 *uvr*$^+$/*rec*$^+$) Blood	Lung	Liver	Spleen	Kidneys	Testes
IQ [b)]	40	4	24 ± 9	27 ± 8	28 ± 10	35 ± 5	48 ± 3	37 ± 1
MeIQ [b)]	40	4	35 ± 9	21 ± 3	20 ± 4	31 ± 2	47 ± 5	41 ± 6
MeIQx [b)]	40	4	48 ± 4	36 ± 5	38 ± 2	51 ± 10	60 ± 3	56 ± 16
Trp-P-2 [b)]	40	4	69 ± 16	45 ± 5	40 ± 6	60 ± 13	61 ± 4	61 ± 2
PhIP [c)]	200	4	47 ± 23	38 ± 12	37 ± 8	47 ± 13	57 ± 11	51 ± 15
NDMA [d)]	40	4	47 ± 8	8 ± 4	6 ± 4	47 ± 8	8 ± 2	13 ± 5
NDELA [e)]	700	4	n.d.[f)]	59 ± 4	66 ± 6	n.d.	87 ± 2	n.d.
NPYR [d)]	360	3	70 ± 20	45 ± 20	10 ± 2	62 ± 5	24 ± 3	31 ± 11
NPYR [d)]	95	4	45 ± 14	47 ± 8	32 ± 8	61 ± 12	40 ± 5	n.d.
NNN [d)]	95	4	46 ± 8	46 ± 7	37 ± 5	57 ± 5	51 ± 7	n.d.
NNK [d)]	360	4	76 ± 16	59 ± 3	40 ± 2	88 ± 5	53 ± 9	n.d.
Control	none	15	115 ± 31	95 ± 12	98 ± 8	101 ± 11	89 ± 14	82 ± 13

a) Male Swiss Albino mice, 25 g were deprived of feed 12 hrs before oral administration of the genotoxins but received water *ad libitum*. A mix of the indicator bacteria (2-4 x 10^8 cells of each strain in 0.2 ml PBS) were given i.v. immediately before the genotoxins.

b) Solvent: PBS, 30% DMSO

c) Aqueous suspension

d) Solvent: PBS

e) Corn oil

f) n.d. - not determined

induction of SCEs by these compounds in V 79 cells[7]. With phenethylisothiocyanate (PEITC), which is contained in *Brassica* species, it has been shown that it diminishes the carcinogenic effects of NDMA and PAHs but it is not known if these anticarcinogenic effects are paralleled by antimutagenic properties[2,3,8,9].

The results obtained with the various putative inhibitors oleic acid (OA), triolein (TO), vitamin A (ROL), and PEITC in animal mediated DNA repair assays and in liquid holding experiments in combination with NDMA and NPYR are summarized in Table 2.

Table 2

Influence of various dietary constituents on the genotoxic effects of NDMA and NPYR

Putative anti-mutagens	***in vivo*** Acute treatment a) Dose (mg/kg)	Effect c)	Repeated treatment b) Dose (mg/kg/day)	Effect c)	***in vitro*** Liquid holding d) Dose (μg/ml)	Effect c)
oleic acid	2000	none	2000	none	10	++ e)
triolein	8000	none	16000	+	10	+/++ e)
vitamin A	250	+	80	none	10	+/++
PEITC	150	++	150	none	10	++

a) Test compounds were given orally 2 hrs before treatment with the nitrosamines (NDMA 80 mg/kg, or NPYR 360 mg/kg i.g.).

b) In repeated treatment experiments test compounds were given consecutively over four days (last treatment 24 hrs before administration of the nitrosamines), nitrosamine doses were 80 mg/kg bw. for NDMA and 360 mg/kg bw. for NPYR.

c) "none" indicates lack of statistical significance (Dunnett´s Test), + indicates enhancement of differential survival ≤ 25 %, ++ indicates enhancement of differential survival > 25 %; In animal mediated assays + and ++ refer only to organs in which most pronounced genotoxicity was measured (liver, lungs, kidneys).

d) Liquid incubation mixtures were rotated for 120 min before testing.The mixture contained 0.8 ml mouse liver S-9 mix, 0.1 ml of a bacterial mix, 0.1 ml of aqueous solutions of two nitrosamines (10mM NDMA, 100 mM NPYR) and the various inhibitors (vitamin A was predissolved in methanol).

e) Strong inhibitory effects (reversion > 25%) were only measured with NDMA.

The influence of the various compounds on the genotoxic effects of both nitrosamines were identical: In contrast to the results obtained in DNA repair assays under *in vitro* conditions with the same *E. coli* strains, in which protective effects were found with all compounds (ranking order PEITC > OA > TO ≥ ROL), only PEITC caused pronounced antigenotoxic effects *in vivo* which only occurred when the compound was given shortly (1 hr) before the nitrosamines. Vitamin A induced moderate effects only at extremely high (almost toxic) doses upon acute treatment. Oleic acid was ineffective under all conditions of test. With triolein a moderare inhibitory effect was measured in combination with NDMA after repeated treatment.

Antimutagenic effects of phenethylisothiocyanate against cooked food mutagens

First evidence for antimutagenic properties of PEITC towards heterocyclic amines was obtained in preliminary *in vitro* experiments with intact rat hepatocytes. Addition of the isothiocyanate resulted in a pronounced reduction of his$^+$ revertants induced in *Salmonella typhimurium* TA 98 with MeIQ (Figure 1). Also in subsequent DNA repair assays with mouse S-9 mix, antigenotoxic effects of PEITC were measured with several cooked food mutagens (effective dose > 10 μg/ml) and in animal mediated assays substantial inhibition of DNA repair induced by IQ and PhIP was found when PEITC (27 mg/kg) was given 60 min before the amines (Figure 2).

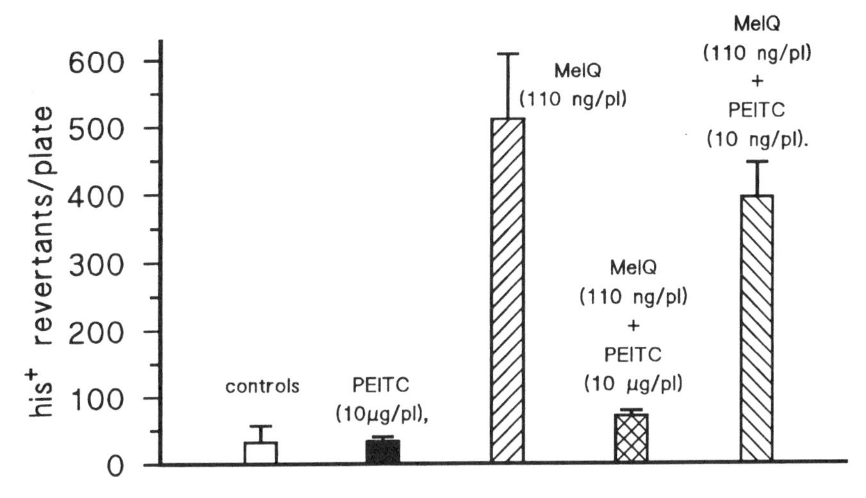

Figure 1 Influence of PEITC on the induction of his$^+$ revertants induced by MeIQ in Salmonella typhimurium TA 98, after activation by rat hepatocytes. Three plates per point.

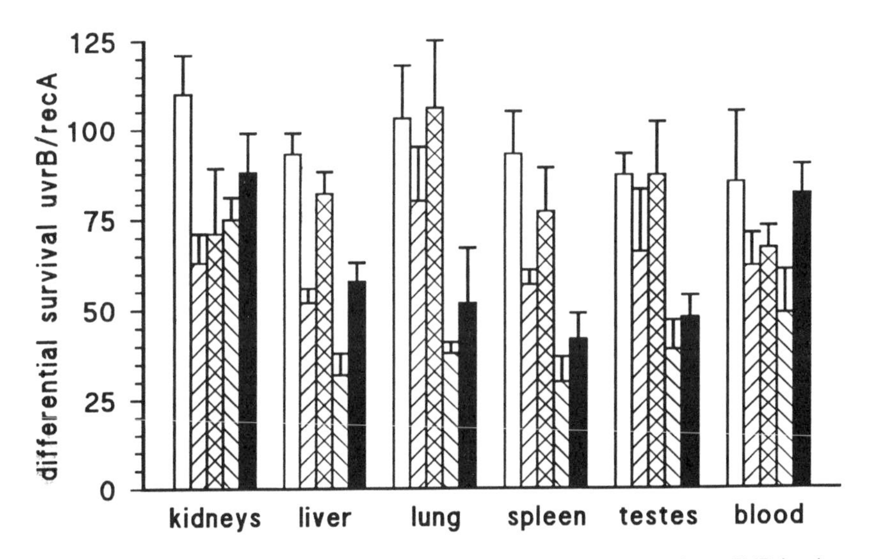

Figure 2 Influence of PEITC on the genotoxic effects induced by IQ or PhIP in vivo. PEITC was given orally (210 mg/kg b.w.) 60 min before i.p. administration of IQ (32 mg/kg b.w.) or PhIP (80 mg/kg b.w.).
Mixtures of the bacteria (2–4 x 10^8 E. coli of each strain in 0.2 ml PBS per animal) were given immediately before administration of the genotoxins. After 120 min the mice were killed and the survival rates of the bacteria per animal determined.
□ –control, ▨ –PhIP only, ⊠ –PhIP + PEITC, ▧ –IQ only, ■ –IQ + PEITC

4. CONCLUSIONS

The differential DNA repair assay with *E. coli* K-12 strains 343/753 (*uvrB/recA*) and 343/765 (*uvr+/rec+*) is a suitable method to measure the genotoxic effects of nitrosamines and cooked food mutagens. It also enables the detection of modifying effects of dietary constituents against these carcinogens in the living animal. Our results show that representatives of classes of antimutagens which are very effective under *in vitro* conditions (oleic acid, vitamin A) are only weakly or not effective in the living animal. Of all compounds tested, PEITC was the most efficient antigenotoxin in combination with nitrosamines and it has been shown that it reduces the carcinogenic effects of NDMA and related compounds[3,8]. The present experiments further demonstrated that the isothiocyanate is also an effective inhibitor of DNA damage caused by IQ and PhIP *in vivo*. This might indicate that PEITC protects against the carcinogenic effects of heterocyclic amines as well. Attempts to prove this assumption are presently in progress.

ACKNOWLEDGEMENTS

The authors are thankful to Edith Zöhrer, Inge Richter, Gerhard Lepschy and Evelyn Kainzbauer for competent technical assistance. Parts of these experiments were sponsored by an EC grant and by an Otto Loewi Stipendium of the Fonds zur Förderung wissenschaftlicher Forschung (to SK).

REFERENCES

1. H. Hayatsu, S. Arimoto, and T. Negishi. *Mutat. Res.*, 1988, 202, 429-446
2. L. W. Wattenberg. *Cancer Res.*, 1988, **45**, 1-8
3. M. A. Morse, K. I. Elkind, S. S. Hecht, and F. L. Kung, *Cancer. Res.*, 1989, **49**, 2894-2897
4. G. R. Mohn., *Arch. Toxicol.*, 1984, **55**, 268-271
5. S. Knasmüller, P. R. M. Kerklaan, and G. R. Mohn. *Mutat. Res.*, 1986, **164**, 9-17
6. W. Parzefall, P. Monschau, and R. Schulte-Hermann. *Arch. Toxicol.*, 1989, **63**, 456-461
7. C. C. Huang. *Mutat. Res.*, 1987, **187**, 133-140
8. G. D. Stoner, D. T. Morrissey, Y.-H. Heur, E. M. Daniel, A. J. Galati, and S. A. Wagner. *Cancer. Res.*, 1991, **51**, 2062-2068
9. L. W. Wattenberg. *Cancer Res.*, 1981, **41**, 2991-2994

INFLUENCE OF SUGAR-LINKED- AND DIALLYL-DITHIOCARBAMATES ON MUTAGENIC AND CARCINOGENIC N-NITROSO COMPOUNDS

B. H. Lee[1], B. Bertram[1], P. Schmezer[2], M. Wießler[1]
[1]Department of Molecular Toxicology, [2]Department of Carcinogenesis and Chemotherapy, German Cancer Research Center, 6900 Heidelberg, Germany

INTRODUCTION

Antigenotoxic and anticarcinogenic properties are probably linked to an inhibition of CytP450 enzymes and to an activation of the glutathione related detoxifying system.
In experiments with tetraethylthiuram disulfide (DSF) and mixed disulfides derived from diethyldithiocarbamate (DDTC), the main metabolite of DSF, namely acetylcysteinyl-DDTC and glutathione-DDTC, we could demonstrate such a relationship.
Several members of the allium family (garlic, onions, leeks, shallots) have also been shown to possess chemopreventive properties, probably because of their main constituents allylsulfide or diallylsulfide. As it seemed promising to combine the antigenotoxic and anticarcinogenic properties of these substances with DDTC and in order to improve cell transport and to direct the substances against specific organs, DDTC and diallyldithiocarbamate (DADTC) were linked to glucose or lactose. Experiments were carried out in rats to elucidate the effects of DADTC, acetylcysteinyl-DADTC, gluc-DDTC, lac-DDTC, gluc-DADTC and lac-DADTC on

1) nitrosamine-dealkylating enzymes,
2) glutathione, glutathione reductase and glutathione-S-transferase,
3) NDEA induced single strand breaks of liver DNA

MATERIALS AND METHODS

A) Chemical Synthesis

Details on chemical synthesis and analytical data of DATC, acetylcysteinyl-DATC, gluc-DDTC, lac-DDTC, gluc-DADTC and lac-DADTC will be published elsewhere (Lee et al., in preparation).

B) In vivo and in vitro experiments

Male Sprague-Dawley rats weighing between 100 and 200 g were used. The animals were fasted overnight (16h) and injected the various substances 1,7mM i.p. (experiments

1 and 2) or 0,5mM p.o. (experiment 3). In experiment 1 and 2 the animals were killed after 4h or 24h, and microsomes and cytosol were prepared from the livers. Glutathione, glutathione-reductase, glutathione-S-transferase and nitrosamine-dealkylating enzymes were determined according to the methods indicated below. In experiment 3 the animals received 1,4 mg/kg NDEA p.o. 2h after the treatment with gluc-DDTC; 1h later hepatocytes were prepared as described (Pool 1990) and DNA single strand breaks determined according to Schmezer 1990.

DETERMINATIONS

1) Glutathione (GSH and GSSG) by the DTNB reductase recycling system according to Griffith, O. W.: Anal. Biochem. 106, 207 - 212 (1980)
2) Glutathione-S-transferase by the Habig method: Habig, W. H. et al., J. Biol. Chem. 249, 7130 - 9 (1974)
3) Glutathione reductase according to Carlberg, J. and Mannervik, B.:J. Biol. Chem. 250, 5475 - 80 (1975)
4) Nitrosamine-dealkylating enzymes according to Janzowski, Ch. et al., Carcinogenesis 3, 155 - 9 (1982)
5) Preparation of hepatocytes: Pool, B. L. et al., Environ. Mol. Mutagen. 15, 24 (1990)
6) DNA Single Strand Breaks: Schmezer, P. et al., Environ. Mol. Mutagen. 15, 190 (1990)

RESULTS

The figures show the effects of gluc-DDTC (1a), lac-DDTC (1b), DADTC (2a), acetylcysteinyl-DADTC (2b), gluc-DADTC (3a) and lac-DADTC (3b) upon cytochrome-P450 related enzymes (NDMA-demethylase and NDEA-deethylase), glutathione (GSH and GSSG) and GSH-related enzymes (GSH-reductase and GSHS-transferase) 4h and 24h after the administration of the test compounds.
1) Nitrosamine-dealkylating enzymes:
All compounds tested had a strong inhibiting effect on nitrosamine-dealkylating enzymes (Fig. 1 - 3). 24 h after administration of the DADTC derived compounds the inhibition is almost as strong as after 4h (Fig. 2 and 3), whereas the DDTC linked sugars had lost their inhibiting activity after 24h (Fig. 1a and Fig. 1b).
2) GSH, GSH-reductase and GSH-S-transferase:
Gluc-DDTC did not influence the content of GSH or GSSG in rat liver but effectively raised the activities of GSH-reductase and GSH-transferase (Fig. 1a). These enzymes were not changed by lac-DDTC (Fig. 1b). In contrast, both DADTC-conjugated sugars had a more or less strong, biphasic effect upon GSH-reductase and GSH: after 4h the values were reduced and after 24h they were raised (Fig. 3a and 3b). Neither DADTC nor the mixed disulfide accys-DADTC had this effect, as GSH-reductase was elevated after 4h and this value

maintained for 24h (Fig. 2a and 2b). GSH-transferase was activated by both gluc-DADTC and lac-DADTC 24h after their administration (Fig. 3a and 3b).

3) DNA Single Strand Breaks

Gluc-DDTC, the only compound out of this series tested up to now, showed a 100% reduction of the clearcut genotoxic effects of NDEA on liver DNA (Table 1).

Table 1: Ex vivo analysis of NDEA-induced single strand breaks in primary rat hepatocytes after pretreatment with gluc-DDTC (0.5 mmol/kg)

	Treatment abs/rel *	vitality in % (M SD; n=6)	%DNA upon filter	C-T in %**
Exp. 1	NaCl/NaCl	60/100	67±7	-
	GlucDDTC/NaCl	82	60±8	7
	NDEA/NaCl	77	31±5	36
	GlucDDTC/NDEA	92	74±3	-7
Exp. 2	NaCl/NaCl	62/100	67±8	-
	GlucDDTC/NaCl	100	58±5	9
	NDEA/NaCl	92	46±5	21
	GlucDDTC/NDEA	106	77±7	-10

* absolute/relative (solvent control = 100%) vitality

** DNA on filter, control (C) minus treated value (T)

CONCLUSIONS

The substances presented here show a more or less pronounced protection against those effects of N-nitroso compounds which are believed to trigger mutagenic and carcinogenic processes in the cell: dealkylation (=activation) of N-nitroso compounds and production of DNA single strand breaks.

Moreover gluc-DDTC activates the glutathione related detoxication system. With respect to their activity upon GSH and GSH-reductase in vivo the compounds derived from diallyldithiocarbamate (gluc-DADTC and lac-DADTC) show an uncommon property. 4 h after administration they **reduce** GSH content and GSH-related enzyme values in the liver and after 24 h they produce an **augmentation.**

When the protective effect of our model compounds against DNA single strand breaks is mainly based on an improvement of detoxication mechanisms we should expect no protection against DNA damage by the diallyl-derived compounds after 4h. The strong inhibitory effect of the model compounds on nitrosamine activating enzymes, however, could nevertheless protect DNA against deleterious effects of NDEA. Further experiments are planned to elucidate the question which of these two effects is responsible for the chemopreventive potency of these compounds.

Fig. 1a, b: Inhibition or activation of enzyme activities (glutathione reductase, glutathione-S-transferase in liver cytosol, and nitrosamine dealkylases in liver microsomes) and of glutathione content in the liver of rats 4h and 24h after i.p. administration of gluc-DDTC and lac-DDTC (1.7 mM).

Glucose DDTC
150
100
50
0
-50
-100
GS-reduct. GS-transf. NDEA-deet NDMA-dem GSH GSSG
4 h 47* 100* -60* -65* 0 0
24 h 80* 100* -4 -3 0 0
%activation or inhibition
4 h
24 h

* p < 0.001

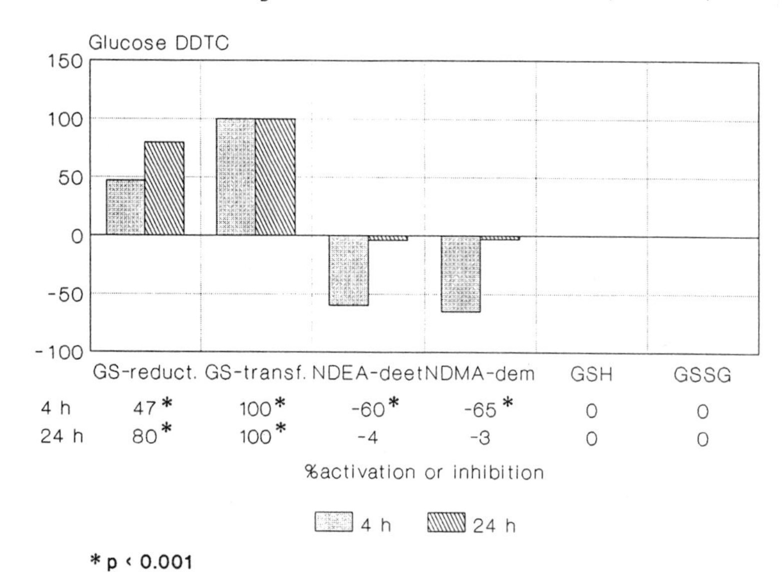

lactose-DDTC
40
20
0
-20
-40
-60
-80
GS-reduct. GS-transf. NDEA-deet NDMA-dem GSH GSSG §
4 h 0 11 -60* -37* 0
24 h 22* 9 -16 0 0
%activation or inhibition
4 h
24 h

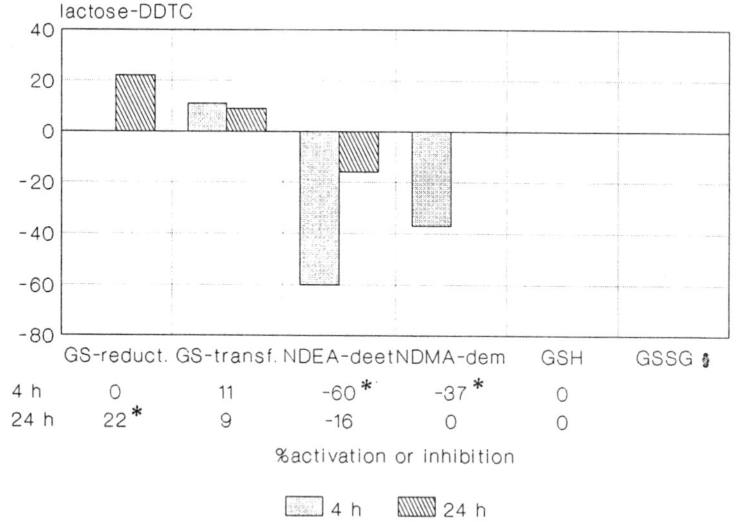

§ = not done

Fig. 2a, b and Fig. 3a, b: Inhibition or activation of enzyme activities (glutathione reductase, glutathione-S-transferase in liver cytosol, and nitrosamine dealkylases in liver microsomes) and of glutathione content in the liver of rats 4h and 24h after i.p. administration of DADTC, Acc-DADTC, gluc-DADTC and lac-ADTC (1.7 mM).

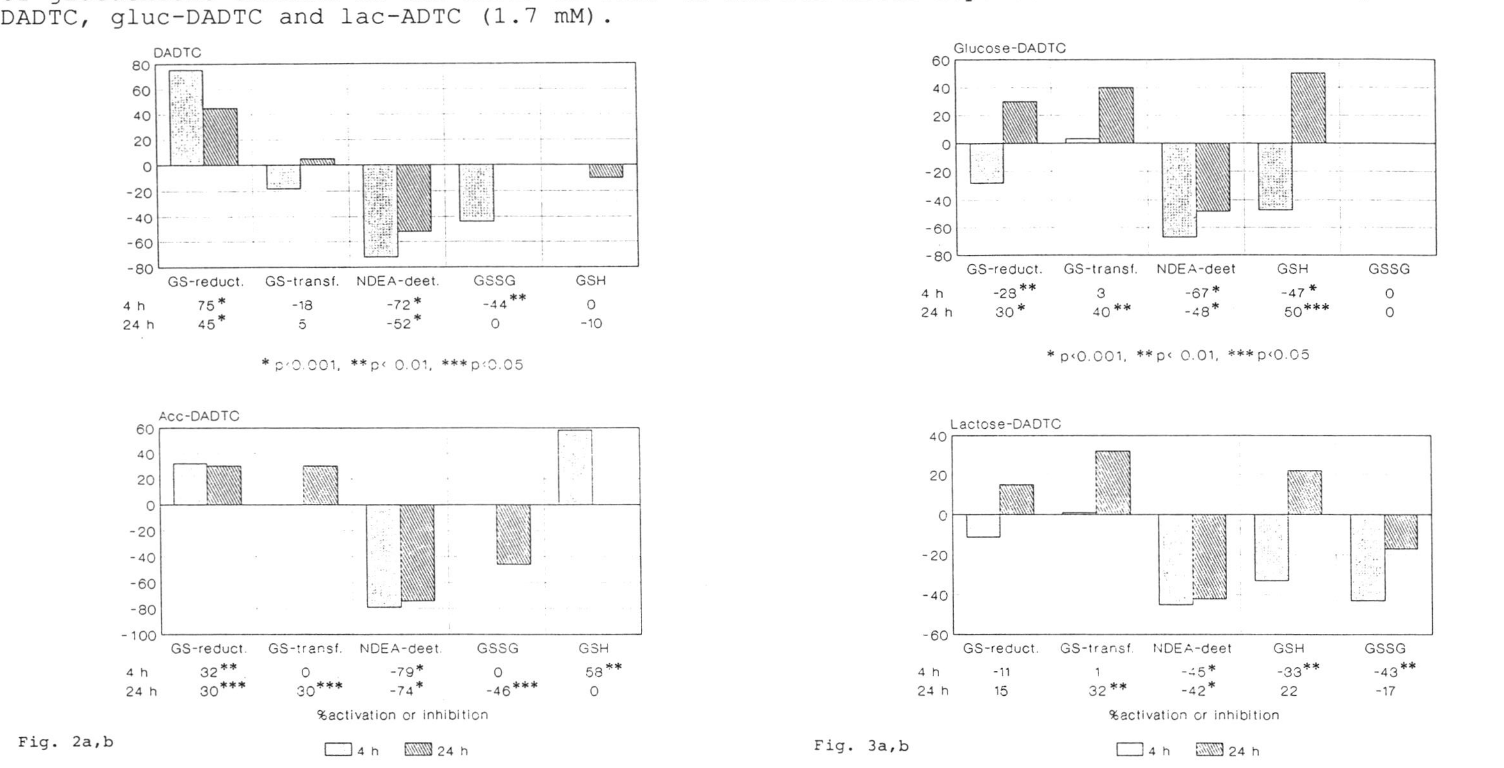

Fig. 2a,b

Fig. 3a,b

IN VITRO GENETIC TOXICOLOGY TESTING OF NATURALLY OCCURRING ISOTHIOCYANATES

S. R. R. Musk and I. T. Johnson

AFRC Institute of Food Research
Norwich Laboratory
Norwich Research Park
Colney
Norwich NR4 7UA

1 INTRODUCTION

One group of compounds in the human diet which have been highlighted as possible anticarcinogens are the isothiocyanates (ITCs) which are present in significant amounts in cruciferous vegetables either as such or more usually as the parent glucosinolate (1). The plants possess an enzyme, myrosinase, which, upon disruption of the tissue, can convert the glucosinolate to the corresponding ITC. A number of ITCs have been shown to protect laboratory animals from the tumourigenic effects of model carcingens such as DMBA, B[a]P, NNK and NBMA (2). Epidemiological data indicates a negative correlation between the consumption of vegetables and specifically of cruciferous vegetables and the incidence of colorectal cancer (3).

The route by which ITCs exert an anticarcinogenic effect remains unclear. PEITC (phenylethyl ITC) has been demonstrated to inhibit the metabolism of a variety of model carcinogens both *in vivo* and *in vitro* (2). Ishizaki *et al.* (4) reported that administration of PEITC to rats resulted in the suppression of P450 IIEI activity but induction of P450 IIBI activity in hepatic microsomes isolated 24 hours later.

Little or no data have been reported in the literature on the possible hazards of consuming BITC or PEITC. Morse *et al.* (5) reported a non-significant increase in pancreatic, mammary and adrenal tumours and in mesotheliomas in F344 rats treated with 3μmol PEITC/g diet. The closely related compound allylITC (AITC) has been the subject of much study in a variety of *in vitro* and *in vivo* assays, and has tested positive in certain short term tests for carcinogenicity (Caldwell, unpublished). The purpose of the present study was to investigate BITC (benzyl ITC), PEITC and PITC (phenyl ITC) for possible clastogenic activity utilizing an SV_{40}-transformed Indian muntjac cell line (SVM).

2 MATERIALS AND METHODS

Details of the phenotype of the SVM cell line and its growth in culture are given by Musk and Johnson (6). For assays of clonal survival cells were harvested from log-phase cultures and plated out in tissue culture flasks at the required low densities 4 hours before exposure to ITCs. The ITCs were dissolved in ethanol at a concentration of 1 mg/ml immediately prior to treatment, further dilutions being made in medium before addition to the cultures. The final concentration of ethanol in the medium was less than 1%, and had no effect on the survival of SVM. After addition of ITC each flask was sealed air-tight to prevent the escape of volatilized ITC. The exposure time was 24 hours following which the cells were given fresh medium and incubated for 10-12 days until colonies were visible with the naked eye. At this point the flasks were fixed, stained with Crystal violet and scored for colonies of over 50 cells. Each experiment was carried out in triplicate.

Induction of chromosome aberrations and SCEs

Cells were plated out at 10^5 per culture flask and left for 24 hours to achieve logarithmic growth. Solutions of ITCs were prepared as above and the cells were exposed for either 24 or 48 hours in sealed flasks. Chromosome preparations were made, stained with Crystal violet or Giemsa (2% in 0.3 M Na_2HPO_4, pH 10.45) and scored for the induction of aberrations or SCEs respectively.

3 RESULTS

Cell killing by isothiocyanates

Table 1 presents the parameters of the survival curves of SVM treated with ITCs. It can be seen that, whilst BITC and PEITC were of similar toxicity, PITC is an order of magnitude less cytotoxic. Data for AITC is also included for comparison: its cytotoxicity was similar to that of BITC.

Induction of chromosome aberrations and SCEs

Table 2 shows the induction of chromosome aberrations and SCEs by ITCs. All three induced both chromosome gaps and triradials in SVM, with the effectiveness of PITC again being approximately one tenth of the other two ITCs. ITCs induced SCEs but only very weakly.

Table 1 Parameters of Survival Curves of SVM Treated with ITCs

	D_q	D_o	D_{37}
		(all in μg/ml)	
BITC	0.11±0.01	0.23±0.03	0.34±0.03
PEITC	0.27±0.02	0.58±0.06	0.85±0.07
PITC	8.30±0.41	7.62±0.49	15.9±0.61
AITC	0.09±0.01	0.21±0.02	0.30±0.02

Table 2 Induction of Chromosome Aberrations and SCEs by ITCs

	Aberrations Induced/100 Cells		SCEs/Cell
	Gaps/Breaks	Exchanges	
CONTROL	2.5±0.3	0.8±0.1	7.5±0.6
BITC			
0.22 μg/ml	3.3±0.3	0.8±0.1	14.1±0.8
0.44 μg/ml	4.7±0.3	2.8±0.5	13.3±2.3
0.88 μg/ml	11.0±0.8	7.2±0.6	
PEITC			
0.44 μg/ml	3.9±0.2	1.5±0.1	10.6±1.0
0.88 μg/ml	8.7±0.9	3.0±0.2	13.4±1.3
1.32 μg/ml	12.6±1.5	6.0±0.5	
PITC			
5.50 μg/ml	2.6±0.4	1.2±0.3	10.0±0.9
11.0 μg/ml	7.0±1.0	2.0±0.4	11.4±1.1
22.0 μg/ml	25.7±4.1	8.5±1.0	
AITC			
0.20 μg/ml	4.1±0.3	1.0±0.3	9.1±0.8
0.40 μg/ml	3.5±0.6	0.5±0.1	10.1±0.9
0.80 μg/ml	3.7±0.7	1.2±0.4	

4 DISCUSSION

All three ITCs showed significant clastogenic activity, with PITC generating as many as 17 aberrant cells per 100 at the D_{37} dose. Whilst no assays of mutagenic activity *per se* have been performed, the present results do indicate that these ITCs should be considered as potential carcinogens. This data contrasts with many of the published studies (7) on AITC and indeed with our own observations which indicate that AITC is either nongenotoxic or at most only very weakly genotoxic, even at highly cytotoxic concentrations.

The lachrymatory nature of ITCs (AITC is the major flavour constituent of mustard) would tend to limit their consumption, as such, to insignificant levels. However, relatively large amounts may be present in the human diet as the parent glucosinolates and, although these are likely to be far less toxic than the corresponding ITCs, it has been reported that certain gastrointestinal flora possess myrosinase activity (8,9). Whilst epidemiological data clearly indicate that consumption of cruciferous vegetables at current levels may well be beneficial, it would be unwise to greatly increase the intake of such ITCs, or their glucosinolate precursors by the use of concentrated dietary supplements, without a thorough investigation of their potential to act as carcinogens in their own right. It may be that the optimum level of consumption of any given ITC in the human diet will be determined by a balance between the beneficial, anticarcinogenic effects and potentially harmful genotoxic activity.

REFERENCES

1. C.H. Van Etten, M.E. Daxenbichler, H.L. Tookey, W.F. Kwolek, P.H. Williams and O.C. Yoder, J. Amer. Soc. Hort. Sci., 1979, 105, 710.
2. G.D. Stoner, D.T. Morrissey, Y.-H. Heur, E.M. Daniel, A.J. Galati and S.A. Wagner, Cancer Res., 1991, 51, 2063.
3. E. Negri, C. La Vecchia, S. Franceschi, B. d'Avanzo and F. Parazzini, Int. J. Cancer, 1991, 48, 350.
4. H. Ishizaki, J.F. Brady, S.M. Ning and C.S. Yang, Xenobiotica, 1990, 20, 255.
5. M.A. Morse, C.-X. Wang, G.D. Stoner, S. Mandal, P.B. Conran, S.G. Amin, S.S. Hecht and F.-L. Chung, Cancer Res., 1989, 49, 549.
6. S.R.R. Musk and I.T. Johnson, Mutagenesis, 1992, in press.
7. IARC Monographs, 1984, 36, 55.
8. N. Tani, M. Ohtsuru and T. Hata, Agric. Biol. Chem., 1974, 38, 1617.
9. ibid., Agric. Biol. Chem., 1974, 38, 1623.

POSSIBLE CLASTOGENIC AND ANTICLASTOGENIC ACTIONS OF FERMENTED MILK "NARINE"

A. K. Nersessian

V.A. Fanardjian Centre for
Oncology Research
Yerevan 37052 Armenia

1 INTRODUCTION

Milk fermented with *Lactobacillus acidophilus* (strain 317/402) and called "Narine" (NN) is widely used as babies' food in Armenia. NN contains live lactobacilli (200-250 million per 1 ml). It is known that many strains of microbes including *Lactobacillus delbrueckii* can induce chromosomal aberrations (CAs) and micronuclei in mice somatic and germ cells,[1,2] though some strains of lactobacilli and yoghurt containing live lactobacilli have anticlastogenic property.[3] The aim of present work was to study possible clastogenic and anticlastogenic actions of NN.

2 MATERIALS AND METHODS

Male Wistar rats (100 g b.w.) were used. An experiment was performed to study the possible clastogenic action of NN. Daily consumption of NN by babies is approximately 50 ml/kg. The animals received oral doses of NN by stomach tube in a volume of 50 ml/kg b.w. (during 1 h) as 1 day (10 rats) and 30 days (10 rats) treatment. 5 rats were used as intact control and they received the same volume of distilled water. 24 h after the last treatment rats were killed with ether and chromosome specimens were prepared. A second experiment was performed to study the possible anticlastogenic action of NN. As clastogens 2 human carcinogens were used - cyclophosphamide (CP) and thiotepa (TT) which act with and without metabolic conversion respectively. Clastogens dissolved in distilled water were used at doses which induced about 20% of aberrant cells in bone marrow 24 h after intraperitoneal injection. CP dose was 17 mg/kg and TT dose was 1.2 mg/kg. 24 h before clastogens administration rats received NN with live or heat-killed lactobacilli (50 ml/mg). Positive control animals received only clastogens. Every group consisted of 10 rats. 5 rats (negative control) received i.p. only distilled water. 24 h after the last treatment rats were killed with ether and chromosome specimens were prepared.

As genetic endpoint CAs were evaluated. Bone marrow specimens were prepared and stained according to the conventional technique.[4] Colchicine injection (1 mg/kg b.w. i.p.) was given 2 h before rats were killed. TT, CP and colchicine were produced in the U.S.S.R. NN was purchased at a local store. Metaphase cells with CAs were scored from 100 well-spread metaphases per rat. Altogether 90 rats were used and 9000 cells were scored. The statistical significance of differences in CA frequency was determined by performing Student's t-test.

3 RESULTS AND DISCUSSION

The results of the first experiment have shown that CAs level in bone marrow cells of rats after NN treatment (1 and 30 days) did not significantly differ from control level. Therefore these data are not presented.

The results of the second experiment are presented in Table 1. CP and TT induced approximately 20% of cells with CAs, cheifly chromatid breaks (75-80%), chromosome breaks and exchanges. In bone marrow cells of rats received NN with live lactobacilli before both clastogens the CAs levels decreased significantly ($p<0.01$). In cells of CP-treated rats the CAs level decreased 2.6 times and CA/cell 5.6 times, in TT-treated rats 1.8 times and 3.2 times respectively. The decrease of CAs in bone marrow cells was followed by an almost proportional decrease of all types of CAs. In bone marrow cells of rats receiving NN with heat-killed lactobacilli the CA levels induced by 2 clastogens did not decrease. As NN with live lactobacilli has anticlastogenic property and NN with heat-killed lactobacilli has not, I suppose that anticlastogenic action is due to live lactobacilli.

Table 1 The influence of "Narine" on clastogenic action of cyclophosphamide and thiotepa in bone marrow cells of rats

Treatment	Aberrant cells (mean ± SE)	CA/cell
CP	21.6±1.6	0.50
NN^1 + CP	8.5±0.9*	0.09
NN^2 + CP	18.9±1.5	0.45
TT	20.6±1.8	0.38
NN^1 + TT	11.4±0.8*	0.12
NN^2 + TT	21.0±1.4*	0.33
Distilled water	0.8±0.2	0.008

*$p<0.01$ as compared with the corresponding positive control
NN^1 with live lactobacilli
NN^2 with heat-killed lactobacilli

Mechanism of anticlastogenic action of live microbes remains unclear, but some investigators suppose that this effect is due to the influence of microbes on a microsomal enzyme activation of chemicals.[3,4]

Hence, NN widely used as babies' food has no clastogenic activity and can decrease the clastogenic action of mutagens which act with and without metabolic conversion. It would be of interest to carry out further investigations of the anticlastogenic effect of milk fermented with lactobacilli in view of the increasing consumption of such food in many countries.

REFERENCES

1. G.K. Manna, Proc. Zool. Soc., 1989, 41, 1.
2. G.K. Manna and A.K. Sakar, Nat. Acad. Sci. Letters, 1989, 12, 331.
3. H.W. Renner and R. Münzner, Mutation Res., 1991, 262, 239.
4. A.K. Nersessian, V.N. Zilfian and V.A. Koumkoumadjian, Mutation Res., 1991, 260, 215.

INFLUENCE OF DIETARY FAT ON METABOLISM OF 2-AMINO-3-METHYL-3H-IMIDAZO[4,5-f]QUINOLINE (IQ)

C.J. Rumney, I.R. Rowland and I.K. O'Neill[1]

BIBRA Toxicology International
Woodmansterne Road, Carshalton,
Surrey, SM5 4DS, Great Britain

[1]IARC, 150 cours Albert Thomas,
69372 Lyon Cedex 08, France

1 INTRODUCTION

Dietary fat, amongst other dietary constituents, has been shown to modulate the risk of human carcinogenesis. In recent years, attention has also focused on pyrolysis carcinogens (or cooked food mutagens), formed during the cooking of proteinaceous foods at high temperatures,[1] as potential initiators of tumorigenesis. One of the most potent of these substances is 2-amino-3-methyl-3H-imidazo[4,5-f]quinoline (IQ[2]), which despite being capable of inducing between 200 and 400 revertants per ng[3] in the *Salmonella* mutagenicity test, requires metabolic activation by cytochrome P450-mediated mixed function oxidases to do so.[4] The major site of such activation is the liver, where detoxification of IQ by the production of a glucuronic acid conjugate also occurs. These conjugates of IQ are excreted via the bile into the gut lumen and reach the colon intact, where they may be subsequently deconjugated by bacterial β-glucuronidase. In addition, IQ has recently been shown to be converted *in vitro* by human gut bacteria to the 7-keto derivative (7-OHIQ[5]), which has been detected in the faeces of volunteers ingesting high levels of IQ-containing fried meat.[6] Unlike IQ, 7-OHIQ does not require metabolic activation for its mutagenic activity and is capable of inducing between 5 and 10 revertants per ng in the *Salmonella* mutagenicity test.[7]

The potential effects of a low *vs* a high fat diet on these mammalian and microbial bioactivation processes for IQ have been compared in human-flora-associated (HFA) rats fed human diets.

2 MATERIALS AND METHODS

Two groups of 5 male Fischer F344 rats were housed in flexible film isolators and weaned at 3 weeks of age on to SDS RM3 expanded diet, sterilised by exposure to 50kGy of γ-radiation from a ^{60}Co source. At 4 weeks of age, the rats were dosed by stomach tube with 1ml of a 5%

(w/v) human faecal suspension and at approximately 7 weeks of age, each group was transferred onto one of 2 isocaloric human diets (sterilised as above). The fat content of the diets differed by 3-fold within normal human intake and was 7.1% of weight (15% of calories) in the low fat diet and 25% of weight (45% of calories) in the high fat diet. Preparation of the human diets has been described previously.[8] After 4 weeks on these diets, the rats were killed and the livers and caecal contents were removed.

Hepatic S9 was prepared[9] and incubated at a concentration of 4mg S9 protein/ml for 30 minutes with IQ (Toronto Research Chemicals, Ontario, Canada; 10ng/plate) in the *Salmonella* mutagenicity test, using *S. typhimurium* TA98 as mutagenicity indicator strain.

Caecal suspensions (10%) from each rat were incubated anaerobically with [^{14}C]IQ (Toronto Research Chemicals, Ontario, Canada) at a final concentration of 5μg/ml, 0.1μCi/ml. Samples taken at 2, 4 and 6h of incubation were analysed by the method of Bashir *et al.*[5] Clarified samples were extracted with blue cotton (copper phthalocyanine cellulose; Sigma Chemicals) into methanol:ammonium hydroxide (50:1) and the extracts subjected to t.l.c. Proportions of [^{14}C]IQ and [^{14}C]7-OHIQ were then determined.

ß-Glucuronidase activity in each 10% caecal suspension was also determined.[10]

Statistical analysis of results was by analysis of variance, using the Minitab Statistical Package (Minitab Inc., University Park, PA, USA).

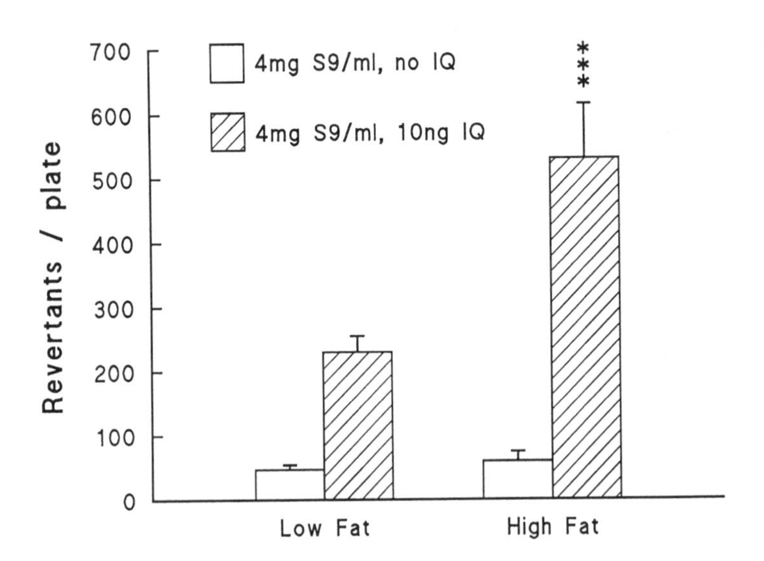

Figure 1 Hepatic activation of IQ (10ng/plate; *** = P<0.001)

3 RESULTS

A reduction in the fat content of the diet resulted in a significant ($P<0.001$) reduction in the hepatic activation of IQ *in vitro*, with an average of 230 revertants per plate from the group of rats fed the low fat diet, compared with 530 revertants per plate from the group fed the high fat diet (Figure 1).

Rates of IQ conversion to 7-OHIQ were significantly ($P<0.05$) lower for caecal contents from rats fed the low fat diet (approximately 10% converted after 6h) compared with those from rats fed the high fat diet (approximately 30% converted after 6h incubation; Figure 2). A highly significant ($P<0.001$) reduction in caecal ß-glucuronidase activity was also observed in rats fed the low fat diet (approximately 10μmol/hr/g caecal contents as opposed to approximately 50μmol/hr/g in caecal contents from rats fed the high fat diet; Figure 3).

4 CONCLUSIONS

The use in this study of a combination of HFA rats and freeze-dried human diets make the results of particular relevance to man.

Hepatic activation of IQ, bacterial deconjugation of IQ conjugates and subsequent conversion of IQ to 7-OHIQ, are three determining factors in the potential risk of IQ

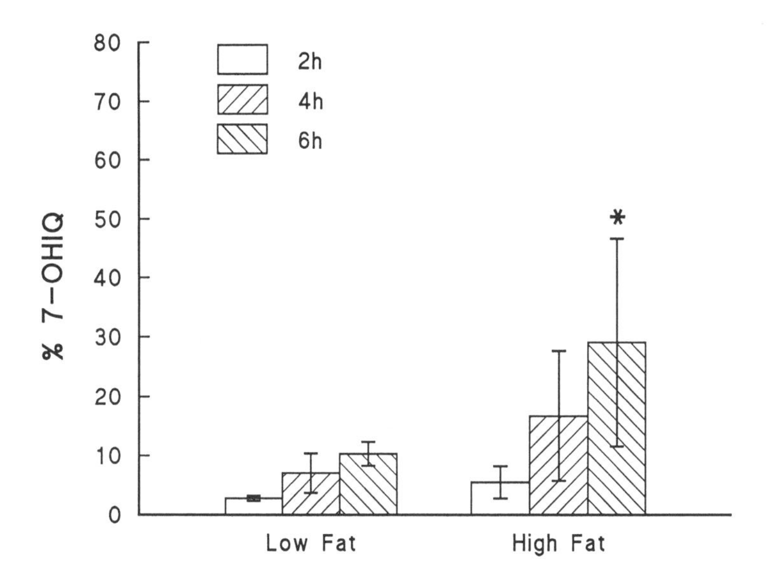

Figure 2 Conversion of IQ to 7-OHIQ by caecal contents (* = $P<0.05$)

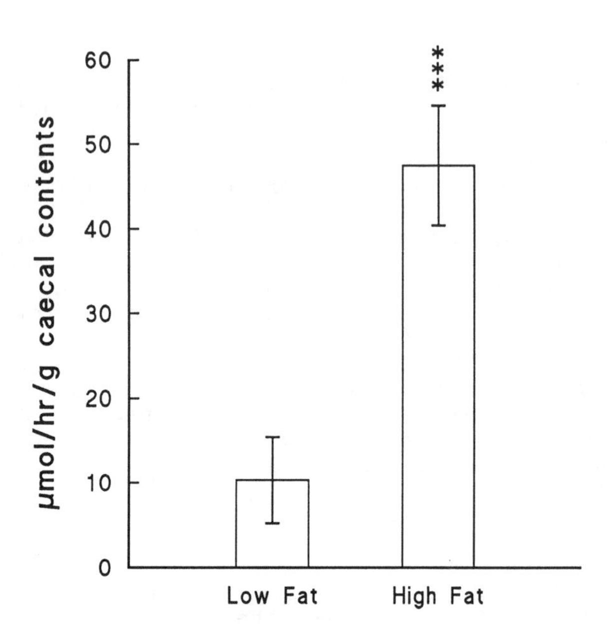

Figure 3 Caecal β-glucuronidase activity (*** = P<0.001)

ingestion. The present results have not only confirmed that dietary fat may modulate the risks associated with ingesting pyrolysis carcinogens, but also suggest that a reduction in dietary fat may concomitantly reduce the risks associated with one such carcinogen, namely IQ.

5 REFERENCES

1. J.S. Felton, M.G. Knize, C. Wood, B.J. Wuebbles, K.S. Healy, D.H. Stuermer, L.F. Bjeldanes, B.J. Kimble and F.T. Hatch, Carcinogenesis, 1984, 5, 95-102.
2. F.T. Htch and J.S. Felton, 'Genetic Toxicology of the Diet', Knudsen, I., Ed, Liss, New York, 1986, p.109.
3. T. Sugimura and S. Sato, Cancer Res., 1983, 43, 2415s-2421s.
4. H. Kasai, S. Nishimura, K. Wakabayashi, M. Nagao and T. Sugimura, Proc. Jpn. Acad. Sci., 1980, 56B, 382-384.
5. M. Bashir, D.G.I. Kingston, R.J. Carman, R.L. Van Tassell and T.D. Wilkins, Mutat. Res., 1987,190, 187-190.
6. R.J. Carman, R.L. Van Tassell, M. Bashir, D.G.I. Kingston and T.D. Wilkins, 'Anaerobes Today', Hardie, J.M. and Borriello, S.P., Eds, Wiley, Chichester, 1988, p.224.
7. R.J. Carman, R.L. Van Tassell, D.G.I. Kingston, M. Bashir and T.D. Wilkins, Mutat. Res., 1988, 206, 335-342.
8. I.K. O'Neill, S. Bingham, A.C. Povey, I. Brouet and J.C. Bereziat, Carcinogenesis, 1990, 11,599-607.
9. A.J. Alldrick, B.G. Lake, J. Flynn and I.R. Rowland, Mutat. Res., 1986, 163, 109-114.
10. A.K. Mallett, I.R. Rowland and C.A. Bearne, Toxicol., 1985, 36, 253-262.

6 ACKNOWLEDGEMENTS

CJR and IRR thank the UK Ministry of Agriculture, Fisheries and Food for financial support. This work has been partially supported by the U.S. National Institutes of Health under grant CA-39417. The HFA rats were housed at the MRC Toxicology Unit, Surrey and we are grateful for the expert technical assistance of Chris Jones and Paul Riemen. We thank Dr Sheila Bingham for provision of human diets and Theresia Coutts and Steve Livens for expert technical assistance.

INFLUENCE OF DIET ON THE CONVERSION OF 2-AMINO-3-METHYL-3H-IMIDAZO[4,5-f]QUINOLINE (IQ) TO THE 7-KETO DERIVATIVE (7-OHIQ)

C.J. Rumney and I.R. Rowland

BIBRA Toxicology International
Woodmansterne Road,
Carshalton,
Surrey, SM5 4DS
Great Britain

1 INTRODUCTION

Cooking proteinaceous foods, particularly meat, at high temperatures results in the production of a number of potent pyrolysis carcinogens.[1] One such compound (shown to be carcinogenic in rodent bioassays[2]) is 2-amino-3-methyl-3H-imidazo[4,5-f]quinoline (IQ), formed as a result of the reaction between creatinine and sugars during cooking[3] and present for example, at levels of 0.19ng/g of grilled beef.[4]

IQ reaching the colon in the form of a glucuronide may be deconjugated by bacterial β-glucuronidase and subsequently converted to 7-hydroxy-2-amino-3,6-dihydro-3-methyl-3H-imidazo[4,5-f]quinoline-7-one (7-OHIQ), the 7-kéto derivative of IQ[5] and a direct-acting mutagen in the ***Salmonella*** mutagenicity test.[6] This conversion has been shown to be carried out by human gut bacteria both *in vitro* and *in vivo*[7] and their release of such a direct-acting genotoxin directly into the colon may lead to DNA damage in the colonic mucosa and ultimately to colon carcinogenesis.

Results from three studies are presented in which the effect of different dietary components on the potential of human gut bacteria to convert IQ to 7-OHIQ has been investigated, using human-flora-associated (HFA) rats, to provide relevance to man.

2 MATERIALS AND METHODS

Diets

Study 1. Three groups of rats (3 male, 2 female per group) were transferred to either a low fat (1% w/w), 25% (w/w) beef dripping or 25% (w/w) olive oil diet.[8]

Study 2. Four groups of rats (3 male, 2 female per group) were fed either SSA[9] (fibre-free) or SSA supplemented with 10% fibre in the form of wheatbran, sugarbeet fibre or oat fibre.

Study 3. Two groups of rats (2 male, 2 female per group) were given a purified casein-based diet into which a preparation of transgalactosylated oligosaccharides (TOS;[10] a mixture of tri-, tetra-, penta- and hexasaccharides of galactose and glucose) was added at 5% (w/w) for one of the groups. TOS is a non-absorbable sugar shown to increase lactic acid bacteria in the gut.

Animals

For all three studies, groups of Lister-Hooded rats were used, which had been born germ-free and then associated with a human faecal flora (by gavaging with 1ml of a 10% suspension of freshly collected human faeces) shortly after weaning. The animals were housed in flexible film isolators and initially fed a stock rodent diet (GR3 EKR20; Special Diet Services, Witham, Essex, UK) which had been sterilized by exposure to 50 kGy of γ-radiation from a ^{60}Co source. Approximately one week after being dosed with a human flora, the rats were transferred onto the experimental diets, sterilized as above. Animals were killed after 4 weeks on the experimental diets and caecal contents used to prepare 20% (w/v) suspensions.

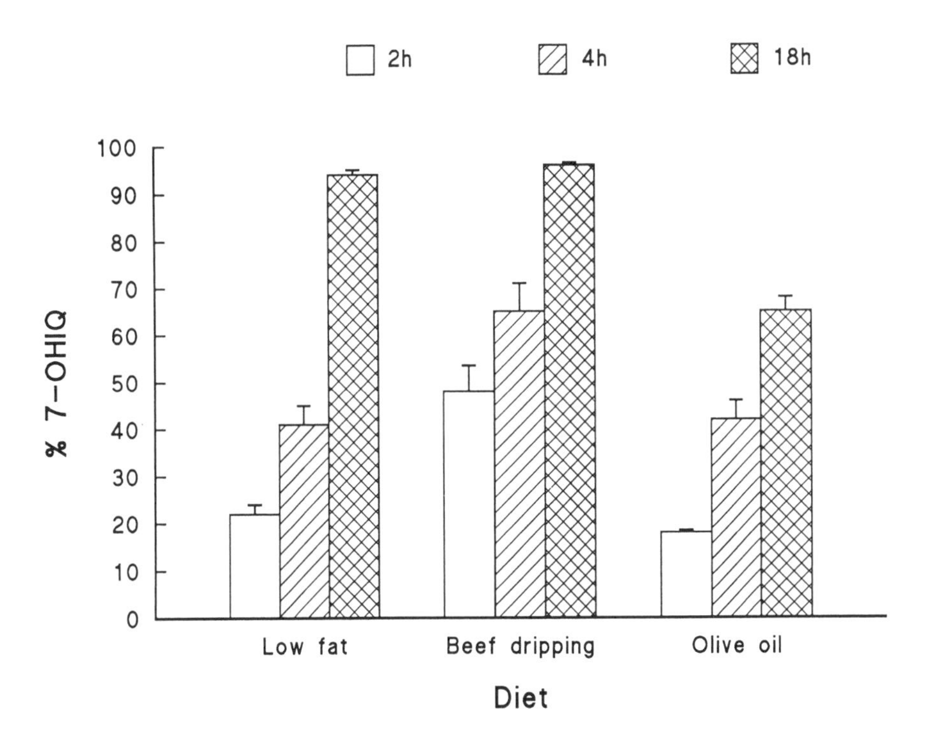

Figure 1 Effect of dietary fat on caecal conversion of IQ.

Measurement of IQ Conversion to 7-OHIQ

Caecal suspensions from individual rats were incubated anaerobically with [^{14}C]IQ (Toronto Research Chemicals, Ontario, Canada) at a final concentration of 5μg/ml, 0.1μCi/ml and samples removed at various time intervals. Clarified samples were analysed for 7-OHIQ content.[5]

3 RESULTS

Study 1

After 2h incubation with [^{14}C]IQ, caecal contents from rats fed either the low fat or 25% olive oil diet exhibited approximately 20% conversion of IQ to 7-OHIQ, compared with approximately 50% in caecal contents from rats fed the 25% beef dripping diet (Figure 1). After 18h incubation however, approximately 95% conversion had occurred in caecal contents from both the control and beef dripping diet fed rats, whilst only 65% conversion had occurred in caecal contents from rats fed the 25% olive oil diet.

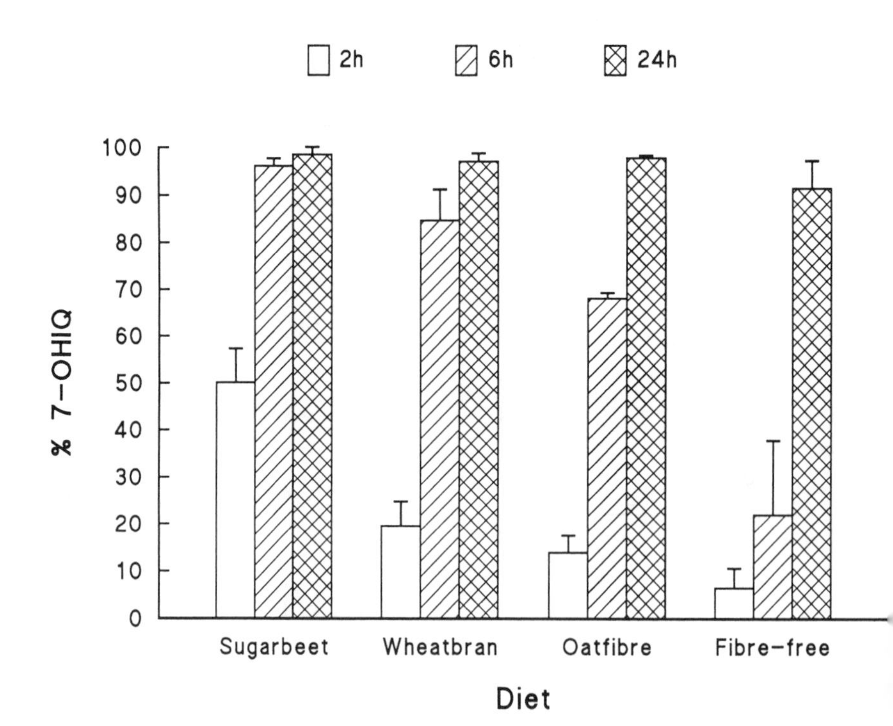

Figure 2 Effect of dietary fibre on caecal conversion of IQ

Study 2

Following 6h incubation with [^{14}C]IQ, caecal contents from rats fed the fibre-free diet showed only 22% conversion to 7-OHIQ, compared with 96%, 85% and 68% for the caecal contents from rats fed the sugarbeet, wheatbran and oat fibre diets respectively (Figure 2). After 24h incubation however, caecal contents from rats fed each of the fibre-containing diets exhibited over 97% conversion of IQ to 7-OHIQ and the caecal contents from rats fed the fibre-free diet showed only a slightly lower level of conversion (approximately 92%).

Study 3

After 4h incubation with [^{14}C]IQ, caecal contents from rats fed the diet supplemented with TOS showed a reduced level of conversion to 7-OHIQ (approximately 22% compared with 36% for caecal contents from the control diet fed rats; Figure 3). A marked difference in the levels of IQ conversion following 24h incubation was also apparent (approximately 77% converted in caecal contents from TOS fed rats compared to approximately 93% in control diet fed rats).

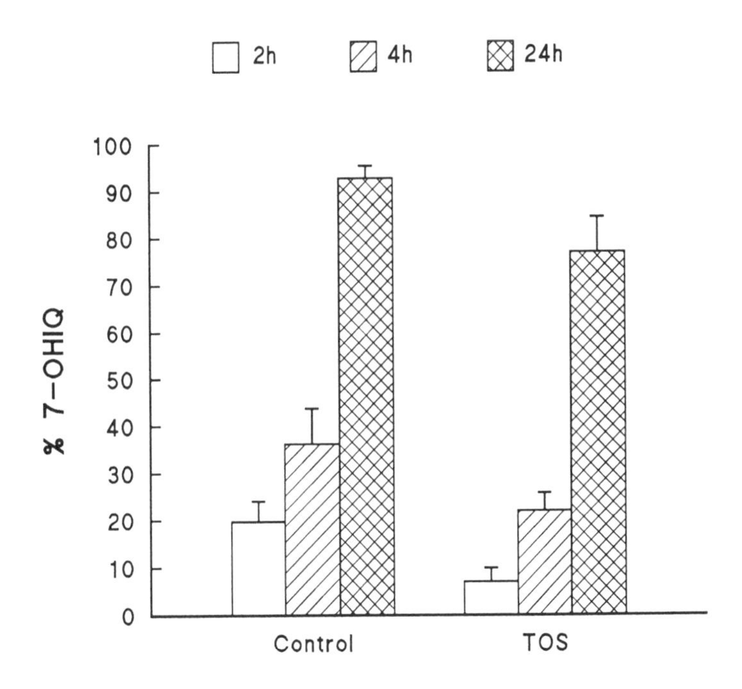

Figure 3 Effect of TOS on caecal conversion of IQ

4 CONCLUSIONS

The results presented confirm that dietary macrocomponents may modulate gut bacterial metabolism in such a way as to influence the release of a direct-acting genotoxin (7-OHIQ) into the colonic lumen. Whilst both fat and fibre *per se* are reputedly important factors in colon carcinogenesis, if genotoxins such as 7-OHIQ are considered likely contenders in tumour induction, the type of fat and fibre in the diet also becomes important, since this appears to have a major influence on their modulatory effects.

Supplementation of a diet with TOS reduced the potential for 7-OHIQ formation in the gut, which may be attributable to the concomitant major changes in caecal microflora observed in these animals (data not shown). In particular, lactic acid bacteria (purported to be beneficial intestinal organisms) were increased.

5 REFERENCES

1. J.S. Felton, M.G. Knize, C. Wood, B.J. Wuebbles, K.S. Healy, D.H. Stuermer, L.F. Bjeldanes, B.F. Kimble and F.T. Hatch, Carcinogenesis, 1984, 5, 95-102.
2. H. Ohgaki, S. Takayama and T. Sugimura, Mutat. Res., 1991, 259, 399-410.
3. M. Jägerstad, A.L. Reuterswärd, R.Öste and A. Dahlqvist, 'The Maillard Reaction in Foods and Nutrition', Waller, G.R. and Feather, M.S., Eds, American Chemical Society, Washington DC, 1983, p.507.
4. K. Wakabayashi, M. Nagao, H. Esumi and T. Sugimura, Cancer Res., 1992, 52, 2092s-2098s.
5. M. Bashir, D.G.I. Kingston, R.J. Carman, R.L. Van Tassell and T.D. Wilkins, Mutat. Res., 1987, 190, 187-190.
6. R.J. Carman, R.L. Van Tassell, D.G.I. Kingston, M. Bashir and T.D. Wilkins, Mutat. Res., 1988, 206, 335-342.
7. R.J. Carman, R.L. Van Tassell, M. Bashir, D.G.I. Kingston and T.D. Wilkins, 'Anaerobes Today', Hardie, J.M. and Borriello, S.P., Eds, Wiley, Chichester, 1988, p.224.
8. W.E. Brennan-Craddock, T.M. Coutts, I.R. Rowland and A.J. Alldrick, Mutat. Res., 1990, 230, 49-54.
9. A. Wise, A.K. Mallett and I.R. Rowland, Xenobiotica, 1982, 12, 111-118.
10. R. Tanaka, H. Takayama, M. Morotomi, T. Kuroshima, S. Ueyama, K. Matsumoto, A. Kuroda and M. Mutai, Bifidobacteria Microflora, 1983, 2, 17-24.

6 ACKNOWLEDGEMENTS

We thank Dr R. Tanaka (Yakult Central Institute for Microbiological Research, Tokyo, Japan) for providing the TOS and financial support. We also thank the UK Ministry of Agriculture, Fisheries and Food for financial support. The HFA rats were housed at Surrey University and we are grateful for the expert technical assistance of Vivyenne Ronaasen. We also thank Theresia Coutts and Steve Livens for expert technical assistance.

ANTIMUTAGENIC ACTION OF BETA CAROTENE, CANTHAXANTHIN AND EXTRACTS OF *ROSMARINUS OFFICINALIS* AND *MELISSA OFFICINALIS*. GENOTOXICITY OF BASIL AND TARRAGON OIL.

Amalia Bianchi-Santamaria[1,3], Fernando Tateo[2] and Leonida Santamaria[1]

[1]Istituto di Patologia Generale "C. Golgi", Centro Tumori, Università degli Studi di Pavia; [2]Dipartimento di Scienze e Tecnologie Alimentari e Microbiologiche (DISTAM), Università degli Studi di Milano; [3]Istituto di Farmacologia Medica II, Università degli Studi di Pavia; 27100 - Pavia - Italy.

1 INTRODUCTION

Epidemiological studies have shown diversities in the incidence of a substantial number of neoplasm in different geographical areas. These differences may, at least in part, be due to changes in some factors protecting people against carcinogens. Moreover, there is considerable evidence that higher plants used in foods contain a variety of molecules with antimutagenic or mutagenic activity[1-3] as well as anticarcinogenic or carcinogenic potential,[4] which can be explanatory for the above epidemiologic findings within definite criteria.

Carotenoids, such as beta-carotene (BC) and canthaxanthin (CX), widely distributed among living world, were experimentally found to be efficient protective agents against photodynamic carcinogenesis induced by benzo(a)pyrene (BP) and even by 8-methoxypsoralen (8-MOP) in mice.[5] Therefore, the properties of carotenoids as radical scavengers and singlet oxygen quenchers must also have played a basic role. The action of BC and CX on photomutagenicity in a UVA (320-400 nm) irradiated 8-MOP-bacteria system was investigated. Briefly, the TA102 strain of *S. typhimurium*, especially sensitive to oxidative mutagenesis was treated as above mentioned under air or bubbled with nitrogen.[6] The results of this experiment demonstrated that under normal aerated conditions 8-MOP was mutagenic after UVA irradiation at a concentration of 1 μg/ml (4.6 μM) as already demonstrated on *E. coli*.[7] This mutation was prevented by BC or CX up to about 60% (i.e. mutation was about 40%), demonstrating the antimutagenic capacity of these carotenoids. The same experiment carried out with the medium saturated with nitrogen showed that photomutagenesis by 8-MOP does occur but to a lower extent, just up to about 40% than in air conditions (100%); furthermore, under anoxia neither BC nor CX played any protective role (Fig. 1).[6] This demonstrated that the above photodynamic reaction takes place through two steps, namely one independent of oxygen followed by another one dependent on oxygen. The latter is apparently responsible for oxygen radical production, whereas, the first step should be consistent with 8-MOP-DNA photo-adduct formation.

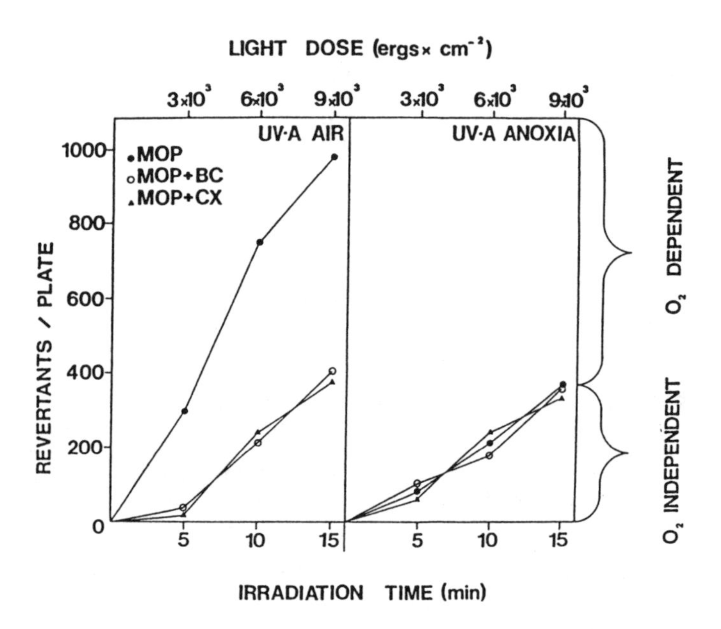

Fig. 1. 8-MOP photomutagenicity on *S. typhimurium* TA 102 in aerated and anoxic conditions and its prevention by carotenoids only in air. Evidence of a two-step reaction.[6]

On the basis of the above findings, a study was carried out to evaluate the mutagenic or antimutagenic activity of other plant extracts using the same experimental model. This should contribute to elucidate the epidemiological findings on anticancer activity of antioxidants naturally occurring and the genotoxic activity of several other botanical compounds as already reported.[1] Thus, it has been observed the antimutagenicity of extracts from *Rosmarinus officinalis* and *Melissa officinalis*, apparently by antioxidant mechanism, whereas, *Tarragon* oil and two basil oils may display genotoxic activity. These results along with their methods and discussion of the original experiments are presented here as follows.

2. MATERIALS AND METHODS

Rosmarinus officinalis extract: it was prepared through an improvement of conventional technology by using CO_2

High Pressure Extraction (HPE) to produce a highly organoleptically "neutral" product.[8] This turned out to be antioxidant as evaluated by measurement of rancidity induction time in highly unsaturated fats using a rancimat apparatus. The components active as antioxidants were mainly carnosol, carnosic and rosmarine acids.

Melissa officinalis extract was prepared as described for *Rosmarinus officinalis* extract.[8] The components active as antioxidants were mainly rosmarine acid and hydroxy-cynnamic derivatives.[14]

Tarragon oil and two basil oils were obtained by steam distillation of *Artemisia dracunculus L.* and *Ocimum basilicum L.*, respectively. Among several other components these oils are similar in their estragole (methyl chavicol) content which is 60%, 8.1% and 16.5%, respectively.[9]

Assay procedure for antimutagenesis by *Rosmarinus officinalis* and *Melissa officinalis* on 8-MOP (Sigma) photomutagenesis and BP (Kodak) mutagenesis was similar to that described by Jose.[10] Cells from overnight culture of *S. typhimurium* TA 102, a strain sensitive to oxidative mutagens,[11] were centrifuged and resuspended in a replacing volume of sodium phosphate buffer pH 7.4. Suspensions were transferred to glass Petri dishes and all the compounds dissolved in DMSO (the latter being not higher than 1% final concentration) were added to this suspension.

The final chemical concentrations were as follows: 1) 8-MOP = 1 μg/ml (4.6×10^{-6} M), 2) crystalline BC = 100 μg/ml (1.86×10^{-4} M), 3) *Rosmarinus officinalis* extract 100 μg/ml, which was the highest soluble dose; 4) *Melissa officinalis* extract 1, 10, 100% of the extract. The suspensions were pre-incubated for 20 minutes at room temperature and then exposed to UV-A radiation; the light source was kept at 12 cm above the culture surface. Irradiation was done with a Philips high pressure mercury vapor lamp HP 125 W emitting radiation between 300-400 nm with maximum emission band at 365 nm. Flux of light, filtered by window glass (to obtain UVA spectrum) measured with a black ray UV meter (UV products S. Gabriel CA) was 1×10^{3} ergs $cm^{-2}sec^{-1}$ (1×10^{-4}J) at the level of the sample.

At appropriate intervals, irradiated cells (0.1 ml) were added to 2 ml of molten 0.6% top agar (containing 0.5 mM L-histidine and 0.5 mM biotin) kept at 45°C and poured into Petri plates containing Vogel minimal salt agar with glucose. After 48 h of incubation at 37°C in the dark, revertant colonies were counted scoring for histidine reversion.

The BP mutagenicity assay was performed as described

by Ames *et al.*[14] with some slight modifications, described by Calle.[12] BP was dissolved in DMSO. In the assay procedure 15 μl or 30 μl of a BP solution (5.5×10^{-4} M or 2 μg or 4 μg/plate), 100 μl of BC or *Rosmarinus officinalis* extract and 100 μl of an overnight culture of TA 98 were added to 2 ml of top agar containing biotin and histine. After these additions, 500 μl of an *in vitro* metabolizing system of rat-liver microsomal fraction (S9 mix) prepared from beta-naphthoflavone and phenobarbital induced male Sprague-Dawley rats were quickly mixed with the top agar and poured over a minimal plate. The number of revertant colonies per plate were scored after 48-h incubation in the dark at 37°C and the number of spontaneous mutants was subtracted.

The genotoxicity evaluation of tarragon oil and two basil oils was carried out using the *Saccharomyces cerevisiae* yeast strain D7 according to Zimmermann.[13] The diploid strain D7 of the yeast *S. cerevisiae* was used. The strain has the following genotype: aα, ade 2-40/ade 2-119, trp 5-12/trp 5-27, ilv 1-92/ilv 1-92. This strain is used for the simultaneous detection of induced reverse mutations, mitotic gene conversion, mitotic crossing overs and other genetic events. Cells were grown in a complete liquid medium at 28°C until they reached a stationary phase. Cells washed and resuspended in distilled water at a concentration of 10^7 cells/ml were incubated in the dark for 30 minutes in the presence of 1, 10, 100 μl/ml of Tarragon oil, or 1, 10μl/ml of basil oil. Suitable dilutions of cell suspension were plated: a) on a isoleucine-free medium; b) on a tryptophan-free medium; and c) on a complete medium. The plates were incubated at 28°C. The plates were scored for the number of survivor and convertant colonies on the fifth day after treatment. Revertants for isoleucine and altered colonies including mitotic crossing-overs were scored after 8 days. Experiments were performed in triplicate. The standard mutagenic substance used was ethylmethanesulphonate (EMS), the incubation time was 5 hours.

In this study, the mutagenicity test has been carried out according to Zimmermann[13] rather than the Ames test[10,11] since in preliminary experiments the oils studied exhibited a high cytoxicity in *Salmonella typhimurium*, thus making it difficult to evaluate possible substrate mutagenicity.

3. RESULTS

In the control tests BC and *Rosmarinus officinalis* extract showed neither mutagenic nor photomutagenic effect; UVA light showed no mutagenic effect by itself. The spontaneous frequencies and background lawns were normal, so no toxicity by BC or *Rosmarinus officinalis* extract was detected. The series of experiments carried out with 8-MOP ± BC or *Rosmarinus officinalis* extract at the same experimental conditions confirmed, the photomutagenic effect of 8-MOP and its protection by BC up to 60% in TA 102;[6] in addition, a protective effect by *Rosmarinus officinalis* extract was detected up to about 30%.

In the series of experiments carried out with BP in the presence of S9 fraction, BC showed a protection against mutagenesis up to about 40% and extract up to 30% in *S. typhimurium* TA 98.

At the dose of 1% *Melissa officinalis* extract (dissolved in DMSO) showed a protective action up to about 50%, whereas, the 10% solution and the undiluted extract showed a complete protective effect against 8-MOP photomutagenesis.

Tarragon oil at the concentration of 1 μl/ml showed a survival of 98% in *S. cerevisiae* D7, whereas, a ten-fold increase in concentration (10 μl/ml) was found to yield only a 21% survival. There is no survival at a concentration of 100 μl/ml. At a concentration of 1 μl/ml the revertants and convertants were 2 x and 4 x higher than the control, respectively, while at a concentration of 10 μl/ml they were 8 x and 10 x higher than the control. At both concentrations, no increase in mitotic recombinations was observed.

The two basil oils (estragole content 8.1% and 16.5%) at a 1 μl/ml oil concentration decreased survival levels up to 64% and 86%, respectively, in *Saccharomyces cerevisiae*. The survival rates decreased to 7% and 18%, respectively, at 10 μl/ml. At all concentrations, no crossing over nor revertant or convertant values (mitotic recombinations or genotoxicity) were detected at the found survival values.

4. DISCUSSION AND CONCLUSIONS

The extract of *Rosmarinus officinalis* at the above dosage showed an antimutagenetic activity as antioxidant, with efficacy somehow lesser than exerted by BC in both tests with 8-MOP and BP. Also the antimutagenic effect of *Melissa officinalis* appeared to be linked to the antioxidant properties of this natural substance.

As far as tarragon oil and basil oils are concerned, it should be pointed out that, in the Zimmerman test, tarragon oil with estragole content 60%, was found to exhibit significant genotoxicity, whereas the two basil oils from *Artemisia dracunculus L.* and *Ocimum basilicum L.*, respectively with estragole contents 8.1% and 16.5%, respectively, did not exhibit any genotoxicity. Nevertheless, the biological activity or potential genotoxicity of any extract should not be predicted only on the basis of a single component (i.e., in this case, estragol).

Furthermore, because of the above results on basil oil, the potential risk associated with the use of basil in foods, as reported by Ames *et al.*,[1] could be misleading. There is no doubt that foods can contain both genotoxic and antigenotoxic substances, nevertheless any consideration about the possible risk associated with the intake of a particular constituent of the diet should be put forward only after a thorough evaluation of all the diet components which are assumed during the entire life in different proportions.

REFERENCES

1. B.N. Ames, R. Magaw and L.S. Gold, Ranking possible carcinogenic hazard, Science, 1987, 236, 271-280.
2. R. Ishii, H. Yoshikawa, H. Minakata, N.T. Komura and T. Kada, Specific of bio-antimutagens in the plant kingdom, Agric. Biol. Chem., 1984, 48, 2587-2591.
3. L.A. Mitscher, S. Drake, S.R. Gollapudi, J.A. Harris and D.M. Shankel, Isolation and identification of higher plant agents active in antimutagenesis assay systems: Glycyrrhiza glabra. In: D.M. Shankel, P.E. Hartman, T. Kada and A. Hollaender (Eds.) "Antimutagenesis and Anticarcinogenesis Mechanisms", Plenum Press, New York, 1986.
4. L. Santamaria, A. Bianchi, L. Andreoni, A.G. A.G. Arnaboldi and P. Bermond, 8-Methoxypsoralen photocarcinogenesis and its prevention by dietary carotenoids, Preliminary results, Med. Biol. Environn., 1984, 12, 533-537.
5. L. Santamaria, A. Bianchi, A. Arnaboldi, L. Andreoni and P. Bermond, Dietary carotenoids block photocarcinogenic enhancement by benzo(a)pyrene and inhibit its carcinogenesis in the dark, Experientia, 1983, 39, 1043-1045.
6. L. Santamaria, L. Bianchi, A. Bianchi, R. Pizzala, G. Santagati and P. Bermond, Photomutagenicity by 8-methoxypsoralen with and without singlet oxygen involvement and its prevention by beta-carotene. Relevance to the mechanism of 8-MOP photocarcinogenesis and to PUVA application, Med. Biol. Environn., 1984, 12(1), 541-549.
7. N.J. De Mol, G.M.J. Beijersbergen Van Henegowenn, G.R. Mohn, B.W. Glickman and P.M. Kleef, On the involvement of singlet oxygen in mutation induction by 8-methoxypsoralen and UV-A irradiation in *E. coli* K 12, Mutat. Res., 1981, 82, 23-30.
8. F. Tateo, M. Fellin, L. Santamaria, A. Bianchi and L. Bianchi, *Rosmarinus officinalis L.* extract production antioxidant and antimutagenic activity, Perfumer and Flavouring, 1988, 13, 48-54.
9. F. Tateo, L. Santamaria, L. Bianchi and A. Bianchi, Basil oil and tarragon oil: Composition and genotoxicity evaluation, Journ. of Ess. Oil Res., 1989, Vol. 1 (3), 111-118.
10. J. Jose, Photomutagenesis by chlorinated phenothiazine tranquillizers, P.N.A.S., 1976, 76,

469-472.

11. D.E. Levin, M. Hollenstein, M.F. Christman, e. Schwiers and B.N. Ames, A new Salmonella tester strain (TA 102) with A.T. base pairs at the site of mutations detects oxidative mutagens, P.N.A.S., 1982, 79, 7445-7449.
12. L.M. Calle and P.D. Sullivan, Screening of antioxidants and other compounds for antimutagenic properties toward benzo(a)pyrene-induced mutagenicity in strain TA 98 of *Salmonella typhimurium*, Mut. Res., 1982, 101, 99-114.
13. F.K. Zimmerman, R. Kern, H. Rosemberger, A yeast strain for simultaneous detection of induced mitotic crossing-over, mitotic gene conversion and reversion mutation, Mut. Res., 1975, 28, 381-388.
14. J.L. Lamaison, C. Petitjean-Freytet, A. Carnat, Lamiacées, médicinales à propriétés antioxidantes, sources potentielles d'acide rosmarinique, Pharm. Acta Helv., 1991, 66(7), 185-188.

NITRITE-FREE MEAT CURING SYSTEMS AND THE N-NITROSAMINE PROBLEM

F. Shahidi and R.B. Pegg
Department of Biochemistry
Memorial University of Newfoundland
St. John's, Newfoundland Canada
A1B 3X9

1 INTRODUCTION

Nitrite is an important meat preservative. Its incidental use dates back to antiquity and as early as 3000 BC in Mesopotamia. Rock salt used for meat preservation contained nitrate impurities which were reduced to nitrite by the post-mortem reducing activity of muscle tissues. Regulated use of nitrite, as such, has been practiced in North America since 1925. Nitrite is responsible for a reddening effect and prevention of meat flavour deterioration as well as development of the characteristic and well-loved flavour of cured meats. More importantly, nitrite acts as an antimicrobial agent and thus retards the germination of spores and toxin formation by Clostridium botulinum.

Despite all of its desirable effects, nitrite has also been the culprit in the formation of carcinogenic N-nitrosamines in certain cured products under high temperatures of pan-frying. N-nitrosopyrrolidine and N-nitrosodimethylamine have been detected at < 100 ppb in fried bacon.[1,2] Residual nitrite in cured meats reacts with amines and amino acids to produce these and other N-nitrosamines. Therefore, it is prudent to develop alternatives to nitrite in the curing of meat products. This is in line with the stated policy of the Canadian government.[3]

Since the likelihood of finding a single compound to mimic all functions of nitrite was remote, we formulated composite non-nitrite curing mixtures for duplicating the cumulative action of nitrite.[4] A summary of the multicomponent systems so prepared and their efficiency in inhibiting N-nitrosamine formation in treated products is presented.

2 COLOUR OF CURED MEATS AND NITRITE SUBSTITUTES

The colour of raw meat is due to its hemoproteins, principally myoglobin.[5] Myoglobin is composed of a protein, globin, and an iron-porphyrin prosthetic heme group. The colour of heat-processed cured meats is due to nitrosyl

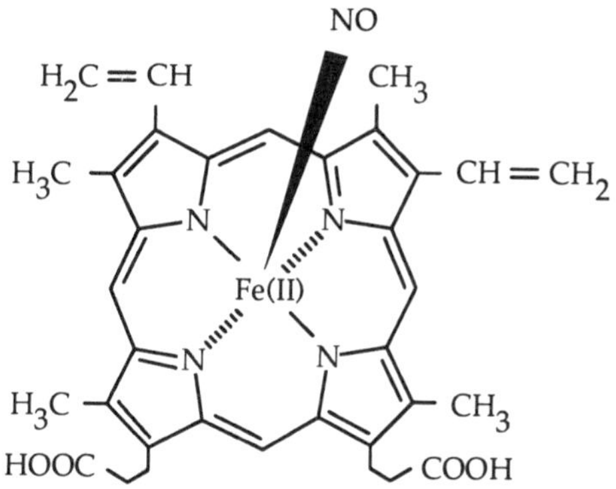

Figure 1 Chemical structure of the cooked cured-meat pigment.

ferrohemochromogen. This pigment may also be produced from bovine or porcine hemoglobin. Preparation of the pre-formed cooked cured-meat pigment (CCMP) from hemoglobin or from hemin has been reported previously (Figure 1).[6,7] The CCMP like the pigment present in the nitrite-cured meats undergoes decomposition. Therefore, its stabilization is crucial.

Stabilization of CCMP by its storage under a modified headspace gas or by microencapsulation has been reported elsewhere.[8] Application of this pigment, either as such or in the encapsulated form, to a variety of emulsion-type muscle foods ranging from cod surimi to seal meat has been accomplished. The amount of CCMP required for duplicating the typical colour of their nitrite-cured counterparts was directly proportional to the amount of hemoprotein originally present in muscle tissues. In general, up to 60 ppm CCMP was required for providing appropriate cured-colours to products as light as cod surimi and as dark as seal meat (Table 1).[9]

Table 1 Effect of Muscle Species and Pigments on the Required Concentrations of CCMP to Obtain a Cured Colour.[a]

Species	CCMP, ppm	Pigments, mg/g
Cod	0	0
Chicken Breast	3-6	0.4
Pork	6-12	1.2
Beef	24-36	4.5
Seal	48-60	48.0
Seal Surimi	18-30	24.0

[a]From reference 9, in parts.

Table 2 Effect of Nitrite Curing or Treatment with Nitrite-Free Mixtures on the Concentration of Selected Carbonyl Compounds of Meat.

Carbonyl Compound	Relative Concentration		
	Uncured	Nitrite-Cured[a]	Nitrite-Free Cured[b]
Hexanal	100	7.0	6.5
Pentanal	31.3	0.5	0.5
Nonanal	8.8	0.5	0.7
2,4-Decadienal	1.1	--	<0.1

[a]Sample contained 550 ppm sodium ascorbate.
[b]Sample contained 12 ppm CCMP, 3000 ppm STPP, 550 ppm sodium ascorbate and 30 ppm TBHQ.

3 FLAVOUR OF NITRITE-CURED AND NITRITE-FREE TREATED MEATS

Only as little as 10-40 ppm of sodium nitrite was found necessary to attain a nitrite-cured colour and flavour in meat products.[10] Lipids make an important contribution towards the overall flavour of meats and are also mainly responsible for meat flavour deterioration. Nitrite, due to its strong antioxidant properties retards the development of warmed-over flavour due to the formation of overtone carbonyl compounds which obscure the true-to-nature flavour of cooked meats. Based on these observations, it was suggested that the true nature of meat flavour may indeed by that of cured meats.[10]

To reproduce the antioxidant effect of nitrite, we have examined a number of synthetic and natural antioxidants and sequestrants as well as their possible combinations. Curing adjunctes, in particular phosphates and ascorbates, were quite effective in retarding lipid oxidation when used in combination. Addition of CCMP, with or without 30 ppm of an antioxidant such as BHA, BHT or TBHQ, to the above systems practically duplicated the flavour effects of nitrite in meats (Table 2).[4,11]

Although presence of yet unreported substances, in minute quantities, may be responsible for the cured flavour, there is no doubt that stabilization of microsomal lipids and heme pigments plays a dominant role in development of cured meat flavour.

4 ANTIMICROBIAL ACTION OF NITRITE AND ITS ALTERNATIVES

Nitrite exerts a concentration-dependent antimicrobial effect in cured meat products.[12] The degree of protection provided to meat depends on the concentration of the residual nitrite, duration of temperature abuse, and extent of contamination. The mechanism(s) by which nitrite inhibits/retards the outgrowth of spores and toxin formation has not been fully elucidated. However, it appears that a reaction with iron-containing enzymes is involved. A better understanding of the exact mechanism(s) of the antimicrobial role of nitrite is still needed.

To take advantage of all positive aspects of nitrite yet to eliminate/reduce the chance of N-nitrosamine formation, use of 10-40 ppm nitrite in meat products possibly together with antimicrobial agents has been tested. Among the antimicrobial agents investigated, para-hydroxybenzoic acid esters (parabens) were found effective in microbiological media.[13] However,their effectiveness in meat against C. botulinum was questionable. Moreover, potassium sorbate at 2600 ppm exhibited antibotulinal activity equivalent to that of nitrite at 156 ppm.[14] In combination with 40 ppm of sodium nitrite, potassium sorbate reduced the extent of N-nitrosamine formation from nearly 100 ppb to less than 5 ppb.

Sodium hypophosphite was another effective candidate which at 3000 ppm alone or at 1000 ppm together with 40 ppm of sodium nitrite provided antibotulinal protection, equivalent to that of 120 ppm nitrite to meats.[15] Esters of fumaric acid at 1250 to 2500 ppm were also found effective.[16]

Lactic acid, its salts, or lactic acid producing bacteria by bacteriocins may be used in meat products to reduce pH of the products. This in turn protects the meat against the formation of botulinum toxin, with or without added nitrite.[17] Wood et al. recently evaluated the antibotulinal activity of some of these compounds in nitrite-free curing systems.[18] The treatment containing 3000 ppm sodium hypophosphite, together with low levels of TBHQ, most closely resembled that of nitrite at 150 ppm. Finally, irradiation at 5 or 10 kGy of meats treated with CCMP not only ensured the microbial quality of products, but it did not have any adverse effects on their colour stability and flavour quality.[19]

5 THE N-NITROSAMINE PROBLEM

Possible presence of N-nitrosamines in muscle foods cured with nitrite or treated with CCMP was monitored. While some samples cured with nitrite showed the presence of N-nitrosodimethylamine, those treated with CCMP were devoid of it, unless nitrite was also present. Therefore, it appears that CCMP-treated samples, under conditions tested, do not contain any of N-nitrosamines (Table 3).

6 CUMULATIVE EFFECTS OF NITRITE ALTERNATIVES

Several nitrite-free combinations consisting of the pre-formed cooked cured-meat pigment, a sequestrant and/or an antioxidant as well as an antimicrobial agent have been formulated for curing of meat products, both comminuted and solid cuts. These mixtures have been effective in reproducing the colour, the oxidative stability and flavour, as well as the antimicrobial effects of nitrite without concerns about N-nitrosamine formation. Formulation of combinations consisting of the pre-formed pigment and all natural ingredients has also been successful.

Table 3 Effects of Nitrite and CCMP on the Formation of N-Nitrosodimethylamine (NDMA) in Selected Muscle Food Systems.

Muscle System	Treatment Mixture, ppm	NDMA, ppb
Cod	Nitrite, 156	0.9
Cod	CCMP, 12	ND
Cod (50%) + Pork (50%)	Nitrite, 156	1.0
Cod (50%) + Pork (50%)	CCMP, 12	ND
Cod (15%) + Pork (85%)	Nitrite, 156	0.3
Cod (15%) + Pork (85%)	CCMP, 12	ND

[a]ND - not detected.

ACKNOWLEDGEMENTS

Financial support from the Natural Sciences and Engineering Research Council (NSERC) of Canada is acknowledged. We are grateful to Dr. N.P. Sen for the analysis of N-nitrosamines in the samples.

REFERENCES

1. J.I. Gray, J. Milk Food Technol., 1976, 39, 686.
2. N.P. Sen, B. Donaldson, S. Seaman, B. Collins and J.R. Iyenger, Can. Inst. Food Sci. Technol. J., 1977, 10, A13.
3. R.A. Holley, Can. Inst. Food Sci. Technol. J., 1981, 14, 183.
4. F. Shahidi and R.B. Pegg, Food Chem., 1992, 43, 185.
5. J.B. Fox, Jr., J. Agric. Food Chem., 1966, 14, 207.
6. F. Shahidi, L.J. Rubin, L.L. Diosady and D.F. Wood, J. Food Sci., 1985, 50, 271.
7. F. Shahidi and R.B. Pegg, J. Food Sci., 1991, 56, 1205.
8. F. Shahidi and R.B. Pegg, J. Food Sci., 1991, 56, 1500.
9. F. Shahidi and R.B. Pegg, J. Muscle Foods, 1991, 2, 297.
10. F. Shahidi, 'ACS Symposium Series 388', American Chemical Society, Washington, DC, 1989, pp. 188-201.
11. F. Shahidi, Trends Food Sci. Technol., 1991, 2, 219.
12. M.D. Pierson and L.A. Smoot, CRC Crit. Rev. Food Sci. Nutr., 1982, 17, 141.
13. M.C. Robach and M.D. Pierson, J. Food Sci., 1978, 43, 787.
14. J.N. Sofos, F.F. Busta and C.E. Allen, J. Food Protec., 1979, 42, 739.
15. M.D. Pierson, K.M. Rice and J.F. Jablocki, 'Proceedings of the 27th European Meat Research Workers Congress', Vienna, Austria, Volume 2, 1981, pp. 651-658.
16. National Academy of Science, 'Alternatives to the Current Use of Nitrite in Foods', National Academy of Science, Washington, DC, p. 43.
17. M.E. Stiles and J.W. Hastings, Trends Food Sci Technol., 1991, 2, 247.
18. D.S. Wood, D.L. Collins-Thompson, W.R. Usborne and B. Picard, J. Food Protec., 1986, 49, 691.
19. F. Shahidi, R.B. Pegg and K. Shamsuzzaman, J. Food Sci., 1991, 56, 1450.

CARBOHYDRATES, ESPECIALLY MONO- AND DISACCHARIDES IN EXCESS INHIBIT THE FORMATION OF MUTAGENIC HETEROCYCLIC AMINES DURING FRYING OF MEAT

K.I. Skog and I.M. Jägerstad

Department of Applied Nutrition and Food Chemistry, Chemical Center, University of Lund, P.O. Box 124, S-221 00 Lund, Sweden

1 INTRODUCTION

During the last decade more than a dozen mutagenic heterocyclic amines(HA) have been isolated from the crust of fried meat and fish[1,2]. All of them so far tested in long-term animal experiments have been shown to be multipotent carcinogens[3-6]. Therefore, though no evidence yet exists that they are carcinogenic to man, IARC regard them as potential human carcinogens and recommend actions that might reduce human exposure to such compounds[7]. Moreover, recent epidemiological studies indicate increased relative cancer risk for persons consuming well-done red meat[8,9].

The heterocyclic amines isolated from fried, broiled, deep-fried or baked meat and fish have also been shown to arise from heating creatine, free amino acids and sugar in model systems at temperatures between 125°C and 200°C[10,11]. These three classes of precursors (creatine, free amino acids and sugar) occur naturally in animal muscles from meat and fish in varying concentrations[10]. Generally, sugar is present in muscles in half the molar amounts of the other precursors. According to recent observations using model systems, mono- and disaccharides in half the molar amounts of those of creatine and/or amino acids give an optimum yield of the heterocyclic amines[12,13]. In contrast, the presence of an increasing proportion of mono- and disaccharides inhibits the formation of HA[12,13].

The fact that sugar in excess compared with the other precursors, inhibits the formation of HA in model systems tempted us to examine if addition of carbohydrates to beef patties could reduce the formation of HA. Minced meat was mixed with either milk powder or starch from potato or golden bread crumbs with and without addition of glucose and lactose and formed to beef patties, that were pan-fried. The formation of HA was monitored using Ames test and compared with the mutagenic activity formed in beef patties without any addition of carbohydrates.

2 MATERIAL AND METHODS

Frying of beef patties

Beef patties were prepared by mixing minced meat (bovine *Musculus longissimus dorsi*) with water and either glucose (1,2 or 4%), lactose (1,2, or 4%) or powdered milk (2,4 o 8%) before frying. In another experiment minced meat was mixed with starch from golden bread crumbs (3%) or potatoes (4%) with and without glucose (1,3 or 4%). The recipe of the patties fried is shown in Table I. Patties, 7 mm thick with a diameter of 10-11 cm, were formed, each weighing 100g. The patties were fried, one at a time in a thermostat-controlled, double-sided and teflon-coated fryer for 3 min at 180°C or 150°C. For each patty, 3 g lard devoid of carbohydrates, was used as frying fat. After frying, the patties were weighed and frozen, and th crusts(1-2 mm thickness from each side) were removed with a scalpel. For each type of patty, the crusts from three patties were pooled.

Table I Experimental design and composition of raw beef patties

		Recipe for 100 g raw patty				
Frying temperature	Sample No.	Meat (g)	Water (g)	Starch (g)	Sugar (g)	
Experiment 1	1	96.2	3.8			0
(180°C)	2	95.2	3.8		Glucose	1.0
	3	94.3	3.8		Glucose	1.9
	4	92.6	3.7		Glucose	3.7
	5	95.2	3.8		Lactose	1.0
	6	94.3	3.8		Lactose	1.9
	7	92.6	3.7		Lactose	3.7
	8	94.3	3.7		Lactose[1]	1.0
	9	92.4	3.7		Lactose[1]	1.9
	10	89.0	3.6		Lactose[1]	3.7
Experiment 2	11	96.2	3.8			0
(180°C)	12	87.7	6.5	3.8[2]		0
	13	87.0	6.1	3.8[2]	Glucose	0.9
	14	84.8	5.9	3.8[2]	Glucose	3.4
	15	87.0	6.1	3.8[2]	Lactose	0.9
	16	84.8	6.9	3.8[2]	Lactose	3.4
Experiment 3	17	96.2	3.8			0
(150°C)	18	93.5	3.7	2.8[3]		0
	19	94.3	3.8		Glucose	1.9
	20	91.7	3.6	2.8[3]	Glucose	1.9

1) Lactose in powdered milk
2) Golden bread crumbs containing 65 % starch
3) Potato starch

Analysis of mutagenic activity

The crusts, about 40 g for each sample, were extracted and purified as earlier described[14]. The mutagenic activity was determined according to Ames et al.[15] using Salmonella typhimurium strain TA 98 with metabolic activation by rat liver homogenate (3mg S-9 protein per plate). Four dose points run in duplicate were used to produce dose-response curves. The mutagenic activity in the crusts, expressed as the number of TA 98 revertants, was calculated from the linear part of the the curves. Synthetic 2-amino-3,8-dimethylimidazo[4,5-f]quinoxaline (MeIQx) used as a positive control yielded around 50 000 revertants/μg.

3 RESULTS AND DISCUSSION

The mutagenic activity in the crusts expressed as the number of TA 98 revertants per 100 gE is shown in Figure 1[16]. (gE denotes uncooked pure meat corrected for the dilution effect of the ingredients added to the meat). When glucose or lactose was added to beef patties, the mutagenic activity in the crusts was depressed in all samples but one (No.19). The inhibitory effect was similar (37-76%) for glucose and lactose in corresponding concentrations, but was weaker (32-66%) for lactose from powdered milk. In samples Nos 12 and 18 containing only starch (from bread or potato), a rather modest inhibitory effect (<25%) on mutagenic activity was observed. In our study, the greatest inhibitory effect on mutagenic activity (54-79%) was obtained when both starch and glucose/lactose were added to the sample (Nos 13-16, 20).

The observed inhibitory effect on mutagenic activity of glucose/lactose when added to meat is in accordance with our previous modelling studies in which we showed that glucose or lactose, in more than equimolar amounts compared with creatine, clearly inhibited the formation of mutagens. The mechanism behind the inhibitory effect of glucose and lactose is still unknown. However, with increasing concentrations of reducing sugars, the Maillard reaction may favour the formation of other Maillard reaction products, thus competing with the formation of mutagenic heterocyclic amines. The Maillard reaction is also known to produce antioxidants, which may inhibit mutagen formation[17].

In conclusion, the present study clearly demonstrates that adding pure glucose or lactose, powdered milk or starch in combination with glucose/lactose to beef patties markedly inhibited the mutagenic activity in the crust after frying at 150 or 180°C. The Maillard reaction has a significant influence on colour formation: more reducing sugars lead to more rapid browning. This result indicates that milder cooking conditions can be used when glucose or lactose is added to beef patties, and that the time and temperature required for patties to achieve an acceptable brown colour can be decreased. We have shown that it is possible to depress mutagenic activity from about 4000 to about 1600 revertants/100 g meat and still obtain a patty with a good taste.

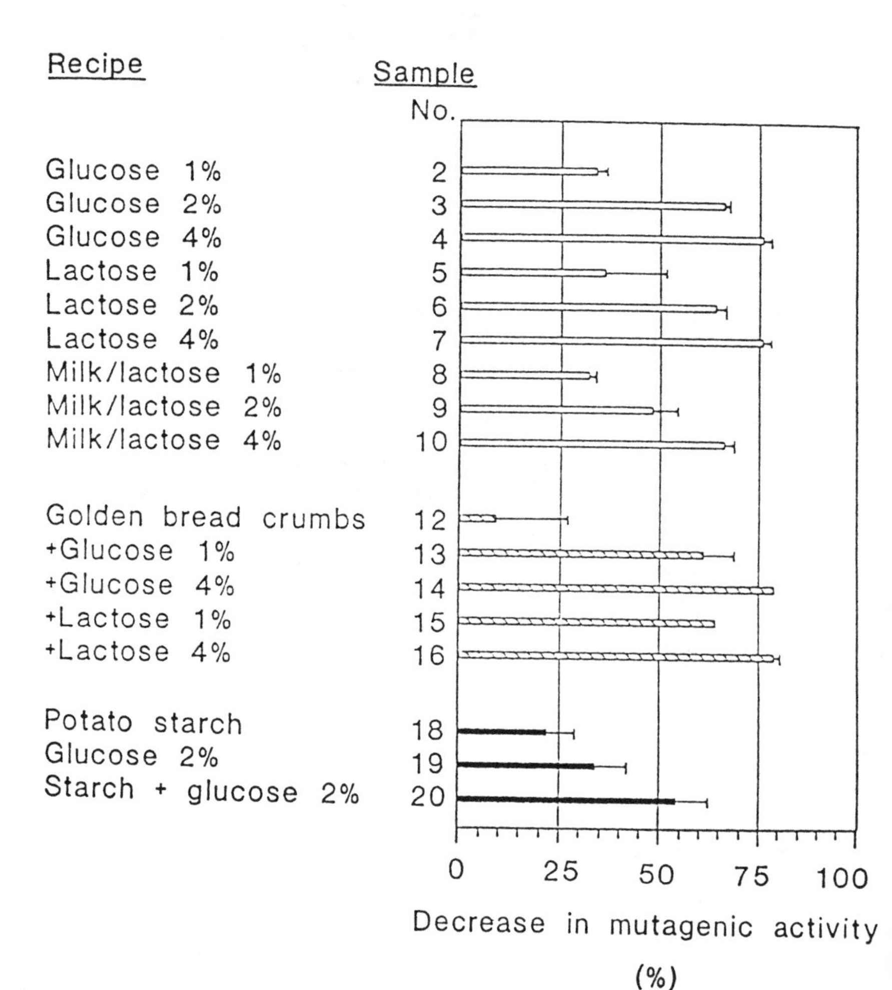

(from K.Skog et al, Fd Chem Tox, 1992, in press)

Figure 1 Inhibition (mean and maximum value of two tests) of the mutagenic activity in the crust of beef patties fried for 3 min in a double-sided fryer. The patties were mixed with additional ingredients before frying. Experiment 1, 180°C, Experiment 2, 180°C, and Experiment 3, 150°C. The percentage of inhibition was calculated in comparison with that of reference patties (0%, sample no 1, 11 or 17).

4 ACKNOWLEDGEMENTS

We thank our technician, Ms Marie Birger, and Ms Cecilia Granström for their excellent assistance. This study was supported finacially by the Swedish Cancer Foundation (1824-B88-06XB) and the Swedish Council for Forestry and Agricultural Research(85/88L-96:3).

5 REFERENCES

1. T.S. Sugimura, S. Sato and K.J. Wakabayashi, 'Chemical Induction of Cancer, Structural Bases and Biological mechanisms', Academic Press, New York, 1988, pp 681.
2. J.S. Felton, Mutat. Res., 1991, 259, 205.
3. T.S. Sugimura and K.J. Wakabayashi, Prog. Clin. Biol. Res., 1990, 347, 1.
4. H. Ohgaki, S. Takayama and T. Sugimura, Mutat. Res., 1991, 259, 399
5. I. Nobuyiki, R. Hasegawa, M. Sano, S. Tamano, H. Esumi, S. Takayama and T. Sugimura, Carcinogenesis, 1991, 12, 1503.
6. M. Ochiai, K. Ogawa, K. Wakabayashi, T. Sugimura, S. Nagase, H. Esumi and M. Nagao, Jpn. J. Cancer Res. 1991, 82, 363.
7. IARC Monogr 40: 1986, p 223
8. M.H. Schiffman and J.S. Felton, Amer. J. Epidemiol., 1990, 131, 376
9. W.C. Willett, M.J. Stampfer, G.C. Colditz, B.A. Rosner and F.E. Speizer, New Engl. J. Med., 1990, 323, 1664.
10. M. Jägerstad, A. Laser Reuterswärd, R. Öste, A. Dahlqvist, S. Grivas, K. Olsson and T. Nyhammar, 'The Maillard reactions in Fods and Nutrition' ACS Symposium Series, Washington DC, 1983, 215, 507.
11. M. Jägerstad, K. Skog, S. Grivas and K. Olsson, Mutat. Res, 1991, 259 219.
12. K. Skog and M. Jägerstad, Mutat. Res., 1990, 230, 263.
13. K. Skog and M. Jägerstad, Carcinogenesis, 1991, 12, 2297.
14. L.F. Bjeldanes, K.G. Grose, P.H. Davis, D.H. Stuermer, S.K. Healy and J.S. Felton, Mutat. Res., 1982, 105, 43.
15. B.N. Ames, J. McCann and E. Yamasaki, Mutat. Res., 1975, 31, 347.
16. K. Skog, M. Jägerstad and A. Laser Reuterswärd, Fd Chem. Toxic., 1992 in press.
17. H. Lignert and K. Eriksson, 'Progress in Food and Nutrition Science. Maillard Reactions in Foods,' 1981, 5, 453.

Effects of ellagic acid, tannic acid and quercetin on the mutagenic activity of cooked food mutagens in the *Salmonella* strain TA98

Michael Strube, Preben Aagaard Nielsen and John C. Larsen

Institute of Toxicology,
National Food Agency,
DK-2860 Søborg, Denmark.

1 INTRODUCTION

During the last decade a number of studies have shown that plant phenols are able to counteract the mutagenic activity *in vitro* of different types of chemicals[1-3]. Especially ellagic acid, tannic acid and the hydroxylated flavonoid quercetin have shown potent anti-mutagenic activities[4-9]. A reduction in the activity of the phase I (activating) enzymes has been proposed as the anti-mutagenic mechanism of action of the plant phenols, resulting in an inhibition of the biotransformation of promutagens to ultimate mutagens[10,11]. Furthermore, a scavenging effect of plant phenols has been demonstrated towards the direct acting diol-epoxide metabolites of PAHs[5,12].

Most often PAHs have been used as the mutagenic compounds in studies on the inhibitory effect of plant phenols, and only a few other food-related mutagens, like mycotoxins and N-nitroso compounds, have so far been used. A few studies have been performed with heterocyclic amines isolated from cooked food. Structurally these cooked food mutagens belong to the amino-imidazo azaarenes, and at least three subclasses have to date been isolated from fried meat[13]: the quinolines (e.g. IQ and MeIQ), the quinoxalines (e.g. IQx, MeIQx and DiMeIQx) and the pyridines (e.g. PhIP).

Ayrton et al.[3,4] have studied the effect of plant phenols on the mutagenic activity of IQ, whereas the effect of plant phenols on the mutagenic activity of IQ, MeIQ and MeIQx has been studied by Alldrick et al.[6]

It is reasonable to assume that nearly the whole human population is exposed to the cooked food mutagens via the diet. As the plant phenols are ubiquitous in e.g. fruits and vegetables as well as in soft beverages like tea and coffee, we have studied the effect of ellagic acid, tannic acid and

---

Abbreviations: PAH: Polycyclic aromatic hydrocarbon; IQ = 2-amino-3-methyl-imidazo[4,5-f] quinoline; MeIQ = 2-amino-3,4-dimethyl-imidazo[4,5-f]-quinoline; MeIQx = 2-amino-3,8-dimethyl-imidazo[4,5-f]quinoxaline; DiMeIQx = 2-amino-3,4,8-trimethylimidazo[4,5-f] quinoxaline; PhIP = 2-amino-1-methyl-6-phenyl-imidazo[4,5-b] pyridine.

quercetin on the mutagenic activity in the Salmonella/microsome assay of MeIQ, DiMeIQx and PhIP, which includes some of the cooked food mutagens occurring in the largest amount in the diet[14,15].

2 MATERIALS & METHODS

Chemicals

Tannic acid, ellagic acid and quercetin were obtained from Sigma (St. Louis, Mo, USA). Tannic acid is a mixture of digallic acid esters of glucose, of which the major one is pentadigalloylglucose with an empirical formula of $C_{76}H_{52}O_{46}$ and a molecular weight of 1701.

MeIQ and DiMeIQx were kindly supplied by Dr. Kjell Olsson, the Swedish University of Agriculture, Uppsala, Sweden. PhIP was the kind gift from Dr. Errol Zeiger, NIEHS, Research Triangle Park, North Carolina, USA. Dimethyl sulfoxide (DMSO) (analytical grade) was from Merck (Darmstadt, Germany). Aroclor 1254 was obtained from Monsanto Industrial Chemical Co., St. Louis, USA.

Mutagenicity Testing

The Salmonella/mammalian microsome assays were carried out by the pre-incubation procedure, as described by Maron and Ames[16], using the strain TA98 kindly provided by Dr. Bruce N. Ames, University of California, Berkeley, California.

One tenth of a ml of different concentrations of plant phenol in DMSO was pre-incubated for 30 min. at 37 °C with 0.1 ml of cooked food mutagen dissolved in DMSO, 0.1 ml of a 7 h nutrient broth (Oxoid) culture of bacteria (1 - 2 x 10^9 cells/ml), and 0.5 ml of S-9 mix (1 mg protein/ml) prepared from Aroclor 1254 induced male Wistar rat livers. After the pre-incubation period the mixture was added 2 ml of top agar at 45 °C before pouring on minimal glucose agar plates. The number of His^+ revertants on each plate was counted by a Biotran II automatic Colony Counter after a 48 h incubation period at 37 °C.

The test results were evaluated statistically using one way analysis of variance (StatPac Gold). In experiments where the plant phenol significantly ($p<0.05$) inhibited the mutagenic activity of the mutagen this effect was quantified by determining the molar ratio of plant phenol to mutagen which resulted in a 50% reduction in the number of mutant colonies observed. This value, I_{50}, was estimated from the dose-response curve, using linear regression analysis (StatPac Gold).

3 RESULTS & DISCUSSION

In preliminary experiments the plant phenols were tested solely, without the presence of the cooked food mutagens. No mutagenicity or toxicity was observed in the experiments with ellagic acid and tannic acid, even at the highest concentration (1000 nmol per plate), whereas quercetin was mutagenic at the higher concentrations (data not shown). This mutagenic activity of quercetin may hide a possible anti-mutagenic effect, and complicate the data interpretation.

The results of the testing of the three plant phenols in the presence of the cooked food mutagens are shown in Figure 1, and the I_{50} values are shown in Table 1.

The effect of the plant phenols on the mutagenicity of MeIQ (Figure 1A)

From Figure 1A it is seen, that all three plant phenols tested showed a concentration dependent significant inhibition of the mutagenic activity of MeIQ, although with different strength, see the I_{50} values in Table 1. The strongest inhibition was observed with tannic acid which at the highest concentrations completely inhibited the mutagenic activity of MeIQ. The shape of the curve for quercetin at the highest concentrations reflects the mutagenicity of quercetin.

The effect of the plant phenols on the mutagenicity of DiMeIQx (Figure 1B)

None of the plant phenols tested showed any inhibition of the mutagenic activity of DiMeIQx. Again, the shape of the curve for quercetin reflects the mutagenic activity of this compound.

The effect of the plant phenols on the mutagenicity of PhIP (Figure 1C)

Compared with the effect of the plant phenols on the mutagenic activities of MeIQ and DiMeIQx, the effect on the mutagenic activity of PhIP

Table 1 I_{50} values[a] for the effect of tannic acid, ellagic acid and quercetin on the mutagenic activity of different cooked food mutagens.

Mutagen	MeIQ (19 pmol/pl)	DiMeIQx (44 pmol/pl)	PhIP (1000 pmol/pl)
Tannic acid	2630	-	125
Ellagic acid	9062	-	844
Quercetin	3947	-	-

Notes: [a]: The I_{50} values (molar ratio plant phenol:mutagen which caused 50% inhibition of the mutagenic activity) were determined as described in Materials and Methods.
A dash (-) indicate that no reproducible, significant inhibitory effect was detected.

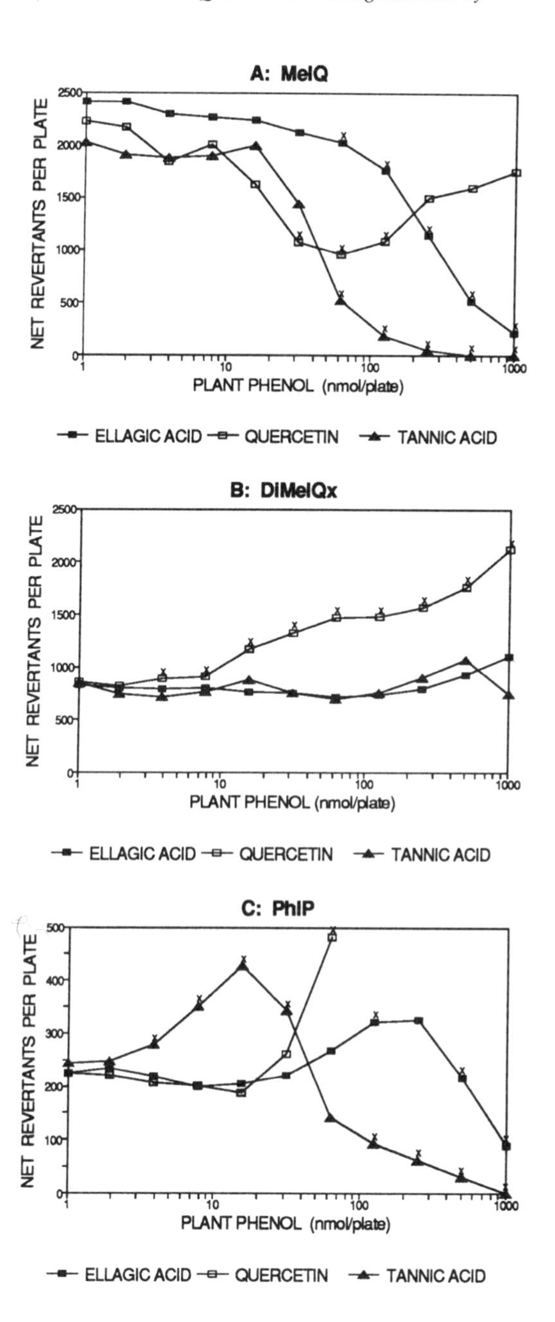

Figure 1, A, B & C The effect of ellagic acid, quercetin and tannic acid on the mutagenic activity of MeIQ (A), DiMeIQx (B) and PhIP (C). The values shown are mean from duplicate experiments. Points marked with an 'x' indicate a significant, reproducible effect of the plant phenol on the mutagenic activity.

seems to be more complicated. For ellagic acid, and especially for tannic acid, an enhancement of the mutagenicity of PhIP was seen at the lower concentrations, whereas at the higher concentrations an inhibition of the mutagenicity was observed. No effect of quercetin was observed on the mutagenicity of PhIP. This stimulating effect of ellagic acid and tannic acid at the lower concentrations on the mutagenicity may be due to a stabilising (antioxidant) effect on the reactive metabolite of PhIP, the N-hydroxy compound (N-OH-PhIP), which is very unstable when exposed to atmospheric oxygen[17,18]. At the higher concentrations of plant phenol this effect may be overruled by the inhibitory effect, possibly acting by an inhibition of the biotransformation of PhIP.

In conclusion, we have detected a strong anti-mutagenic effect of ellagic acid and especially tannic acid on the mutagenicity of MeIQ and PhIP, and an anti-mutagenic effect of quercetin on MeIQ, but no effect of any of the plant phenols on the mutagenicity of DiMeIQx. These differences in the inhibiting activities on chemically closely related compounds are now subject to further studies.

REFERENCES

1. **Stich, H.F. & M.P. Rosin**, Adv. Exp. Med. Biol., **1984**, 177, 1.
2. **Tervel, L. & J.C.M. van der Hoeven**, Mutation Res., **1985**, 152, 1.
3. **Ayrton, A.D.**, C. Ioannides and R. Walker, Mutation Res., **1988**, 207, 121.
4. **Ayrton, A.D.**, D.F. Lewis, R. Walker and C. Ioannides, Fd. Chem. Toxic., **1992**, 30, 289.
5. **Wood, A.W.**, M.-T. Huang, R.L. Chang, H.L. Newmark, R.E. Lehr, H. Yagi, J.M. Sayer, D.M. Jerina and A.H. Conney, Proc. Natl. Acad. Sci., USA, **1982**, 79, 5513.
6. **Alldrick, A.J.**, J. Flynn and I.R. Rowland, Mutation Res., **1986**, 163, 225.
7. **Shimoi, K.**, Y. Nakamura, I. Tomita, Y. Hara and T. Kada, Mutation Res., **1986**, 173, 239.
8. **Huang,M-T.**, A.W. Wood, H.L. Newmark, J.M. Sayer, H. Yagi, D.M. Jerina and A.H. Conney, Carcinogenesis, **1983**, 4, 1631.
9. **Huang, M-T.**, R.L. Chang, A.W. Wood, H.L. Newmark, J.M. Sayer, H. Yagi, D.M. Jerina and A.H. Conney, Carcinogenesis, **1985**, 6, 237.
10. **Del Tito, Jr., B.J.**, H. Mukhtar and D.R. Blickers, Biochem. Biophys. Res. Comm., **1983**, 114, 388.
11. **Das, M.**, H. Mukhtar, D.P. Blik and D.R. Blickers, Cancer Res., **1987**, 47, 760.
12. **Sayer, J.M.**, H. Yagi, A.W. Wood, A.H. Conney and D.M. Jerina, J. Am. Chem. Soc., **1982**, 104, 5562.
13. **Övervik, E. & J.-Å. Gustafsson**, Mutagenesis, **1990**, 5, 437.
14. **Ushiyama, H.**, K. Wakabayashi, M. Hisako, H. Itoh, T. Sugimura and M. Nagao, Carcinogenesis, **1991**, 12, 1417.
15. **Nielsen, P.A.**, M. Vahl and J. Gry, manuscript in preparation.
16. **Maron,D. & B.N. Ames**, Mutation Res., **1983**, 113, 149.
17. **Frandsen, H.**, E.S. Rasmussen, P.A. Nielsen, P. Farmer, L. Dragsted and J.C. Larsen, Mutagenesis, **1990**, 6, 93.
18. **Frandsen, H.**, S. Grivas, R. Andersson, L. Dragsted and J.C. Larsen, Carcinogenesis, **1992**, 13, 629.

ANALYSIS OF HUMAN SERA FOR AFLATOXIN

A.P. Wilkinson, D.W. Denning,[a] H.A. Lee, C.M. Ward and M.R.A. Morgan.

Department of Food Molecular Biochemistry
AFRC Institute of Food Research
Norwich Laboratory
Colney
Norwich NR4 7UA
UK

[a] Department of Infectious Diseases
Hope Hospital
Salford
M6 8HD
UK

1. INTRODUCTION

The aflatoxins are a group of potent toxins formed by certain species of Aspergillus fungi, moulds that commonly infest a wide range of food components, particularly nuts and cereals. Aflatoxins are of concern because of their toxicity and carcinogenicity at very low concentrations, often parts per billion, in a large number of animal species including primates.[1]

Acute illness and death in humans resulting from ingestion of high levels of aflatoxin are rare, but because of their potency, it is possible that regular ingestion of aflatoxin at sub-acute levels may pose a threat to human health particularly in cancer development.[2] To assess such a possibility, two strategies may be employed;

(a) Test food destined for human consumption

(b) Analyse human body fluids and tissues.

For both approaches, the ability to rapidly and cost effectively quantify low aflatoxin levels in large sample numbers of foods, body fluids and tissues is necessary.[3]

The Biorecognition and Immunotechnology group at IFR has developed enzyme-linked immunosorbent assays (ELISAS) to determine aflatoxin in a wide range of foodstuffs.[4] One of these assays was adapted to measure aflatoxin in human serum.[5] The test procedure is simple, requiring the addition of methanol to samples to precipate interfering substances prior to assay.

The figure below shows a standard curve for aflatoxin B_1 diluted with methanol-treated aflatoxin free control serum. The limit of detection of the assay, dotted line, is 1 pg.well^{-1} giving an assay sensitivity of 20 pg.ml^{-1} of original serum. Also shown in the diagram is the analysis of 27 serum samples obtained from U.K. blood donors. None of the samples had aflatoxin above 20 pg.ml^{-1}.[6] In contrast Figure 2 shows that the blood of some Nigerian [7] and all of the Nepalese [8] subjects studied were contaminated with aflatoxin.

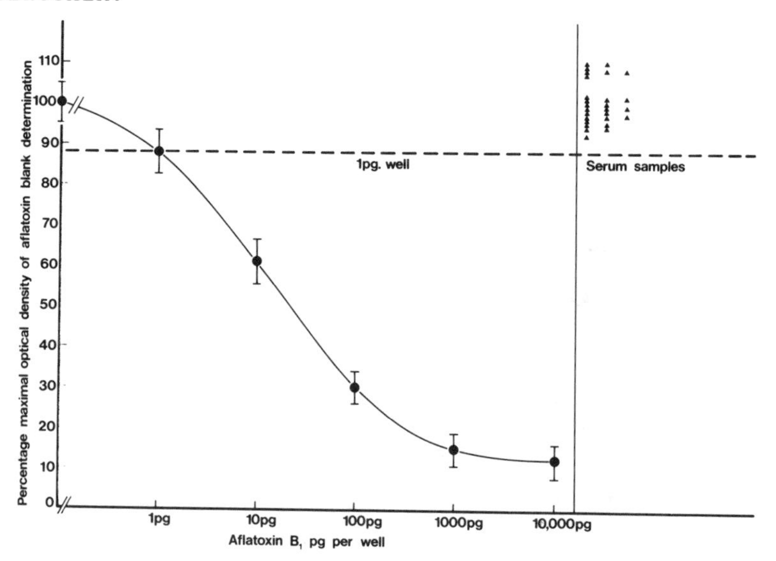

Fig.1 An ELISA standard curve for aflatoxin B_1 in human serum. Points are plotted ± 2 s.d.

For the Nigerian study, 19 samples (24%) had no detectable aflatoxin, whilst 59 samples (76%) were positive. The positive samples ranged from 20 pg.ml^{-1} to 3.1 ng.ml^{-1} with a mean of 665 pg.ml^{-1}. All these subjects were apparently healthy. The aflatoxin levels detected in the 28 Nepalese subjects ranged from 60 pg.ml^{-1} to 10 ng.ml^{-1}. Of these donors, 16 were hospitalized and 12 were healthy hospital workers. There was no correlation between the health of the donors at time of sampling and the level of aflatoxin in their blood.

Though these three studies have examined a small sample size, the results reflect the risk of exposure to aflatoxin in different areas of the world. In the U.K., the most likely source of aflatoxin is from imported foods, particularly nuts, and the results seem to show that voluntary and statutory regulations

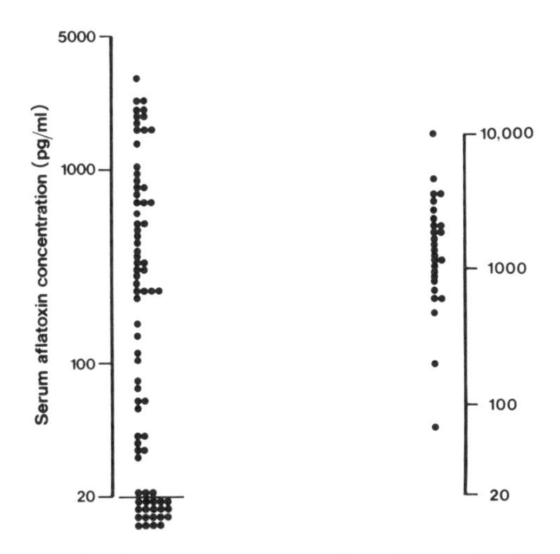

Fig.2 Aflatoxin concentration in sera from 78 Nigerian and 28 Nepalese subjects.

governing aflatoxin levels in foods and animal foodstuffs have been effective in limiting the exposure of the U.K. population to aflatoxin. Unlike the U.K., tropical and sub-tropical countries such as Nigeria and Nepal, have climates and food storage systems that favour aflatoxin production by toxigenic moulds that commonly infest foods. Thus local produce becomes contaminated by aflatoxin particularly during or just following the wet season. Our studies of Nigerian and Nepalese subjects were made at such time and the higher risk of consuming aflatoxin contaminated food is reflected in the data.

High levels of aflatoxin consumption during pregnancy might have mutagenic, carcinogenic or immunosuppressive effects on the human fetus if transplacental transmission of aflatoxin occurs. Such toxic effects have been demonstrated in other species.[9] Fig. 3 shows the results of our study of blood from 35 paired samples of Thai mothers and neonates.[9] The blood was collected from the cord at birth and from the mother immediately afterwards. Seventeen (48%) of the cord sera and two of the maternal sera (6%) contained detectable aflatoxin.

The low contamination of the maternal blood samples possibly reflects the absence of food intake prior to delivery as well as the timing of the study which was made during the dry season when aflatoxin contamination of food has been observed to be low.[10] The results show

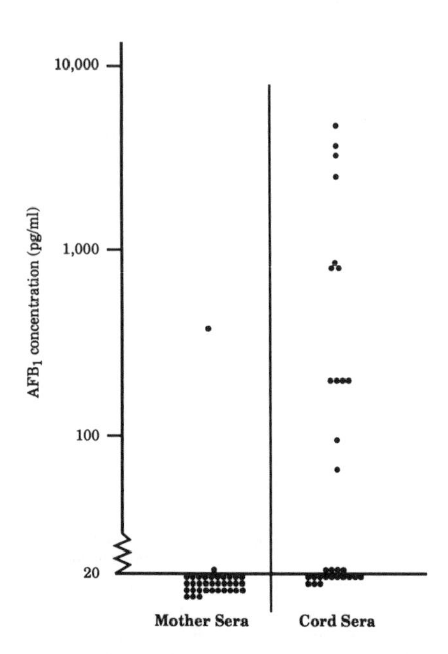

Fig.3 Aflatoxin concentration in sera of paired samples of Thai mothers and neonates.

clearly transplacental transfer of aflatoxin and it would also appear that the feto-placental unit is capable of concentrating aflatoxin, as a result of excretion of aflatoxin into the amniotic fluid and re-ingestion of the toxin.

2. CONCLUSIONS

(1) The ELISA is a simple and sensitive technique for monitoring aflatoxin exposure at the individual level.

(2) Aflatoxin levels in U.K. plasma is low.

(3) The high levels of aflatoxin in the sera of Nigerian and Nepalese subjects indicate that populations in tropical and sub-tropical countries can be exposed to considerable amounts of aflatoxin in their diets.

(4) Aflatoxin can cross the human placental membrane and may be concentrated by the developing feto-placental unit.

ACKNOWLEDGEMENTS

This work was sponsored by the Ministry of Agriculture, Fisheries and Food.

REFERENCES

1. W.F.Busby and G.N.Wogan, 'Chemical Carcinogens', C.E.Searle (ed), American Chemical Society, Washington D.C., 1985, Vol.2, p.945.
2. D.W.Denning, *Adverse Drug React. Acute Poison Rev.* 1987, *4*, 175.
3. J.D.Groopman and K.F.Donahue, *J. Assoc. Off. Anal. Chem.*, 1988, *71*, 861.
4. M.R.A.Morgan, A.S.Kang and H.W-S.Chan, *J. Sci. Food Agric.*, 1986, *37*, 908.
5. A.P.Wilkinson, D.W.Denning, and M.R.A.Morgan, *Food Add. Contam.*, 1988, *5*, 609.
6. A.P.Wilkinson, D.W.Denning and M.R.A.Morgan, *Hum. Toxicol.*, 1988, *7*, 353.
7. D.W.Denning, J.K. Onwubalili, A.P.Wilkinson and M.R.A.Morgan, *Trans. R. Soc. Trop. Med. Hyg.*, 1988, *82*, 169.
8. A.P.Wilkinson, D.W.Denning and M.R.A.Morgan, *J. Toxicol. Toxin Rev*, 1989, *8*, 69.
9. D.W.Denning, R.Allen, A.P.Wilkinson and M.R.A.Morgan, *Carcinogenesis*, 1990, *11*, 1033.
10. R.C.Shank, J.E.Gordon, G.N.Wogan, A.Nondasuta and B.Subhamini, *Food Cosmet. Toxicol.*, 1972, *10*, 71.

WORKSHOP REPORT: DIETARY CARCINOGENESIS - WHAT ROLE IN HUMAN CANCER?

W. Jongen

ATO-DLO
Haagsteeg 6
Postbus 1
6700AA Wageningen
The Netherlands

The Workshop dealt with two major subjects: 1) the occurrence and 2) the significance. Within these subjects priority was given to the following topics.

1a. Naturally occurring carcinogens.

1b. Role of food preparation and endogenous formation.

2a. The use of experimental systems.

2b. Markers of exposure.

2c. Epidemiological approaches.

1a. Naturally occurring carcinogens.

There was a general consensus that the major naturally occurring carcinogens have been identified. There is not one dominating factor and the relationship between diet and cancer comes from an interplay between a large number of contributing factors, although there are examples in certain regions of a specific compound being implicated in a specific type of cancer, such as aflatoxin in liver cancer. Future research should be aimed at the extrapolation. Compounds are generally tested in isolation, at maximally tolerated doses, and such approaches were felt not to be appropriate for food associated compounds. The food matrix is a major modulating factor and should be included in future experiments.

Dr Schlatter presented some of his work on risk estimation using data from experimental animal studies. He pointed out that caloric intake is a major determining factor in tumour occurrence and that caloric intake should be controlled in these types of studies.

1b. Role of food preparation and endogenous formation

There is no evidence for a role of food contaminants and additives in Western societies. With regard to food preparation there are two groups of compounds which are candidates to be implicated in human cancer. For the heterocyclic amines, relationships were suggested between the occurrence and the incidence of breast and colon cancer.

With regard to the N-nitroso compounds it was felt that there is good experimental evidence for the carcinogenic potential of these compounds. There is a lack of appropriate epidemiological data on this subject. Factors to be considered are: 1) mode of action 2) organ specificity 3) nitrite-counterpart 4) appropriate controls.

2a. Use of experimental systems

1. Isolated Compounds

Advantages:

- Can very easily be tested in *in vitro* mutagenicity, carcinogenicity or promoter tests.

- Are very easy to handle in pre-screening tests and mechanistic studies.

- Can be concentrated for use in dose-response studies.

- Fit quite well in standard toxicological protocols to establish guidelines (ADI, permissible levels).

Disadvantages:

- Sometimes so many different compounds are formed (e.g. pyrolysates, Maillard reaction products due to heating) that it is extremely difficult or impossible to predict the final effect, due to unknown interactions and the presence of unknown compounds. Another example is the transgenic plant where, by changes in metabolic routes and pleotropic effects, unknown compounds may be formed.

- The effect of the food matrix in the toxicity and the bioavailability of individual constituents is often unknown (e.g. flavonoids-glycosides, cell wall constituents, binding to proteins).

- Nutritional influences are missed, like effects on pH, intestinal uptake, digestion, interaction with micro- and macronutrients.

2. Whole food

Advantages:

- Combined effects, effects of the matrix and nutritional influences are all involved.

- Testing whole food in animals makes extrapolation to human diet and human cancer easier.

Disadvantages:

- *In vitro* testing is limited, extraction and fractionation procedures are necessary.

- Concentration of particular food factors is limited, or impossible.

- Normally used safety factors (100) for assessing ADI's can not be applied.

- Experiments are time-consuming and more expensive.

Testing individual compounds can give an over-or under-estimation of the real risk (e.g. the carcinogenic risk of baking or frying). On the other hand whole food without or with limited concentration of the carcinogenic compound(s), may miss weak effects of the compound due to the limited number of test animals and the lack of sensitivity of this type of approach.

2b. Markers for exposure

The concept of biomarkers provides a useful framework to structure these metabolic routes and pathophysiological processes.

Three main categories of biomarkers can be distinguished: (i) biomarkers of dietary exposure, reflecting recent or time-integrated longer-term intake; (ii) biomarkers of disease or outcome, such as tumour markers, or biomarkers of early stages in the disease process, like activated oncogenes, bronchial or cervical dysplasia, colon polyps; (iii) susceptibility markers, indicating whether an individual will react more sensitively to the compound of exposure, like lipids or fibre, or has an innate genetic trait which prediposes to, e.g. carcinogenesis or atherogenesis. Susceptibility markers may help to trace high risk groups who might benefit most from, e.g. chemoprevention. Objectives of the application of biomarkers are:

- To improve sensitivity and specifity of exposure measures, to increase validity and strengthen weak associations between dietary factors and health outcomes.

- To allow for more etiologically relevant disease classification.

- To identify (individual) susceptibility and thus effect modification.

- To enhance understanding of the mechanisms of disease occurrence to the extent that biomarkers are part of the causal chain between exposure, susceptibility and disease.

2c. Epidemiological approach

There is evidence from epidemiologic studies that cooked meat and fish are associated with the occurrence of colon and pancreatic cancer. During the cooking process mutagenic heterocyclic amines may be formed. These pyrolytic products can be metabolically activated by humans both through N-oxidation and O-oxidation to produce highly reactive metabolites that form DNA adducts. In rats these compounds readily lead to induction of tumours. Turesky and co-workers concluded that these genotoxins should be distinctly regarded as potential human colo-rectal carcinogens. One limitation of epidemiological studies in this field is that there is no appropriate control, so that no distinction can be made between the suspected heterocyclic amines and other unknown intrinsic factors.

PART 3 FREE RADICAL REACTIONS AND ANTIOXIDANT NUTRIENTS IN THE ETIOLOGY OF HUMAN CANCERS

CHEMICAL ASPECTS AND BIOLOGICAL MECHANISMS OF ANTICANCER NUTRIENTS IN PLANT FOODS

D.I. Thurnham

MRC Dunn Nutrition Centre,
Milton Road,
Cambridge CB4 1XJ

1 INTRODUCTION

The importance of lifestyle and particularly diet in the aetiology of cancer is widely accepted. Analyses of cancer mortality statistics in the United States suggest that dietary factors contribute to as much as 35% (range 10 to 70%) of cancer risk.[1,2] However, in addition to foods like fat, meat, salt etc which may increase the risk of cancer, diet also contains foods which appear to reduce the cancer risk. High intakes of vegetables and fruits which are major sources of fibre as well as several vitamins, are frequently protective.[3-5] The principal nutrients in plant foods which are believed to have anticancer properties are vitamins C[5,6] and the precursors of vitamin A namely the pro-vitamin A carotenoids.[4,7] Vitamin E[8,9], riboflavin[10,11] and folic acid[12] have also attracted a certain amount of interest as have specific elements; selenium[3], zinc, molybdenum, manganese[5,13,14] and magnesium.[15]

Epidemiological studies suggest that certain nutrient deficiencies may be site-specific with respect to protection against cancers.[16] In particular, good vitamin C status is associated with a lower risk for gastric and oesophageal cancer[6] and β-carotene with protection against lung[17,18], oral[19] and to a lesser extent cervical cancer[20]. Vitamin E is effective *in vitro* against mutagenesis and can suppress chemically-induced cancer in animals[6] but no definite links with human cancer have been established except a possible protection against lung and breast cancer in Finnish non-smokers[8,9]. Retinol and retinoids in general protect against carcinogenesis *in vitro* and good vitamin A status is associated with a lower risk of many epithelial cancers in man. Circulating vitamin A however is carefully controlled in mammals and it is widely accepted that vitamin A or retinol may be acting as a proxy for β-carotene or carotenes in general.[21] Links between selenium deficiency and cancer of the breast[3], riboflavin or zinc deficiency with oesophageal cancer[14] and folate deficiency with cancer of the cervix[12] are less well established.

The hypothesis which may link most of these nutrient deficiencies with an increased risk of cancer stems from accumulating evidence that oxidative damage is implicated in the transformation of normal to neoplastic cells and the fact that most of the nutrients have antioxidant properties or are associated in some way with antioxidant defences in the tissues. I propose to discuss the general role which antioxidant defences may exert against cancer and the interactions which may exist between nutrients, for although specific links between nutrients and cancers have been identified, the possibility also exists that the nutrients identified may be proxies for other substances with similar food distributions. Most risk estimates of the links between diet and cancer tend to be weak. This may be due to the inherent difficulties in epidemiological studies which will tend to underestimate relationships[22] but it may also mean the wrong substance has been studied.

2 ANTIOXIDANT PROTECTION AGAINST CANCER

Oxidant stress and antioxidant defences in tissues

There are three main sources of reactive oxygen species in mammalian tissues: normal oxidative metabolism, the mixed function oxidase system (P_{450} enzymes) and infection and inflammation. The main oxygen free-radical produced by these systems is believed to be superoxide but this is probably the least damaging of potential radical products as there is a well-developed, enzymic, endogenous antioxidant system to deal with it. Superoxide dismutase which is zinc and manganese-dependent, is present in all aerobic tissues to convert superoxide to hydrogen peroxide. Likewise, hydrogen peroxide is rapidly removed by the widely distributed cytoplasmic, selenium-dependent, glutathione peroxidase enzyme. Furthermore there is evidence that these enzymes are inducible, e.g. in the lung exposed to ozone,[23] and therefore that production can be varied to meet demand. The P_{450} enzymes also actively respond or adapt to other environmental stresses such as smoking,[24] alcohol, food toxins, products of pyrolysis, xenobiotic drugs etc[25].

However, the endogenous antioxidant system in the body is not able to respond to rapid increases in oxygen stress. For example in infection, stimulated macrophages produce powerful radicals to combat invading organisms as part of the inflammatory reponse with a varying degree of tissue breakdown and disruption.

Tissue integrity is an important component of the antioxidant properties of tissue for any tissue break-down will be associated with the release of iron. Iron is a particularly powerful free-radical generator[26] which is normally tightly bound in the plasma (transferrin) and in the tissues (ferritin). It has been recognised for nearly half a century that mammals with neoplasms, infection or other conditions that stimulate inflammation, develop a profound hypoferremia.[27] Changes in plasma concentrations of several acute phase proteins assist in the shift of iron from plasma to storage[28]. This pathological response to trauma is evidence that free iron is released in such conditions and has to be removed to prevent any further stimulation of free radical damage.

If oxidant stress occurs then lipid peroxidation may be initiated but all tissue components eg DNA, protein etc will be exposed to attack. A limiting factor which may control the extent of damage may be the level of exogenously-derived antioxidant vitamins in the tissues. Vitamin E is widely distributed in tissue membranes and vitamin C in the cytoplasm. Both vitamins are important radical-quenching antioxidants. The carotenes also possess antioxidant properties[29] and may be particularly useful at low oxygen tensions.

Cancer Initiation, DNA damage, DNA repair and Mutagenesis

There is evidence that much of the damage to DNA in the cells of the body may result from free-radical attack.[30-32] Active oxygen radicals (mainly superox-ide) arise in normal aerobic metabolism and in spite of the wide distribution of superoxide dismutase, some damage may be unavoidable. Ames and colleagues suggest that oxidative products of thymin measured in urine are equivalent to several thousand oxidative DNA hits per cell per day in man.[33] Other free radicals may arise from xenobiotic substances following metabolism by the mixed function oxidase system (P_{450} enzymes) of the liver and other tissues. Likewise a hypermetabolic state associated with inflammation or hyperplasia will elevate levels of oxygen free radicals and increase the risk of DNA damage.

Oxidative damage to the DNA bases has been studied *in vitro* by exposure of tissue to ionising radiation and has been shown to take many forms. Virtually all this damage can be dealt with by repair processes within the cell. The process can be summarised as follows[34]:

1 damaged bases excised by a glycosylase
2 the apurinic or apyrimidinic site is recognised by an AP endonuclease

3 a small gap in the backbone of DNA is formed, new DNA is synthesised and the patch ligated into the helical structure

However, the repair processes are relatively slow and if DNA replication should take place on a template containing unrepaired damage, mispairing is possible. For such a mispairing to become heritable within the stucture of DNA, the defect must be capable of DNA replication and cell division. The chances of this happening will be higher where cell proliferation is rapid. This will obviously depend on the type of tissue but also on accompanying factors such as inflammation or hyperplasia.[35]

Fortunately most DNA is not expressed in a given cell and most mutations have little or no effect on cell function. Thus a single assault by a carcinogen is very unlikely to induce cancer. However continuous exposure of a cell to cancer-initiating factors increases the frequency of the mutagenic process and the probability of a viable mutation affecting growth and becoming a cancer.

Cancer Protection by Antioxidants

The transformation of a normal cell into a neoplastic cell is of course a multi-step process comprising initiation, promotion and progression and a variety of different factors will affect the different stages of development. Thus initiation of a cancer will depend on the frequency of carcinogenic exposure, the metabolic state of the tissues and the degree of hyperplasia. Antioxidants can modify this stage by preventing the escalation of radical production by blocking lipid peroxidation. Additionally, antioxidants will improve the resistance of tissues to oxidative damage and promote healing, and so reduce hyperplasia.

Initiation is a permanent alteration of the genetic information in the cell and while a mutation does not necessarily lead to cancer, it is indicative of increased risk of neoplasia. There are methods of measuring some non-lethal mutations eg alterations to the *hprt* gene in lymphocytes to assess exposure to exogenous risk factors but the influence of nutrition on their occurrence has not yet been examined.[36] The second step, cancer promotion, can be a slow process in humans. Estimates of the latency period for prostatic cancer have suggested that it may be more than 40 y and is generally reckoned to be 10-30 y for many common cancers[7]. The latency period may be long because promotion may be suppressed and reversed. Premalignancy is regarded as a part of the promotional phase and as such could include a whole range of events leading up to the development of the neoplasm eg the formation of DNA adducts, micronuclei and sister chromatid exchanges but, conventionally, premalignant lesions are defined as 'atypical intraepithelial proliferation, architectural abnormalities, atypical nuclei and general dysplasia'.

3 CANCER CHEMOPREVENTION

β-Carotene and other carotenoids

There is considerable interest in the possibility of using cancer-chemopreventive agents to regress or sufficiently slow the process of conversion to neoplasia to prevent its development in the lifetime of a subject.[20] The only successful intervention studies reported to date have been those involving oral cancer. Intervention studies need an endpoint to assess their success. Mortality is of course the ultimate endpoint but such studies require a very long experimental period.[37]

In the case of oral cancer, Stich and colleagues used two premalignant lesions viz micronuclei and oral leukoplakia against which to assess the effects of supplements. Initial studies done in India with betel nut/tobacco chewers suggested that supplements of retinol and/or β-carotene reduced the prevalence of both lesions at 3 and 6 mth.[38] Unfortunately the design of the study made it impossible to distinguish between an affect due to an improvement in vitamin A status or to antioxidant protection from the carotene. However another study done on Philippino subjects with similar chewing habits who were given β-carotene and the non-provitamin A carotenoid, canthaxanthin (both 180 mg/wk) for 9 wk, found no protection to be given by the canthaxanthin and therefore that antioxidant properties _per se_ were not responsible for the protective properties of β-carotene.[39]

The antioxidant properties of β-carotene were demonstrated by experiments in which the azo-initiated peroxidation of linoleic acid was reduced when tested at low oxygen pressures.[29] Canthaxanthin is a food colour which has also been shown to inhibit azo-initiated lipid peroxidation *in vitro*[40]. It is not a natural dietary carotenoid however, therefore the possibility exists that it may not penetrate those cells where it may be needed to exert its antioxidant effects. Therefore, similar studies still need to be done using non-provitamin carotenoids which are known to be present in human tissues. Lutein would be an appropriate choice. It is the major non-provitamin A carotenoid in our diet and is as abundant as β-carotene in most green and yellow vegetables. Our own studies have shown lutein to be a better inhibitor of azo-initiated peroxidation *in vitro* than β-carotene.[41]

Vitamin C

Theoretically there are several possible ways by which vitamin C may act as a cancer-chemotherapeutic agent. It can influence the activity of microsomal P_{450} enzymes and therefore the potential formation of some carcinogens. It is important for maintaining integrity of tissues by its active involvement in the hydroxylation of proline and lysine for collagen biosynthesis and basement membrane integrity[22] and it may also be important to maintain vitamin E in a reduced state.[42] However, the strong epidemiological associations between low vitamin C status and gastric and oesophageal cancer suggest that a main function of vitamin C is associated with protection against nitrosamine formation.[5,43]

It is now more than 25 y since Magee and Barnes first showed that dimethylnitrosamine was a potent liver carcinogen[44] and since that time many more nitrosamines and susceptible animal species have been identified. There is no proof that nitrosamines cause cancer in man but they do occur in human tissues and were implicated in the causation of gastric cancer by Correa and colleagues.[45] These workers suggested that the elevated bacterial colonisation associated with gastritis or achlorhydria would favour increased nitrate to nitrite conversion and the formation of nitrosamines. Ohshima and Bartsch[46] subsequently reported that nitrosamines could be formed in man when they administered nitrate and proline and showed that nitrosoproline (NPRO) was excreted in the urine but could be suppressed by simultaneously administering vitamin C or E with the proline.

Ascorbate reacts readily in the aqueous phase with nitrite at pH 3-5 (range within the stomach after a meal is ingested) reducing it to nitric oxide (NO). NO is lipophilic so it is conceivable that it may migrate into the lipid phase where it could be reoxidised to nitrogen dioxide (NO_2). NO_2 can nitrosate amines or amides in the lipid phase to form N-nitroso compounds. It may be fortuitous that α-tocopherol is lipid soluble and will also reduce nitrite to NO thus a combination of the two vitamins is especially useful in inhibiting nitrosamine formation in lipid-water mixtures.[5]

It has been suggested by Mirvish that dietary nitrate is positively related to the risk of gastric cancer. This is surprising when one realises that 80% of gastric nitrite is formed endogenously by bacterial reduction of nitrate in the saliva and that this source of nitrate is present in the gut at all times.[5] In this connection, some interesting information emerged a couple of years ago on the vitamin C concentrations in gastric juice which was reported to be approximately 3 times higher than that in the plasma. Furthermore, in patients with gastritis, the concentration of active (ie reduced) ascorbate was negligible.[47]

The high gastric ascorbate concentrations indicate that an active gradient of ascorbate must be present across the gastric mucosa to maintain the higher concentration in gastric juice. The existence of the gradient suggests it has physiological functions one of which may be to prevent nitrosamine formation. There is some evidence for this from some studies by Halling and colleagues who showed slightly lower excretion of endogenously-formed NPRO in vegetarians compared with omnivores.[48] Additional ascorbate supplements further suppressed NPRO excretion in both groups but the difference between the groups remained very similar at each level of the supplement.

Much of the work on nitrosation and the role of vitamin C has been restricted to the stomach but it should be born in mind that vitamin C is widely distributed in the tissues where concentrations are generally higher than those in plasma. NO_2 is present in polluted air but probably more importantly, it is toxic to bacteria and is actively produced by stimulated macrophages which are a potent source of nitrite and nitrate.[49-51] In tissues where there is chronic inflammation, stimulated macrophages will infiltrate, produce NO_2 and nitrosation reactions are therefore possible. It has been suggested that some of the rarer cancers found in the Third World associated with parasite infestation, may be caused by such mechanisms eg cholangiocarcinoma in areas where liver fluke is a problem in NE Thailand.

4 CONCLUSIONS

Most of the nutrients in plants which appear to offer protection against cancer are antioxidants. Oxidative stress, inflammation and hyperplasia may be important factors in cancer initiation and promotion. β-Carotene and vitamin C are the nutrients with the strongest association with cancer protection and they are both radical-quenching antioxidants. However, the mechanism by which β-carotene protects has not been clearly differentiated from that of vitamin A. Evidence suggests that vitamin C protects against nitrosamine formation but there is still no clear evidence that nitrosamines cause cancer in man. The reason for the site specificity of different nutrient antioxidants is not immediately apparent except possibly for vitamin C. The usually weak associations between nutrient and cancer risk may be due to underestimations and the fact that nutrients may be acting as proxies for other substances in vegetables and fruits.

REFERENCES

1. R. Doll and R. Peto, J.Natl Cancer Inst. 1981, 66, 1192-1308.

2. E.L. Wynder and G.B. Gori, J. Natl Cancer Inst., 1977, 58, 825-832.

3. W.C. Willett and B. MacMahon, New Engl.J.Med., 1984, 310, 697-703.

4. C.H. Hennekens, New Engl.J.Med., 1986, 315, 1288-1289.

5. S.S. Mirvish, Cancer, 1986, 58, 1842-1850.

6. L.H. Chen, G.A. Boissonneault and H.P. Glauert, Anticancer Res., 1988, 8, 739-748.

7. V.N. Singh and S.K. Gaby, Am.J.Clin.Nutr., 1991, 53, 386S-390S.

8. P. Knekt, A. Aromaa, J. Maatela, et al., Am.J.Epidemiol., 1988, 127, 28-41.

9. P. Knekt, Ann.Med. 1991, 23, 3-12.

10. H. Foy and A. Kondi, J.Natl Cancer Inst., 1984, 72, 941-948.

11. M. Crespi, N. Munoz, A. Grassi, et al., Lancet, 1979, ii, 217-221.

12. N. Potischman, L.A. Brinton, V.A. Laiming, et al., Cancer Res., 1991, 51, 4785-4789.

13. M.H. Mellow, E.A. Layne, T.O. Lipman, M. Kaushik, C. Hostetler and J.C. Smith, Cancer, 1983, 51, 1615-1620.

14. D.I. Thurnham, N. Munoz, J-B, Lu, et al., Eur.J.Clin.Nutr., 1988, 42, 647-660.

15. S.J. Van Rensburg, J.Natl Cancer Inst., 1981, 67, 243-251.

16. Committee on Diet Nutrition and Cancer. 'Diet, Nutrition, and Cancer', Washington D.C., National Academy Press, 1982:1-39.

17. N.J. Wald, S.G. Thompson, J.W. Densem, J. Boreham and A. Bailey, Br.J.Cancer, 1988, 57, 428-433.

18. J.E Connett, L.H. Kuller, M.O. Kjelsberg, et al., Cancer, 1989, 64, 126-134.

19. H.F. Stich, K.D. Brunnemann, B. Mathew, R. Sankaranarayanan and M. Krishnan Nair, Prev.Med., 1989, 18, 732-739.

20. P.N. Magee, R. Montesano and R. Preussmann, 'Chemical Carcinogens', Searle CE, (ed.), Washington,D.C.: Ammerican Chemical Society, 1976, pp 491-625.

21. R. Peto, R. Doll, J.D. Buckley and M.B. Sporn, Nature, 1981, 290, 201-208.

22. G. Block, Am.J.Clin.Nutr., 1991, 53, 270S-282S.

23. J.M. Howarth, J.A.Gliner and L.J. Folinsbee, Am.Rev.Respir.Dis., 1981, 123, 496-499.

24. J.F. Schneider, D.A. Schoeller, B.D. Schreider, A.N. Kotake, D.L. Hachey and P.D. Klein, 'Proceedings of the Third International Conference on Stable Isotopes', E.R. Klein and P.D. Klein (eds), New York: Academic Press, 1974, pp 507-516.

25. A.J. Paine, Biochem.Pharmacol., 1978, 27, 1805-1813.

26. B. Halliwell and J.M.C. Gutteridge, Biochem.J., 1984, 219, 1-14.

27. E.D. Weinberg, Nutr.Cancer, 1983, 4, 223-233.

28. D.I. Thurnham, Proc.Nutr.Soc., 1990, 48, 247-259.

29. G.W. Burton and K.U. Ingold, Science, 1984, 224, 569-573.

30. P.A. Cerutti, Science 1985, 227, 375-381.

31. S.A. Lesko, R.J. Lorentzen and P.O.P Ts'o, Biochemistry, 1980; 19:3023-3028.

32. P.R. Armel, G.F. Strinste and S.S. Wallace, Radiat.Res., 1977, 69, 328-338.

33. B.N. Ames, R.L. Saul, E. Schwiers, R. Adelman and R. Cathcart, 'Molecular Biology of Aging: Gene Stability and Gene Expression', R.S. Sohal et al. (eds), New York: Raven Press, 1985:137-144.

34. B. Vogelstein, E.R. Fearon, S.R. Hamilton, et al., New Engl.J.Med., 1988, 319, 525-532.

35. S.M. Cohen and L.B. Ellwein, Science, 1990, 249, 1007-1011.

36. J. Cole, A.P.W. Waugh, D. Beare, M. Sala-Trepat, G. Stephens and M.H. Green, 'New Horizons in Biological Dosimetry', London: Wiley-Liss,Inc, 1991, pp 319-328.

37. C.H. Hennekens, M.J. Stampfer and W. Willett, Cancer Detect.Prev., 1984, 7, 147-158.

38. H.F. Stich, M.P. Rosin, A.P. Hornby, B. Mathew, R. Sankaranarayanan and M. Krishnan Nair, Int.J.Cancer, 1988, 42, 195-199.

39. H.F. Stich, W. Stich, M.P. Rosin and M.O. Vallejera, Int.J.Cancer, 1984, 34, 745-750.

40. J. Terao, Lipids, 1989, 24, 659-661.

41. M. Chopra and D.I. Thurnham, 'Food and cancer prevention', London, Royal Society of Chemistry, 1992: this volume.

42. J.E. Packer, T.F. Slater and R.L. Willson, Nature, 1979, 278, 737-738.

43. S.R. Tannenbaum, Lancet, 1983, i, 629-632.

44. P.N Magee and J.M. Barnes, Br.J.Cancer, 1956, 10, 114.

45. P. Correa, W. Haenszel, C. Cuello, S.R. Tannenbaum and M. Archer, Lancet, 1975, ii, 58-60.

46. H. Ohshima and H. Bartsch, Cancer Res., 1981, 41, 3658-3662.

47. B.J. Rathbone, A.W. Johnson, J.I. Wyatt, J. Kelleher, R.V. Heatley and M.S. Losowsky, Clin.Sci., 1989, 76, 237-241.

48. H. Halling, B-G. Osterdahl and J. Carstensen, Food Add. Contam., 1989, 6, 445-452.

49. M. Miwa, D.J. Stuehr, M.A. Marletta, J.S. Wishnok and S.R. Tannenbaum, Carcinogenesis, 1987, 8, 995-958.

50. D.J. Stuehr and J. Marletta, Immunol., 1987, 139, 518-525.

51. R. Iyengar, D.J. Stuehr and M.A. Marletta, Natl Acad.Sci. USA, 1987, 84, 6369-6373.

ANTIOXIDANT AND PRO-OXIDANT ACTIONS OF DIETARY COMPONENTS

O.I. Aruoma and B. Halliwell

Pharmacology Group
University of London King's College
Chelsea Campus
Manresa Road
London SW3 6LX UK

1 INTRODUCTION

Non-enzymic peroxidation of food lipids is a major problem for food manufacturers. For example, the warmed-over flavour in cooked-reheated meat and the deterioration of ground beef patties involve lipid peroxidation[1]. Such deterioration is minimised by the use of antioxidants[2,3,4]. Food manufacturers are becoming increasingly interested in the use of 'natural' antioxidants in the preservation of food materials[2,4]. The antioxidant potencies of synthetic and natural antioxidant additives such as propyl gallate, butylated hydroxytoluene (BHT), butylated hydroxyanisole (BHA), flavonoids and rosemary plant extracts (containing carnosic acid and carnosol as active constituents), are currently tested only in lipid systems. Evidence exists that several of these 'antioxidants' can exert pro-oxidant (accelerating free radical reaction) effects upon non-lipids such as DNA, proteins or carbohydrates under certain circumstances[5,6,7]. The authors have therefore suggested that in testing putative antioxidant activity, reactions involving biologically-relevant reactive oxygen species should be used[4,7,8]. Several assays including the deoxyribose and bleomycin assays have been adopted for the assessment of the antioxidant (protection against reactive oxygen species, ROS) versus pro-oxidant (acceleration of ROS activity) effects of proposed food antioxidants[4,5-8].

DNA Damage and Free Radicals

DNA is a constituent of foods. A key mechanism of the toxicity of oxidative stress is the metal-ion dependent formation of the highly reactive hydroxyl radical. The type of damage induced and what can be subsequently measured depends on the substrate damaged and on what is causing the damage. DNA is prone to oxidative attack. Two mechanisms (which are not mutually exclusive), involving the Fenton system and nuclease activation have been suggested to account for the damage to DNA that occurs[9]. Oxidative stress[10,11] could cause the release of catalytic copper or iron within cells which could bind to DNA. Increased generation of hydroxyl radical upon DNA by reaction of hydrogen peroxide with the transition metal ions would lead to strand breakage, base modification and deoxyribose fragmentation[9]. The technique of gas chromatography-mass spectrometry with selected ion monitoring GC/MS/SIM, allows for the identification and measurement of some of the products derived from the pyrimidines and purines in DNA[9,12,13]. The technique has been adapted to investigate the ability of nutrient components and food additives to act as pro-oxidants in vitro mediating DNA base modifications and/or mediating increases in the markers of oxidative attack upon DNA following reactions involving free radicals in human diseases[9]. Such measurements could also be relevant in assessing, for example, whole body exposure to ionising radiation or for the detection of irradiated foods[12].

The Deoxyribose Assay

'Antioxidants' that have been shown to protect lipids against the free radical chain reaction of peroxidation can be evaluated for their ability to damage carbohydrates using 2-deoxy-D-ribose as a substrate. A mixture of $FeCl_3$-EDTA, hydrogen peroxide (H_2O_2) and ascorbic acid at pH 7.4, generates hydroxyl radicals (·OH) (equations 1 and 2) which can be detected by their ability to degrade the sugar deoxyribose into fragments that, on heating with thiobarbituric acid at low pH generate a pink chromogen[14].

$$Fe^{3+}\text{-EDTA} + \text{Ascorbate} \longrightarrow Fe^{2+}\text{-EDTA} + \text{Oxidized Ascorbate} \quad (1)$$

$$Fe^{2+}\text{-EDTA} + H_2O_2 \longrightarrow Fe^{3+}\text{-EDTA} + {}^{\bullet}OH + OH^- \quad (2)$$

When Fe^{3+}-EDTA is mixed with H_2O_2 in the absence of ascorbate, a slow rate of ·OH generation results. Addition of ascorbic acid greatly increases the rate of ·OH generation by reducing iron and maintaining a supply of Fe^{2+} (equation 1). This ability to reduce Fe^{3+} and stimulate deoxyribose degradation has been adopted as one measure of the pro-oxidant properties of actual and proposed food additives[4,7]. Recent investigations have probed the possibility that proteins could provide protection against the pro-oxidant actions of some food additives or constituents, hence acting as secondary antioxidants. The plant phenolics quercetin, fisetin, gossypol and myricetin have antioxidant properties in lipid systems, but they also have pro-oxidant actions, as illustrated in Table 1. Table 1 also shows the protection provided by albumin (of course it may be that the albumin is itself being oxidatively damaged in the reaction mixtures).

Table 1 Inhibition of flavonoid-induced deoxyribose damage by human serum albumin (HSA)

Additions	HSA (mg/ml)	Deoxyribose degradation at 532 nm	% inhibition
Quercetin	0	2.00	-
	1.125	1.68	17
	0.50	1.28	36
	1.00	0.96	52
	4.00	0.39	80
	10.00	0.19	90
Fisetin	0	0.68	-
	0.125	0.52	24
	0.50	0.39	43
	1.00	0.30	56
	4.00	0.16	76
	10.00	0.11	84
Gossypol	0	2.46	-
	0.125	2.22	10
	0.50	2.16	12
	1.00	1.84	25
	4.00	0.58	76
	10.00	0.09	96
Myricetin	0	2.70	-
	0.125	2.36	13
	0.50	1.94	28
	1.00	1.51	44
	4.00	0.73	73
	10.00	0.36	87

The plant phenolics gossypol, myricetin, fisetin and quercetin were dissolved in 120 mM-KH_2PO_4-KOH buffer pH 7.4 and sonicated to ensure complete solubilization. They were used at a final concentration of 0.10 mM. Human serum albumin was used at the final concentrations (mg/ml) shown. Mean values of absorbance at 532 nm from triplicate experiments are shown. These varied by no more than 10%.

In the presence of ascorbic acid, typical scavengers of hydroxyl radicals yield a characteristic plot (Figure 1) when varying concentrations are assessed for their ability to protect deoxyribose against degradation by •OH. A linear plot indicates a direct competition between deoxyribose and the additive for reaction with •OH.

In Figure 1, carnosic acid (a constituent of rosemary extract, courtesy of Nestec Research Centre, Switzerland) protected deoxyribose and a rate constant for its reaction with •OH was calculated as $5.8 \times 10^{10} M^{-1} s^{-1}$. K_2 is given by slope (line B) x K_{DR} x [DR] x A^{o} where K_{DR} is the rate constant for the reaction between •OH and deoxyribose, calculated by pulse radiolysis studies to be $3.1 \times 10^9 M^{-1} s^{-1}$, [DR] is the concentration of deoxyribose and A^{o} is the initial A_{532} in the absence of the antioxidant.

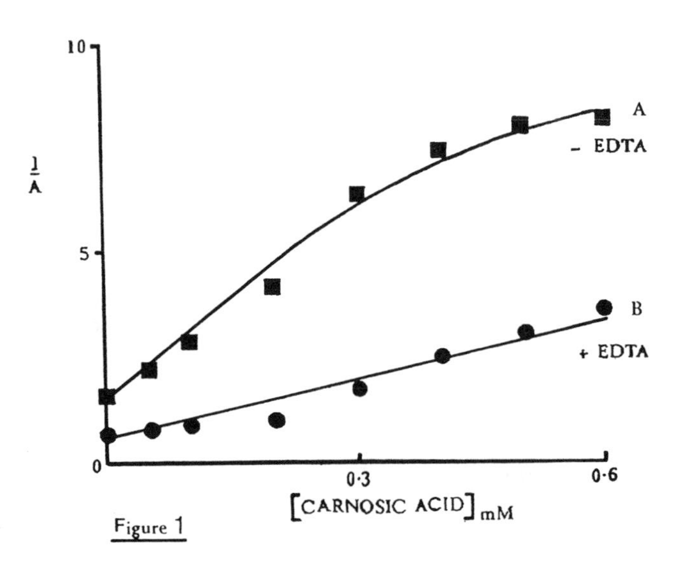

Figure 1

The Bleomycin Assay

The bleomycin assay was introduced in 1981[15] and has been applied in biomedical research to study the presence of non-transferrin bound iron, apparently catalytic for free radical reactions in patients with a variety of diseases including iron overload, rheumatoid arthritis and leukaemia patients undergoing chemotherapy.

Bleomycin binds iron ions and the bleomycin-iron complex will degrade DNA in the presence of O_2 and a reducing agent such as ascorbic acid. The bleomycin-iron(III) complex itself is inactive in inducing damage in DNA. Recent studies have shown that ·OH is not the major DNA-damaging species in the bleomycin system[16]. Ability to promote DNA damage by bleomycin-Fe^{3+} has been adapted as another measure of pro-oxidant action since, any such additive that can reduce iron(III)-bleomycin will cause DNA damage (see refs 4,5-7). Table 2 shows typical data. The ability of albumin to protect DNA against damage by bleomycin-Fe^{3+} promoted by fisetin, propyl gallate, carnosol and carnosic acid supports the observations in Table 1 that this protein might provide antioxidant protection to biological targets. This might have some commercial application in food processing.

Table 2 Bleomycin-dependent DNA damage in the presence of iron ions

Additions at a final concentration of 0.05 mM	Extent of DNA damage (absorbance at 532 nm)		
	Without albumin	With albumin	% inhibition
None	0.00	0.00	-
Propyl gallate	0.30	0.06	80
Carnosol	0.24	0.05	77
Carnosic acid	0.22	0.06	74
Myricetin	1.02	0.90	12
Quercetin	0.97	0.79	18
Fisetin	0.86	0.44	49
Gossypol	0.20	0.19	9
Ascorbate	0.43	0.37	13

Dietary components were dissolved in ethanol. Ethanol itself has no effect on the assay. Albumin (data for BSA [bovine serum albumin] alone are shown here, HSA behaved similarly) was tested at a final concentration of 5 mg/ml. This concentration of albumin consistently produced more than 50% inhibition of pro-oxidant effects for propyl gallate, carnosol, carnosic acid and morin. Values quoted are the means from three separate determinations that varied by no more than 10%.

2 CONCLUDING REMARKS

One important suggestion emanating from our studies (ref. 4-8) is that it may be prudent for food manufacturers to avoid adding both iron and EDTA to foods if certain antioxidants have also been added (Ca^{2+}-EDTA is added to food so as to avoid possible calcium depletion if only EDTA is added). In certain foods such as cornflakes and bread, iron as well as Ca^{2+}-EDTA may be added. H_2O_2 is widely found in the environment and in food materials (examples being vegetable oils, tap water, coffee, urine and exhaled air). Hence reaction of H_2O_2 (hydrogen peroxide) with ferric-EDTA to produce damaging $\cdot OH$ is feasible.

The pro-oxidant actions of nutrient components and/or proposed food antioxidants must be fully characterized[4,7,8]. Until these data become available, care should be taken in the fortification of food with flavonoids and other plant-derived phenolic compounds (often proposed as 'natural' replacements for synthetic antioxidants, the assumption being that natural is necessarily safer) in conditions where iron and Ca^{2+}-EDTA salts are employed.

Proteins fortunately might afford secondary antioxidant protection. Further work is required to aid safer introduction of new antioxidants of plant origin in food processing, and to investigate what happens to the proteins chemically when they act as antioxidants.

REFERENCES

1. V.R. De Vore, J.Food Sci., 1988, 53, 1058.
2. B.J.F. Hudson, 'Food Antioxidants', Elsevier, Amsterdam, 1990.
3. H.W-S. Chan, 'Auto-oxidation of Unsaturated Lipids', Academic Press, London, 1987.
4. O.I. Aruoma and B. Halliwell, 'Free Radicals and Food Additives', Taylor & Francis, London, 1991.
5. M.J. Laughton, B. Halliwell, P.J. Evans and J.R.S. Hoult, Biochem. Pharmacol., 1989, 38, 2859.
6. O.I. Aruoma, P.J. Evans, H. Kaur, L. Sutcliffe and B. Halliwell, Free Radical Res. Commun., 1990, 10, 143.
7. O.I. Aruoma, B. Halliwell, R. Aeschbach and J. Lolliger, Xenobiotica, 1992, 22, 257.
8. B. Halliwell, Free Radical Res. Commun., 1990, 9, 1.
9. B. Halliwell and O.I. Aruoma, FEBS Lett., 1991, 281,
10. H. Sies, 'Oxidative Stress: Oxidants and Antioxidants Academic Press, London, New York, 1991.
11. B. Halliwell and J.M.C. Gutteridge, 'Free Radicals in Biology and Medicine', Clarendon Press, Oxford, 1989.
12. O.I. Aruoma and B. Halliwell, Chem. Brit. February 1991, 149.
13. A.F. Fuciarelli, B.J. Wegher, E. Gajewski, M. Dizdaroglu and W.F. Blakely, Radiat. Res., 1989, 119, 219.
14. B. Halliwell, J.M.C. Gutteridge and O.I. Aruoma, Anal. Biochem., 1987, 165, 215.
15. J.M.C. Gutteridge, D.A. Rowley and B. Halliwell, Biochem. J., 1981, 199, 263.
16. E. Gajewski, O.I. Aruoma, B. Halliwell and M. Dizdaroglu, Biochemistry, 1991, 30. 2444.

IN VITRO ANTIOXIDANT ACTIVITY OF LUTEIN

M. Chopra and D. I. Thurnham

MRC Dunn Nutrition Centre
Milton Road
Cambridge CB4 1XJ

1 INTRODUCTION

Oxidative stress has been implicated in the aetiology of cancer and cardiovascular disease and it has been suggested that β-carotene may play a beneficial role in these diseases.[1,2] β-Carotene has been shown to have antioxidant properties[3] but studies by Japanese workers suggest that some of the xanthophyll carotenoids, which are used as food colours, are more efficient antioxidants than β-carotene.[4] Lutein is one of the most common xanthophyll carotenoids in our diet, and is as abundant as β-carotene in most green and yellow vegetables.[5] In the human body, plasma lutein forms from 20-40% of the total carotenoid components and is one of the five easily identifiable carotenoids in human blood which also include β-cryptoxanthin, lycopene and α and β-carotene. The structures are very similar. In each case the carotenes comprise a conjugated system of double bonds separating two β-ionone rings, except lycopene which is a straight chain compound (figure 1). All appear to have antioxidant properties but the additional hydroxyl groups in the terminal rings of the xanthophyll carotenoids may improve antioxidant properties and this may also apply in vivo.

All carotenoids are lipophilic and may protect against oxidants within or close to the membrane. Three oxidants are important in this respect, peroxy radicals are produced within the membrane, hydrogen peroxide (H_2O_2) and hypochlorus acid (HOCl) are membrane permeable.[6,7,8]. In this study we have examined the ability of lutein to react with these oxidants and in some experiments, compared it with some of the other carotenoids (β-cryptoxanthin, β-carotene, lycopene) and Trolox (vitamin E analogue).

Figure 1

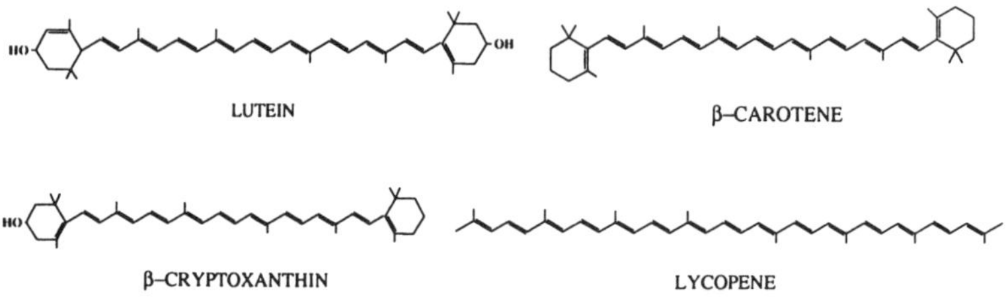

LUTEIN β–CAROTENE

β–CRYPTOXANTHIN LYCOPENE

2 EXPERIMENTAL

Materials

Sources of materials were as follows: Lutein ester (donated by Inexa CA, Quito, Equador), β-carotene, lycopene and methyl linoleic acid (LA) (Sigma), Trolox (Aldrich Biochemicals), β-cryptoxanthin (donated by Hoffman La Roche), 2,2-azo-bis-2,4-dimethylvaleronitrile (AMVN) (Polysciences Inc. Nottingham) and H_2O_2 & sodium hypochlorite, (BDH).

Methods

Lutein ester was hydrolysed at room temperature overnight in ethanolic KOH, extracted into ether and redissolved in ethanol after evaporation under vacuum. This solution was stable at 4° for at least three months. Trolox was prepared fresh in ethanol for each experiment. Stock solutions of β-carotene and β-cryptoxanthin were prepared in hexane:dichloroethane (4:1) and of lycopene in dichloroethane. Working dilutions were made in ethanol or hexane.

The Effect of Carotenoids on Azo-initiated peroxidation of Methyl Linoleic acid. Azo-initiated peroxidation of LA was followed by measuring oxygen consumption in a Rank oxygen electrode. All experiments were carried out at 50° C in ethanol. Final concentrations in electrode cell were 133 mmol/L LA, 13.3 mmol/L AMVN, 5-10 µmol/L carotenoids and 50 µmol/L Trolox. Oxygen consumption was measured every minute in the presence and absence of antioxidant.

Reactivity of Lutein with Hydrogen Peroxide. Stock H_2O_2 was standardised against 0.02 mmol/L potassium permanganate. Working solution was methanol:water (75:25). Lutein (10 µmol/L final) was incubated at 37°C with H_2O_2 (1 mmol/L final) and decrease in absorbance was monitored at 445 nm over 1 hour.

Reactivity of Carotenoids with Hypochlorous acid. HOCl (250 µmol/L) was prepared by adjusting the pH of sodium hypochlorite to 6.2 with sulphuric acid (molar extinction coefficient of aq. HOCl at 235 nm = 100). Each carotenoid (10 µmol/L) was incubated at 37° C with HOCl and their bleaching was monitored spectrophotometrically at their lambda maximum. Similar experiments with Trolox and HOCl were not successful since they both absorbed at the same wavelength.

3 RESULTS

Figure 2 shows the rate of oxygen consumption in the presence and absence of lutein (final concentration 5 and 10 µmol/L). LA on its own consumed oxygen slightly. AMVN consumed approximately 20% oxygen at 8 min. On combining AMVN with LA, the rate of oxygen uptake more than doubled. Lutein inhibited oxygen uptake by the AMVN/LA mixture even at concentrations as low as 5 µmol/L.

Figure 3 summarises the effect of four carotenoids - lutein, β-carotene, β-cryptoxanthin and lycopene (final concentration of each 5 µmol/L) and Trolox(final concentration 50 µmol/L) on oxygen consumption by the AMVN/LA mixture.

Figure 2

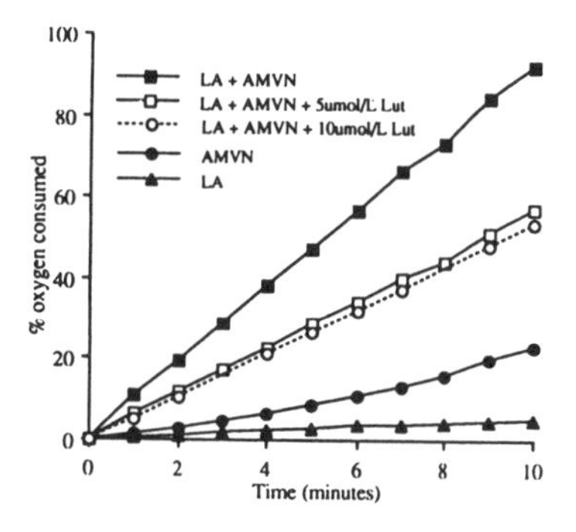

Figure 3

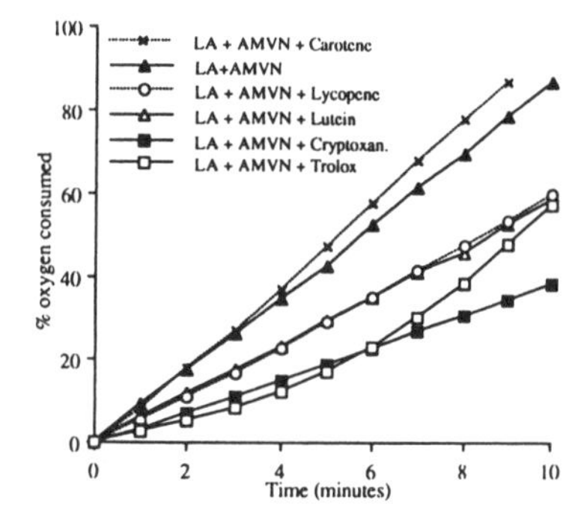

Figure 4 shows the reactivity of carotenoids with hypochlorous acid. The order of reactivity was lycopene > β-carotene > β-cryptoxanthin > lutein.

Figure 4

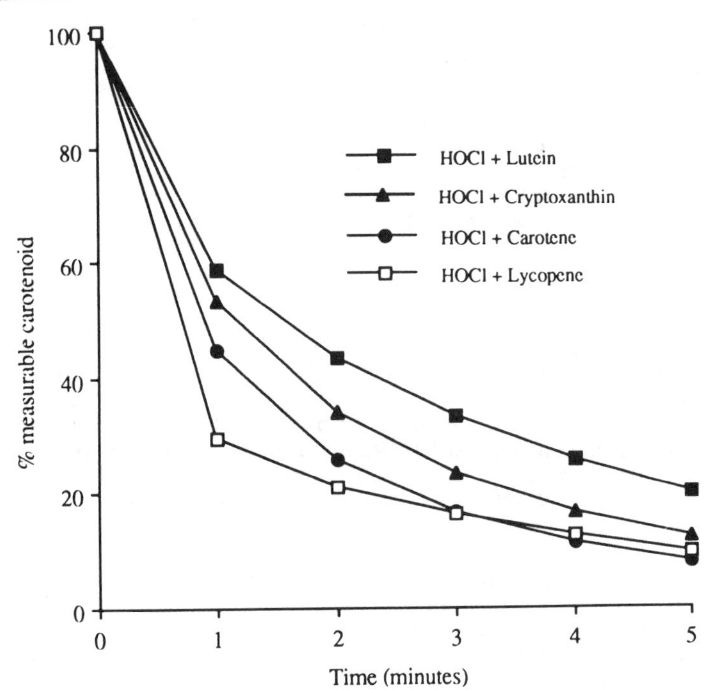

4 DISCUSSION

Results of this study show that lutein and related carotenoids can protect linoleic acid against peroxidation. All carotenoids (except β-carotene) reduced the rate of peroxidation at concentrations lower than that of Trolox. In agreement with Burton and Ingold[3] we find that β-carotene slightly augments the peroxidation of linoleic acid at atmospheric oxygen concentrations whereas the xanthophyll carotenoids (lutein, β-cryptoxanthin as well as lycopene) inhibit peroxidation at this oxygen pressure. The xanthophyll carotenoids also inhibited the oxidation of linoleic acid differently from Trolox or vitamin E.[4] The latter show a lag phase after which peroxidation resumes at the rate seen in the AMVN/LA control (Fig 3). In the case of the carotenoids, in all cases the rate of inhibition remained constant for the entire duration of the experiment, remaining unchanged even after the carotenoids appeared visually bleached within the oxygen electrode well. It is therefore possible that products produced after reaction of xanthophyll carotenoids with free radicals can also inhibit peroxidation. If carotenoids exhibit similar behaviour *in vivo*, they may reduce the rate of peroxidation in tissues and so reduce or 'spare' vitamin E requirements.

H_2O_2 (10 mmol/L) had no significant effect on lutein even after 60 minutes incubation. Lutein therefore is not very reactive towards this species. In contrast, incubation of 10 µmol/L lutein and the other carotenoids with HOCl (250 µmol/L) led to 60% bleaching of lycopene (most reactive of all) and 40% bleaching of lutein (least reactive of all) within 30 seconds. Reaction of carotenoids with HOCl was dependent on the solvent used (highest in methanol:water, lowest in ethanol) for the incubation mixture. These are however preliminary findings and they only indicate that carotenoids can react with HOCl. Whether they can react fast enough to protect biological membranes against damage caused by this species is not yet known.

In conclusion xanthophyll carotenoids supersede β-carotene in their peroxy radical scavenging abilities at atmospheric pressure and perhaps can provide a longer protection than vitamin E or reduce the requirements for vitamin E in the body. Future experiments with liposomes or microsomes may provide a better understanding of their ability to protect membranes against oxidants such as peroxy radicals and hypochlorous acid.

5 ACKNOWLEDGEMENTS

This work was supported by a grant from Nestec Ltd, Lausanne, Switzerland.

6 REFERENCES

1. J.E. Connet, L.H. Kuller, et al., Cancer, 1989, 64, 126-134.
2. D. Kritchevsky. Nutrition Today, 1992, Jan/Feb, 30-33.
3. G.W. Burton and K.U. Ingold, Science, 1984, 224, 569.
4. J. Terao, Lipids, 1989, 24, 659.
5. M.I. Heinonen, V. Ollilainen et al., J. Agric. Food Chem., 1989, 37, 655.
6. C.G. Cochrane, Mol. Aspects Med. 1991, 12, 137.
7. S.J. Weiss, New Engl.J.Med., 1989, 320, 365.
8. I.U. Schaeufstatter, K. Brown et al., J. Clin. Invest., 1990, 85, 554.

Effect of vitamin A dietary intake on DNA damage induced in vitro by AFB1

S. Decoudu, P. Cassand, V. Colin, B. Koch & J.F. Narbonne,

Laboratoire Toxicologie Alimentaire, Université Bordeaux I, Avenue des Facultés, 33405 Talence cedex, France. Réseau Toxicologie Alimentaire et Nutritionnelle, MRE.

I INTRODUCTION

We have previously shown that the genotoxicity of AFB1 was modulated by vitamin A both in vivo and in vitro[1]. Some antimutagenic effects of vitamin A was found to be at the microsomal and cytosolic levels. In order to investigate the protective mechanisms at the nuclear level, incubations of nucleus isolated from livers of rats fed different vitamin A dietary levels were carried out in the presence of S9 from control or vitamin A deficient animals. The DNA damage induced in vitro by AFB1 was evaluated in term of single-strand DNA breaks (SSBs) measured by alkaline elution method.

II MATERIALS AND METHODS

Four groups of wealing SD rats were fed ad libitum for 8 weeks with diets containing either 0 IU, 5 IU (control diet) or 500 IU vitamin A/g as previously described [1]. Rat liver nuclei from vitamin A deficient and supplemented diets, isolated with hypertonic sucrose[2], were incubated 15 min with a post-mitochondrial (S9) fraction, coenzyme factors (NADP, G6P) and AFB1[3]. For the detection of DNA damages induced in vitro by genotoxic AFB1, we have adapted the alkali elution technique described by Parodi et al.[4]. The incubations were conducted with control, vitamin A deficient S9 fractions of which microsomic cytochrome P-450 dependent activities, Ethoxyresorufin-O-Deethylase (EROD), Benzphetamin-N-Demethylase (BzND), Erythromycin-N-Demethylase (ERMD) and cytosolic Glutathion-S-Transferase (GST) activity were determined[1]. Evaluation of DNA damages was expressed as the percentage of double-stranded DNA remaining on the filter.

III RESULTS AND DISCUSSION

The activities of enzymes involved in AFB1 metabolism (Table 1) were significantly decreased by vitamin A deficiency in microsomes (about -20% for BzND and ERMD activities and cytochrome P-450 level) while GST activity was increased in cytosol (+ 35%). When nucleus from supplemented group were incubated with S9 from deficient animals AFB1 induced DNA alterations were decreased by 35% compared with the value obtained with control S9. This decrease seems to be related with decreased cytochrome P-450 dependent activities in microsomes from deficient group .

Inversely when nucleus from deficient group were incubated with S9 from deficient animal AFB1, induced DNA damages were increased by 58% compared to incubations with control S9.

Moreover, the DNA remaining on the filter was 2.6 times lower when incubation was carried out with nucleus from deficient animal than with nucleus from supplemented one's (S9 fraction from deficient group).

Thus, the increase in DNA damages induced by some carcinogens in vitamin A deficient conditions seems to be related to lake of protective effect of chromosome constituents by this vitamin.

Table 1 : Microsomal and cytosolic parameters related to biotransformation activities measured in liver from control and vitamin A deficient rats

EXPERIMENTAL GROUP	DEFICIENT		CONTROL
Microsomes			
Proteins (MP) (mg/g)	19 ± 0.9		20.0 ± 2.3
Cytochrome P-450 (pmol./min/mg MP)	831 ± 44	*	1060 ± 52
EROD (pmol./min/mg MP)	188 ± 19		206 ± 30
BzND (nmol./min/mg MP)	5.9 ± 0.7	*	7.3 ± 0.8
ERMD (pmol./min/mg MP)	721 ± 40	*	935 ± 48
Cytosol			
Proteins (CP) (mg/g)	76.0 ± 3.7		80 ± 4.1
GST (pmol./min/mg CP)	116 ± 7.7	*	86 ± 4.5

* : significantly different from control groups

Table 2 : AFB1 DNA damages measured in vitro by cross incubation carried out with S9 from either control and deficient animals and with nucleus from deficient and supplemented rats.

S9	NUCLEUS	% DOUBLE-STRANDED DNA
control	supplemented	20.5 ± 1.4
deficient	supplemented	27 ± 2.9
control	deficient	23.8 ± 1.7
deficient	deficient	10.5 ± 1.3

REFERENCES

1- S.Decoudu, P. Cassand, M. Daubeze, C. Frayssinet and J.F. Narbonne, Mutation Res., 1992, in press.

2- T.Yu, Biochim. Biophys. Acta, 1975, 395, 329.

3- U.Yu, W Bender and I.H. Geronimo, Carcinogenesis, 1988, 9, 533.

4- V.Parodi, M. Taningher, L. Santi, M. Cavana, L. Sciaba, A. Maura and G. Brambilla, Mutation Res., 1978, 54, 9.

AVAILABILITY OF SOLUBLE ALL-TRANS VERSUS 9-CIS β-CAROTENE

G. Levin and S. Mokady

Department of Food Engineering & Biotechnology
Technion-Israel Institute of Technology
Haifa 32000, Israel.

1 INTRODUCTION

High serum or tissue levels of β-carotene were found, in several epidemiologic and basic studies, to be protective against cancer[1] or cardiovascular diseases.[2] The unicellular alga *Dunaliella bardawil* was previously shown to contain a high concentration (more than 10% of the algal dry weight) of β-carotene, composed of almost equal amounts of the all-trans and 9-cis isomers.[3] Liver analysis of rats or chicks fed diets containing high levels (0.1%) of *Dunaliella* carotenes showed markedly higher carotene accumulation compared to those fed synthetic all-trans β-carotene.[4] This effect was related to the presence of the 9-cis β-carotene in the *Dunaliella*. The higher oil solubility of this isomer was suggested to be responsible for this effect.[5] However, the possibility that the 9-cis β-carotene possesses a unique ability to enhance the absorption of this carotene mixture could not be excluded.

In order to evaluate this hypothesis, rats were fed an oil soluble all-trans β-carotene preparation or preparations differing in their all-trans to 9-cis isomer ratio. Liver β-carotene stores and isomer composition were compared.

2 MATERIALS & METHODS

Carotene Preparations. Synthetic all-trans β-carotene (Sigma Co., type I) was solubilized in soybean oil to a final concentration of 0.7 mg/ml. An extract of carotenes from *Dunaliella bardawil* (N.B.T., Eilat, Israel), in which the 9-cis isomer was 75% of the total β-carotene, was diluted in oil to the same concentration. Mixtures of these two carotene solutions, containing varying amounts of the 9-cis isomer, were prepared (Figure 1).

Animals and Diets. Weanling female rats of the Charles River CD strain (animal colony, Dept. of Food

Engineering & Biotechnology, Technion, Haifa, Israel) were housed in wire cages in a room maintained at 24°C with light-dark cycles of 12 h. The animals were fed ad-libitum AIN-76 diets[6] supplemented with 15% of the β-carotene oily solutions at the expense of the recommended 5% corn oil and sucrose. Two experiments consisting of 30 rats, divided into six groups, were performed:
Exp. 1: The animals were fed diets containing soluble synthetic β-carotene (Figure 1A) or *Dunaliella* extract (Figure 1F). Dietary carotene levels were 35, 70 or 105 mg/kg.
Exp. 2: The diets contained 105 mg β-carotene/kg. β-carotene isomer mixtures shown in Figure 1 were used.

At the end of a 1 week feeding period the animals were killed by CO_2 asphyxiation. The livers were removed and stored at -20°C, for further analysis.

β-carotene Analysis. Livers were lyophilized for 36 h and assayed as described.[4] The β-carotene isomeric composition of the dietary mixtures and of the liver extracts were determined by high performance liquid chromatography (HPLC), using CM 4000 multiple solvent delivery system and SM 4000 programmable wavelength detector, Milton Roy, LDC division. Column and solvents were described before.[4]

Statistical Analysis. Differences between means were analysed by one-way analysis of variance followed by least significant difference test. Differences were considered significant at $p<0.05$ level.

3. RESULTS

No effect on mean body weight of the level of β-carotene in the diet or its isomeric composition was observed.

Liver β-carotene content of the animals of exp. 1 is presented in Figure 2. Rats fed diets containing all-trans β-carotene accumulated in their livers more β-carotene than those given the 9-cis β-carotene enriched mixture. This effect was most pronounced in the livers of the animals consuming the highest dietary carotene level.

All inverse correlation between the 9-cis isomer concentration in the dietary carotene preparation and total hepatic β-carotene content was observed (Figure 3). The level of the 9-cis β-carotene in the livers was positively related to its dietary concentration (Figure 4). However, analysis of liver extracts by HPLC showed that in all the dietary groups all-trans β-carotene was the predominant isomer accumulated. Even when 9-cis β-carotene was the main isomer in the feed, the all-trans isomer was preferentially accumulated.

4. DISCUSSION

The higher bioavailability of *Dunaliella* β-carotene

compared to the synthetic one, when high levels of β-carotene are consumed, was explained in previous studies by the striking difference between the 9-cis and the all-trans β-carotene in their physicochemical properties. The all-trans isomer has a low solubility in vegetable oil and is easily crystallized, while the 9-cis isomer is much more soluble in fats, and can serve as a solvent to the all-trans isomer, thus enhancing its absorption in the gut.[5] However, another effect of the 9-cis β-carotene, independent of its high oil solubility, has not been ruled out. The purpose of this study was to examine this issue. If the higher solubility of the *Dunaliella* carotenes was the only reason for its increased hepatic accumulation, it is conceivable that feeding rats with diets containing oil soluble synthetic all-trans β-carotene would bring about comparable liver carotene stores as would all-trans and 9-cis β-carotene mixtures. In contrast, occurrence of another beneficial property of the 9-cis β-carotene would have been accompanied by higher accumulation of carotene in the liver even when the synthetic all-trans β-carotene was in a soluble state. Surprisingly, the dietary soluble all-trans β-carotene accumulated better in rats liver than did the isomer mixture. Moreover, an increase in the dietary 9-cis isomer level resulted in a decrease in the hepatic β-carotene stores.

The amount of each of the β-carotene isomers stored in the liver is a net result of several mechanisms: a) absorption rate, b) conversion to vitamin A, and c) hepatic secretion into the blood stream. The two last processes are not likely to be responsible for the decreased hepatic accumulation of the 9-cis isomer observed in the present study, since it was shown that this isomer has a lower vitamin A biopotency compared to all-trans β-carotene.[7] In addition, Jensen *et al.*[8] demonstrated that prolonged consumption of equal amounts of all-trans and 9-cis β-carotene isomers by humans resulted in a lower increment in the serum of the latter. This observation suggests that hepatic secretion of the 9-cis isomer is lower than that of the all-trans β-carotene. Therefore, it is conceivable that the preferential hepatic accumulation of the all-trans isomer is due to differences between the two isomers in their absorption rates. It is known that there are species related differences in the ability to absorb various carotenoids. In view of the present concept of lipid absorption in the form of micelles, carotenoid absorption might well be due to one species being able to form suitable micellar solutions in the intestine lumen with one carotenoid but not with others.[7] Similarly, it might be that the all-trans isomer is more suitable than the 9-cis isomer for incorporation into the rat lipid micelles, due to the difference in their configuration. Thus its absorption in the rat intestine is enhanced.

This study clearly indicates that the 9-cis β-carotene

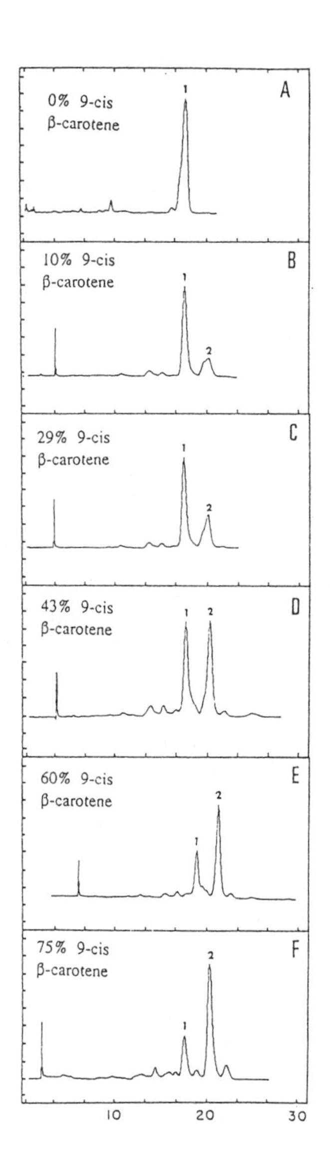

Figure 1 HPLC analysis of the β-carotene mixtures used in Exp. 2 Peak identification: 1. all-trans β-carotenes, 2.9-cis β-carotene.

has no unique ability to enhance hepatic carotene accumulation. It confirms the hypothesis that in diets containing high levels of β-carotene, *Dunaliella* carotenes are absorbed better than synthetic carotene only because of the higher solubility of the 9-cis β-carotene and not because of other unique properties of this isomer.

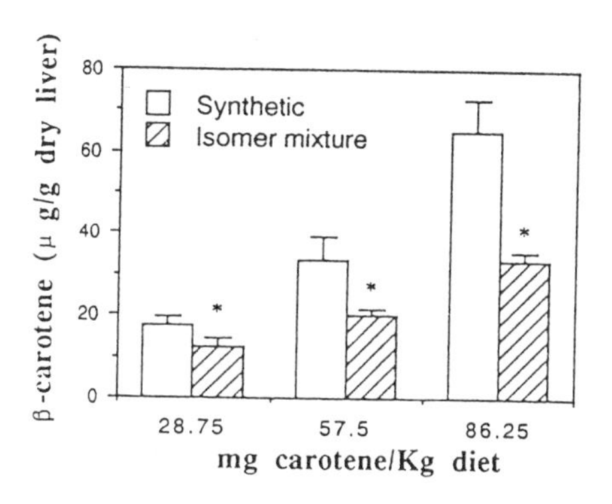

Figure 2 Liver accumulation of soluble β-carotenes.

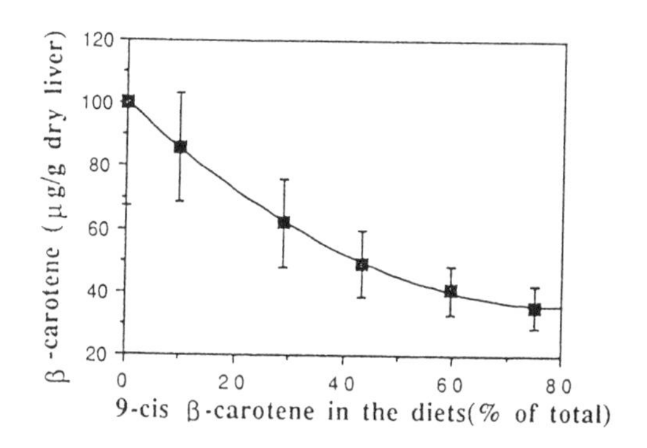

Figure 3 Effect of dietary concentration of the 9-cis isomer on liver total β-carotene accumulation.

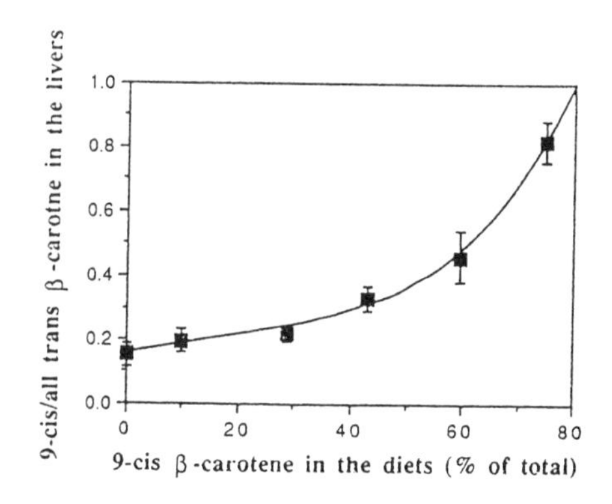

Figure 4 Dietary concentration of the 9-cis isomer and the ratio of 9-cis to all-trans β-carotene in the liver.

REFERENCES

1. R.G. Zeigler, J. Nutr., 1989, 119, 116.
2. H. Gerster, Internat. J. Vit. Nutr. Res., 1991, 61, 277.
3. A. Ben Amotz and M. Avron, Trends in Biotechnology, 1990, 8, 121.
4. A. Ben Amotz, S. Mokady, S. Edelstein and M. Avron, J. Nutr., 1989, 119, 1013.
5. S. Mokady, M. Avron and A. Ben-Amotz, J. Nutr., 1990, 120, 889.
6. Report of the american institute of nutrition ad hoc committee on standards for nutritional studies, J. Nutr., 1977, 107, 1340.
7. J.C. Bauernfeind, 'Carotenoids as Colorants and Vitamin A Precursors', Academic Press, New York, 1981, Chapter 6.
8. C.D. Jensen, T.W. Howes, G.A. Spiller, T.S. Patteison, J.H. Whittam and J. Scala, Am. J. Clin. Nutr., 1986, 43, 689.

EFFECTS OF DIETARY ANTICARCINOGENS ON RAT HEPATIC AND INTESTINAL GLUTATHIONE S-TRANSFERASES.

W.A. Nijhoff and W.H.M. Peters

Department of Gastroenterology,
St Radboud University Hospital,
PO Box 9101, 6500 HB NIJMEGEN,
THE NETHERLANDS.

1 INTRODUCTION

The human diet contains a number of compounds that may affect carcinogenesis. Apart from carcinogens our food contains a wide variety of compounds which prevent tumorigenesis. Among them are minor non-nutrient constituents of vegetables and fruits, such as phenols, flavones and aromatic isothiocyanates. Their mechanism of action is unclear. However, the induction of drug-metabolizing enzymes seems to be crucial. Knowledge about the protection mechanisms of dietary anticarcinogens may be of importance for devising appropriate strategies for prevention of tumours.

2 OUTLINE OF THE STUDY

The response of hepatic and intestinal glutathione S-transferases (GSTs) on dietary anticarcinogenic constituents was investigated. Male Wistar rats received either normal or supplemented lab chow for two weeks. Total GST activity was measured and GST isozyme-expression was quantified by densitometric analysis of Western blots, after incubation with monoclonal antibodies.

3 RESULTS

In Table 1. ratios (Treated over Control) of mean intestinal and hepatic glutathione S-transferase activity are given.

Table 1. The effects of dietary anticarcinogens on rat intestinal and hepatic glutathione S-transferase activity.

Anticarcinogen	Small intestine			Large intestine	Liver
	Proximal	Middle	Distal		
Quercetin	1.2*	1.3*	1.6*	1.8*	1.0
α-Angelicalacton	2.9*	2.1*	3.0*	1.4*	2.0*
Coumarin	1.8*	1.7*	1.6*	1.2	2.4*
Ferulic acid	1.1*	1.2	1.2	1.1	1.4*
Ellagic acid	1.9*	1.7*	1.4*	1.2*	1.4*
Curcumin	1.5*	1.4*	1.1	1.0	1.1
Flavone	1.9*	1.6*	1.1	1.2*	3.1*
Brussels Sprouts	1.7*	1.6*	1.4*	1.2	1.5*

* $P<0.05$, Wilcoxon rank sum test.

Concomittant changes in glutathione S-transferase isozympatterns were observed.

4 CONCLUSION

Induction of hepatic and intestinal glutathione S-transferases may result in a more efficient detoxification of cytotoxic or carcinogenic compounds, and as a consequence could be of significance in the prevention of carcinogenesis.

QUANTITATION OF PROVITAMIN-A AND NON-PROVITAMIN-A CAROTENOIDS IN THE FRUITS MOST COMMONLY CONSUMED IN SPAIN

B. Olmedilla, F. Granado, I. Blanco and E. Rojas-Hidalgo.

Nutrition Service, Clínica Puerta de Hierro.
28035-Madrid (Spain).

1 INTRODUCTION

For over a decade, carotenoids have been studied epidemiologically for their possible carcinogenesis-inhibiting effect[1-3]. Our carotenoid intake comes mainly from fruits, vegetables and food additives. At present, the importance of the carotenoids, and the foods that contain them, is mainly based on two factors: their provitamin A activity and their antioxidant capacity. Given the lack of data on carotenoid content in current Food Composition Tables[4-6], we have carried out this study as a part of an effort to determine the carotenoid content in vegetables[7] and fruits most commonly consumed by the Spanish population. The results of these studies will provide useful information for establishing possible relationships between carotenoid content in diet and in human serum, leading to a better interpretation of the epidemiologic studies dealing with diet and health.

2 MATERIAL AND METHODS

High Performance Liquid Chromatography

A Waters model ALC/GPC 201 liquid chromatograph equipped with a programmable multiwavelength detector (model 409E) was employed. A 220x4.6mm Spheri-5-ODS column (Brownlee, Appl.Biosys.,Inc.) was used with two solvent systems: System I with acetonitrile-dichloromethane-methanol (70:20:10) pumped at a flow rate of 1.8ml/min; and System II with acetonitrile-methanol (85:15) at a gradient rate of 1.8-3.5ml/min. Detection: 450nm or maxplot. The chromatographic procedure has been described in greater detail elsewhere[8,9].

Sampling and Extraction Procedures. Ten of the fruits most commonly consumed by the Spanish population were analyzed[10,11]: orange (Citrus sinensis, L), lemon (Citrus limonis, Osbeck), apple (Pyrus malus, L), banana (Musa paradisiaca, L), pear (Pyrus communis, L), peach (hybrid Prunus persica, Sieb.), watermelon (Citrullus vulgaris, Schered), strawberry (Fragaria elatior, Ehrh.), apricot (Prunus armeniaca, L), and cherry (Prun avium, L). The fruits were sampled during one of the mont corresponding to the season for each product in Spain. A 500-1000g sample of each fruit was purchased in each of three markets in different points of the city of Madrid. The three subsamples were pooled and only the part of the fruit customarily eaten (all were peeled except strawberr apricot and cherry) was analyzed immediately. They were chopped into small pieces and homogenized in a blender. T determination of moisture was performed in triplicate in vacuum desiccation oven at 48±2 ºC until the weight of th sample was constant.

The analyses were performed in quadruplicate in aliquots whose size (25-50g) depended on the intensity of th color of the sample. The extraction method was that reported by Bushway & Wilson[12] with slight modifications. Echinenone was added to two of the aliquots as internal standard (IS). Samples were extracted with tetrahydrofura (THF) with BHT (.01%) until the resulting filtrate was co orless. The extracts were evaporated and then reconstitut with THF. Two aliquots, one of which had been saponified[1 were injected (7.5μl) into chromatographic system I. An aliquot of each was evaporated and reconstituted with TH EtOH (1:3) and injected into chromatographic system II (t separate lutein from zeaxanthin).

Identification and Quantification. The carotenoids were identified by comparing their retention times with those of authenthic standard, by simultaneous injection o standards and sample and, in some cases, by stop-flow sca and wavelength ratio at the top of the peak. Two daily ca ibration curves (one saponified) that included all the ca rotenoids to be assessed in each sample was prepared. The concentrations of stock standard solutions were determine spectrophotometrically on the basis of the published absorptivity value[14].

The mean, standard deviation and coefficient of vari ation (CV) were calculated from the data of quadruplicate analysis. The mean CV was 29% (range 5-53) and 26% (range 0.11-52) for samples without and with saponification respectively. The individual carotenoid values were convert into retinol equivalents (RE) (μg/100g), according to the guidelines of the Food and Nutrition Board[15].

3 RESULTS AND DISUSSION

The carotenoid content, expressed as μg/100g of edible po tion (wet weight) of fresh fruit, is shown in Table I. An yses were performed both with and without saponification; when both results are compared, we generally observe a marked increase in the concentration of carotenoids quantied following saponification of the sample. We consider the process of saponification to be an interesting step to eliminate substances which might interfere with the de termination of carotenoids or to release them from their ester forms, as in the case of fruit.

To assess the possible losses in carotenoid concentration due to handling of the sample, but not related to the efficiency of the extraction method, we have added echinenone at the beginning of the extraction process as IS. This was a useful IS, except in orange, lemon and watermelon where it interferes with other peaks of the chromatogram. Echinenone was added only to half of the subsamples of each fruit, which provoked an increase in the CV (Table I).

The predominant carotenoids in these fruits were lutein and β-carotene -as in vegetables[7]- and β-cryptoxanthin which is present in all of them except banana and strawberry. The highest β-cryptoxanthin concentration was found in orange, and only in this fruit did we quantify a carotenoid reported in serum as "pre-β-cryptoxanthin"[16] and identified later as α-cryptoxanthin[17]. We have detected pre-β-cryptoxanthin in the majority of the samples of control serum analyzed in our laboratory.

The lutein values were higher (watermelon and orange) in fruits with red-orange colored edible portion than in the rest, the edible portion of which is yellowish-white. The joint presence of lutein and zeaxanthin is found in all the fruits, except banana, watermelon and pear, where only lutein was detected. Normally, the amounts of lutein are considerably greater than those of zeaxanthin, but we have quantified similar concentrations for both compounds in orange sample and higher levels of zeaxanthin than lutein in peach (hybrid).

Other non-provitamin carotenoids quantified in fruits are lycopene (in watermelon and cherry) and phytoene (in apricot, watermelon, orange, peach and pear). In addition, we have detected, but not quantified, ξ-carotene and phytofluene in orange and watermelon. Moreover, the use of a polymeric column for these analyses has allowed us to detect cis-isomers. In banana extracts, we have tentatively quantified 9-cis and 13-cis-β-carotene; all-trans and two cis-lycopene were detected in watermelon extracts.

With respect to the carotenoids with provitamin A activity, we have quantified β-carotene in all the fruits, β-cryptoxanthin in all but banana and strawberry; α-carotene in orange, banana, cherry and peach; γ-carotene in apricot. The fruits with greatest provitamin A activity are orange, watermelon and apricot, and those with the lowest are pear and strawberry. This provitamin A activity is mainly due to β-carotene (and in the strawberry, exclusively to this carotenoid), except in the case of citrus fruits, where the RE provided by β-cryptoxanthin are almost five times greater than those of β-carotene in the orange and two times greater in the lemon. The sum of the provitamin A carotenoids quantified surpasses that of the non provitamin A in banana, lemon and apple.

Table I.- CAROTENOID CONTENT EXPRESSED AS μg/100g OF EDIBLE PORTION (WET WEIGHT) OF FRESH FRUIT

FRUIT	MARKET SEASON	MOISTURE %	Provitamin-A			Non-provitamin-A				OTHERS	RE
			β-CRYPT.	α-CAROT.	β-CAROT.	LUTEIN	ZEAXANTHIN	LYCOPENE	PHYTOENE		
ORANGE	Nov-March	85.9	58.84	89.08	42.48	11.24	12.41	---	834.00	ζ-carot. phytofluene	19.41
" (*)			448.25	12.80	48.42	67.98	65.63	---	1065.66	"	49.11
CHERRY	May-June	84.3	2.68	---	14.28	2.60	---	12.87	---		2.60
" (*)			4.79	1.62	13.20	44.28	4.06	10.20	---		2.73
WATERMELON	June-Aug.	91.9	63.15	---	62.63	35.33	---	2489.00	1150.66	ζ-carot. phytofluene	15.70
" (*)			62.25	---	77.07	39.80	---	2454.00	1122.00	"	18.03
PEACH	June-Sept.	86.5	15.88	3.21	69.23	1.45	10.09	---	521.00		13.13
" (*)			73.52	3.47	64.02	15.65	31.45	---	523.83		17.09
STRAWBERRY	March-June	90.9	---	---	5.49	14.45	0.91	---	---		0.92
" (*)			---	---	3.71	13.60	0.56	---	---		0.62
LEMON	Jan.-Dec.	89.4	11.70	---	3.24	1.13	0.62	---	---		1.52
" (*)			14.40	---	0.41	2.54	1.15	---	---		1.27
APPLE	Jan.-Dec.	85.9	---	---	18.66	1.49	---	---	---		3.11
" (*)			7.93	---	20.45	6.22	0.62	---	---		4.38
BANANA	March-June	72.7	---	57.67	69.00	---	---	---	---	9-& 13-	16.31
" (*)			---	63.13	77.33	7.35	---	---	---	cis-β-car.	18.15
PEAR	July-Oct.	83.0	0.42	---	0.65	2.37	---	---	12.05		0.14
" (*)			2.88	---	2.54	11.29	---	---	28.43		0.66
APRICOT	June-July	85.3	11.13	---	132.00	tr.	tr.	tr.	2942.25	γ-carot.	24.25
" (*)			27.52	---	140.00	tr.	tr.	tr.	3151.40	(15.9 & 16.4)	26.99
$\bar{x}$ % C.V.			22	30	24	30	45	24	29		
" (*)			24	36	30	25	32	6	30		

(*): Saponified extracts.

The values for RE presented here fall within the range of the concentrations reported in Food Composition Tables provided by Paul & Southgate[4], and are slightly below those reported by Souci et al[6], while they are higher than those of the Spanish Tables[5]. In our analysis, the RE of the orange are far higher than those provided for this fruit in any of the aforementioned Tables.

There are many factors that influence the concentration of these compounds (ex. variety, season, ripeness, method of analysis). Moreover, one of these, method of analysis, provides information on the distribution of the individual carotenoids. When our results are compared with those obtained by Bureau & Bushway[18] using HPLC, we observe similar concentrations for α and β-carotene in orange and peach, but detected markedly higher levels of β-cryptoxanthin. When our data is compared with those of Heinonen et al[19], we observe a broad discrepancy both in the quantification of individual carotenoids and the calculation of the RE, the latter probably due to these authors quantified β-cryptoxanthin only in few fruits.

REFERENCES

1. R.G. Ziegler, J.Nutr. 1989, 119, 116.
2. G.W.Comstock; K.Helzlsouer; T.L.Bush, Am.J.Clin.Nutr, 1991, 53,260S.
3. R.W.Harris; T.J.A.Key; D.B. Silcocks; N.J. Wald, Nutr.Cancer, 1991, 15, 63.
4. A.A. Paul; D.A.T. Southgate, 'The Composition of Foods' HMSR: London, 1978.
5. Instituto de Nutrición,'Tablas Composición Alimentos' (CSIC), 1980.
6. S.W.Souci; W.Fachmann; H.Kraut, 'Food Composition & Nutrition Tables 1989/90' Wissenschaftliche Verlagsgesellschaft: Stuttgart 1989.
7. F.Granado; B.Olmedilla; I.Blanco; E.Rojas-Hidalgo, J.Agric. Food Chem. (under revision).
8. B.Olmedilla; F.Granado; E.Rojas; I.Blanco, J.Liq.Chromatog, 1990, 13, 1455.
9. F.Granado; B.Olmedilla; I.Blanco; E.Rojas-Hidalgo, J.Liq.Chromatog, 1991, 14, 2457.
10. 'Consumo alimentario en España' Ministerio Agricultura, Pesca y Alimentación. Madrid (Spain), 1988.
11. O.Moreiras; A.Carbajal; I.M.Perea. 'Evolución de los hábitos alimentarios en España' Mto Salud y Consumo. Madrid (Spain), 1990.
12. R.J.Bushway & A.M.Wilson, Can.Inst.Food Technol.J. 1982, 15, 165.
13. 'Methods for the determination of vitamins in food', G.Brubacher, M.Müller-Mulot, D.A.T.Southgate (eds). Elsevier Appl.Sci,Publ.Ltd, Essex (England), 1986, chap.3, p.39.
14. E.De Ritter; A.E.Purcell, 'Carotenoids as colorants and vitamin A precursors' Academic Press: London, 1981, chap.10, p.883.
15. Food and Nutrition Board, 'Recommended Dietary Allowances', National Academic of Sciences: Washington, 1989, p.78.
16. J.G.Bieri; E.D.Brown; J.C.Smith. J.Liq.Chromatog, 1985, 8, 473.
17. F. Khachik; G.R. Beecher; M.B. Goli; W.R. Lusby, Pure & Appl.Chem, 1991, 63, 71.
18. J.L. Bureau & R.J. Bushway, J.Food Science, 1986, 51, 128.
19. M.I. Heinonen; V. Ollilainen; E.K. Linkola; P.T. Varo; P.E. Koivistoinen, J.Agric.Food Chem. 1989, 37, 655.

Seasonal variation of serum levels of β–carotene and α–tocopherol

M. Rautalahti[1], D. Albanes[2], J. Haukka[1], E. Roos[1], J. Virtamo[1]

1) National Public Health Institute, Helsinki, Finland
2) National Cancer Institute, Bethesda, USA

We studied the degree of seasonal variation in the serum levels of β-carotene and α-tocopherol (determined by HPLC) among 16 942 participants of the Alpha-tocopherol, Beta-carotene Lung Cancer Prevention Trial (ATBC–Study)[1]. At the time of this study these men were all smokers, 50–69 years old and free of cancer.

Month of blood sampling was a statistically significant determinant of serum level of β-carotene in a logistic regression model including as covariants age, BMI, alcohol and fat intake, total serum cholesterol, and daily cigarettes. These variables were chosen based on prior studies[2,3]. The mean serum β-carotene levels were lowest in April–June (0.32 μmol/l) and highest in October–November (0.46 μmol/l). The 1.5–fold increase in the serum level of β-carotene during the fall is consistent with the seasonality of many foodstuffs rich in carotenoids in Finland[4].

In contrast, the serum levels of α-tocopherol demonstrated no seasonal variation whatsoever, and remained close to 27.6 μmol/l throughout the year.

The results of this study indicate that the serum concentration of β-carotene can be dependent on the month of blood sampling. The possibility of seasonal variation should be taken into account when conducting long term studies in which comparison of groups or individuals is based on serum levels.

References

1. D. Albanes, J. Virtamo, M. Rautalahti et al., *J Nutr Growth Cancer*, 1986, 3, 207.

2. S. Stryker, L. Kaplan, E. Stein et al., *Am J Epidemiol*, 1988, 127, 283.

3. D. Albanes, J. Virtamo, M. Rautalahti et al., *Eur J Clin Nutr*, 1992, 46, 15.

4. M. Heinonen, PhD Thesis, University of Helsinki, 1990.

Supported by Public Health Service Contract No. N01-CN-45165 from the Division of Cancer Prevention and Control, National Cancer Institute of the United States.

ANTIOXIDANT VITAMINS OR LACTULOSE AS CHEMOPREVENTIVE AGENTS FOR COLORECTAL CANCER

L. Roncucci and M. Ponz de Leon

Istituto di Patologia Medica, Policlinico, via Del Pozzo, 71, University of Modena, 41100 Modena, Italy

1 INTRODUCTION

Colorectal adenomas are the natural precursors of most cancers of the large intestine.[1,2] Adenomas are usually removed during colonoscopy, but they frequently recur.[3]

Recently several compounds have been proposed as chemopreventive agents for various human tumours.[4] Among them some vitamins and unabsorbable carbohydrates might be suitable for intervention studies in colon cancer prevention. In particular, vitamins A, C and E are well-known antioxidants and inhibit carcinogenesis in experimental models.[4,5] Lactulose lowers the pH of the intestinal environment,[6] thus reducing the rate of production of toxic secondary bile acids.[7]

Thus we evaluated the effect of vitamins A, C and E or lactulose on the recurrence rate of colorectal adenomas after endoscopic polypectomy.

2 METHODS

Patients and Study Design

Two hundred and fifty-five subjects were randomized in 3 endoscopic units into 3 groups after colonoscopic removal of one or more polyps of the large intestine. Group 1 was given vitamin A (30,000 I.U./die), C (1 g/die) and E (70 mg/die). Group 2 was administered lactulose (20 g /die). Group 3 did not receive any treatment. After enrolment, subsequent endoscopic examinations were planned at 6-8, 12-18 and 24-36 months. Index and subsequent colonoscopies allowed the examination of the entire large intestine in all individuals. Recurred polyps were removed and processed for pathological examination: colonic subsite, hystotype and maximum diameter of adenomas were recorded. Compliance to the treatment was assessed by asking individuals during and at the end of the follow-up whether they continued to take the scheduled treatments. No attempt was made in order to change the dietary habits of the study population.

Data Analysis

Only subjects with adenomas at index colonoscopy were included in the analysis, according to the "intention to treat" criterion, though 40 individuals did not complete the scheduled treatment. Only adenomas recurred after 1 year since the last colonoscopy were considered not missed by the endoscopist.

Kaplan-Meier survival curves were used to estimate the probability of remaining free of adenomas, and the statistical significance among groups assessed with the log-rank test.[8] Univariate stratified survival analyses were carried out to identify clinical and morphological variables of adenomas at index colonoscopy which could have affected adenoma recurrence. Furthermore a Cox's multivariate regression model was used to adjust for those variables.

3 RESULTS

Of 255 randomized subjects, 46 were excluded from the analysis because their polyps were not adenomas. Two hundred and nine individuals were actually evaluated with an average follow-up time of 18 months. The probability of remaining free of adenomas was significantly different among the 3 groups (log-rank $X^2 = 17.138$, $p<0.001$). In multivariate analysis treatment was the only variable which contributed significantly to the model. The recurrence rate of adenomas was reduced both in vitamins and in lactulose groups, as compared to controls, though the result was more favourable with vitamins (Table 1).

Table 1 Number of subjects with adenoma recurrence, by treatment group

Treatment	Total no. of subjects evaluated	No. of subjects with recurrence
Vitamins	70	4 (5.7%)
Lactulose	61	9 (14.7%)
None	78	28 (35.9%)
Total	209	41

Overall $X^2 = 22.608$ ($p<0.001$).

Subsite of recurrence, histotype and diameter of recurred adenomas were similar in the 3 treatment groups.

4 DISCUSSION

The results of the present randomized controlled study show that either antioxidant vitamins or lactulose are effective in reducing the recurrence rate of colonic adenomas after endoscopic polypectomy. Since adenomas are considered precursor lesions of the large majority of colorectal cancers, these findings are consistent with a putative chemopreventive role for these compounds.

The anticancer effect of antioxidant vitamins is largely unknown. These vitamins, especially retinoids, are inhibitors of carcinogenesis in several experimental models.[4] Furthermore, vitamins C and E reduced the recurrence rate of adenomas in some clinical trials.[9,10] Finally, antioxidant vitamins can reverse the upward expansion of the proliferative compartment of normal colonic crypts, observed in patients with colorectal tumours.[11] Intracolonic bile acids are promoters of experimental colon carcinogenesis.[12] Lactulose can acidify the intestinal content, because it enhances the production of short chain fatty acids. At pH below 6 the degradation of primary to secondary (more toxic and cancer-promoters) bile acids is reduced because the bacterial 7-alpha-dehydroxylase is inhibited.[13] As we did not assess the dietary habits of the study population, we cannot exclude the influence of other dietary factors on the results of the present study, although they should have had the same weight in the 3 treatment groups.

Vitamin A may cause liver damage.[14] However, we observed only one case of toxicity in the vitamins group (pruritus with no skin damage). Moreover, vitamin E seems to be protective against retinol-induced injury to cells.[15] Lactulose may cause diarrhoea, but it is possible to control this side effect adjusting the daily dose. In our study only 3 subjects had to withdraw the intake of lactulose because of diarrhoea.

In conclusion the results reported here suggest an effect of antioxidant vitamins or lactulose as chemopreventive agents for colorectal cancer. A large-scale use of these substances is not justified yet. However they can be proposed to subjects at high risk for malignancy of the large intestine, as members of families with hereditary non-polyposis colorectal cancer or familial adenomatous polyposis, or subjects with large, villous, multiple or frequently recurrent colonic adenomas. Larger numbers of subjects and further studies are needed to validate these results, and to test chemopreventive agents in groups of individuals at increased risk for cancer of the large intestine.

REFERENCES

1. B.C. Morson, Cancer, 1974, 34, 845.
2. C.M. Fenoglio, et al., Pathol. Annu., 1975, 12, 87.
3. J.D. Waye and S. Braunfeld, Endoscopy, 1982, 14, 79.
4. J.S. Bertram, et al., Cancer Res., 1987, 47, 3012.
5. P.M. Newberne and V. Suphakarn, Cancer, 1977, 40, 2553.
6. C. Florent, et al., J. Clin. Invest., 1985, 75, 608.
7. G.P. van Berge Henegouwen, et al., Gut, 1987, 28, 675.
8. R. Peto, et al., Br. J. Cancer, 1977, 35, 1.
9. H.J.R. Bussey, et al., Cancer, 1982, 50, 1434.
10. G. McKeown-Eyssen, et al., Cancer Res., 1988, 48, 4701.
11. G.M. Paganelli, et al., J. Natl. Cancer Inst., 1992, 84, 47.
12. B.I. Rainey, et al., Br. J. Cancer, 1984, 49, 631.
13. J.R. Thornton, Lancet, 1981, 1, 1081.
14. A.P. Geubel, et al., Gastroenterology, 1991, 100, 1701.
15. J.N. Hathcock, et al., Am. J. Clin. Nutr., 1990, 52, 183.

CAROTENOIDS PLUS VITAMIN A IN CANCER PREVENTION, ADJUVANT THERAPY, AND MASTALGIA TREATMENT (*)

Leonida Santamaria and Amalia Bianchi-Santamaria

Camillo Golgi Institute of General Pathology
(**) Tumor Center; °Institute of Pharmacology II
University of Pavia - 27100 Pavia, Italy

1 INTRODUCTION

Carotenoid (CARs: beta-carotene BC and/or canthaxanthin CX) supplementation have been shown by the authors, since 1980, to be chemopreventive in animals against direct or indirect chemical carcinogenesis/photo-carcinogenesis of the skin, breast, and stomach; by others against salivary glands, colon-rectum, urinary bladder carcinogenesis and transplanted tumors. The mechanism of this action was found to be either independent of or dependent on pro-vitamin A activity of BC. The independency of pro-vitamin A property of BC against photochemical carcinogenesis pointed out the relevance of the high antioxidant action of BC. *In vitro*, both BC and CX as antioxidants proved to be antimutagenic and to have anti-malignant transformation properties in cell cultures. In a few experimental instances, such as against urinary bladder cancer, the retinoid potential of BC was responsible for this effect, since CX was inactive.

Pilot interventions in humans with BC±CX, as first attempted by the authors since 1980, prevented the onset of second primary tumors in lung, colon, urinary bladder, and head and neck after radical excision of their first primary tumors.

The current development of the above investigations on CARs action in the Pavia University Tumor Center has so far achieved the following data: 1) anticlastogenicity in humans as demonstrated by the reduction of the micronuclei induced by bleomycin in cultured lymphocytes from subjects supplemented with CARs; 2) stimulation of the immunoresponse by BC in mice, thus lengthening survivals after transplantation of ascites tumors along

---

(*) Revised data from a lecture delivered at the 1st International Congress on Vitamins & Biofactors, Kobe, Japan, 1991.
(**) *Convenzionato* with the Unità Socio-Sanitaria Locale (USSL 77), Pavia.

with a dramatic increase in liver mastocytes; 3) demonstration of a synergism between BC and retinol in humans as shown in the treatment of pre-menstrual mastalgia, with benign breast disease (BBD) or otherwise, thus obtaining marked relief and sometime recovery from breast pain in cyclical mastalgia, with no side effects at all in 20-42 yr aged women; 4) adjuvant effect by BC 80 mg/day in non-surgically treatable human lung cancer cases leading to an increase (1.5 - 3 times more) in overall survival with respect to expected median survival.

All the above data, in an abridged and updated presentation, are reported below.

2. BASIC REFERENCES OF EXPERIMENTAL CANCER CHEMOPREVENTION BY SUPPLEMENTAL CAROTENOIDS

A first experimental trial in 1973 demonstrated that a diet rich in red carrots delayed the onset of tumors induced by dymethyl-benzo-(a)-anthracene in mice and rats. This effect was related to vitamin A production from CARs.[1] In 1977 intraperitoneal injection of beta-carotene delayed skin tumor induction in hairless mice exposed to UV-B (290-320 nm) irradiation.[2] Finally, in 1980, an experimental trial demonstrated that beta-carotene (BC) or canthaxanthin (CX), two carotenoids with and without pro-vitamin A activity respectively, when supplemented at high dosage by diet to albino mice, markedly prevent (up to about 60%) skin cancer induced by benzo(a)pyrene (BP).[3] *In this experiment, care was taken to start carotenoid supplementation one month before carcinogenic induction and to continue this supplementation to the diet throughout the entire experiment*. Strikingly, both CARs completely controlled the marked BP photocarcinogenic enhancement (BP-PCE) obtained as reported in the 1960s.[4] Apparently, this effect was due to a quenching of reacting oxygen intermediates (ROIs), including oxygen radicals, produced by photodynamic process. This effect was independent of provitamin A activity, whereas it was highly dependent on the antioxidant property of CARs. Significantly, the low rate of skin cancer induced by long term exposure to UV light (300-400 nm) alone was thoroughly controlled by carotenoid supplementation. Furthermore, the skin cancer inhibition by BC and CX *was also observed in animals kept in the dark*, apparently through the scavenging and/or quenching of oxyradicals and/or $^1O_2$ endogenously produced through BP metabolization to its diol-epoxy derivatives.

On the whole, these results can be taken as the first clearcut experimental evidence that dietary carotenoid supplementation can control the oxygen radical pathology involved in skin cancer inductions by an *indirect* carcinogen, thus preventing tumor onset, likely at the initiation stage.

In the same year (1980), Mathews-Roth also reported the first of her experiments demonstrating that dietary CARs (BC or CX) can act as antioxidants delaying skin tumors induced in mice either with UVB light, DMBA ± croton oil or with DMBA ± UVB light.[6]

In 1981 and 1982, Seifter *et al.* proved that BC is active against transplanted tumors, by preventive and therapeutic mechanisms, interpreting the effects as due to vitamin A production and immunostimulation.[7,8]

In 1984 and 1985, the same methodology used in the above experiment with BP was adapted to prevent both *indirect* breast photocarcinogenesis induced in albino Swiss mice, strain 955, by 8-methoxypsoralen (8-MOP) topical application plus long UV light (P-UVA)[9] and *direct* gastric carcinogenicity induced by N-methyl-N'-nitro-N-nitrosoguanidine (MNNG) in rats. Breast cancer was prevented at 60% probably at the promotion stage. Also gastric cancer was prevented at 60-70%, but clearly at the progression stage, thus demonstrating that even direct carcinogenesis can be prevented by CARs.[10]

All these results prompted investigations by others on different carcinogenic models, such as salivary glands by DMBA in rats;[11,12,13] DMBA induced cheek pouch squamous cell carcinoma in hamster;[15,16,17,18] chromosomal breaks in mice induced by BP or mitomycin;[14] colon cancer by DMH in mice; urinary cancer induced by OH-BBN in mice.[20] The mechanisms of action of these effects of CARs are primarily consistent with antioxidant and retinoid potentials, the latter being the production of retinal ↔ retinol → retinoic acid from BC. In the case of chemoprevention against urinary bladder, as observed by Mathew-Roth *et al.*,[20] BC was active, whereas CX was not, thus indicating that BC retinoid potential was responsible for this mechanism of action.

These activities are responsible for many combined effects other than anticarcinogenesis, i.e. immunostimulation, antiatherosclerosis, antiageing, antimutagenesis, anticlastogenesis, antiviral effects. In this connection, it is worth recalling that BC and CX proved to be also antimutagenic on *S. typhimurium* TA 102 and to exert anti-malignant transformation in cell cultures.[21,22]

3. CLINICAL TRIAL TO PREVENT SECOND PRIMARY NEOPLASMS

All the above animal experiments are in keeping with the concept of cancer chemoprevention[23] consisting in the reversion of precancerous lesions. Thus, when cancer chemoprevention was applied to human interventions, it was called *primary* when preventing primary malignancies; it was called *secondary* in any post radical surgery condition preventing the expression of second primary malignancies in districts where a latent initiation is presumed to persist.

Following this rationale for secondary chemoprevention, a first pilot clinical case report of 15 cases was published in 1988[24] and updated in 1990,[22] relative to cancers radically removed in compartments including mammary gland, lung, urinary bladder, colon-rectum, head and neck. Here the data demonstrated that in all patients supplementation with BC+CX 40 mg/day prevented second primary malignancies well beyond their expected disease free intervals, with no toxic side effects at all.

4. SYNERGISM BETWEEN BC AND RETINOL TO TREAT PREMENSTRUAL MASTALGIA WITH BENIGN BREAST DISEASE

The potential use of retinoids for chemoprevention of experimental breast carcinomas as reported in a 1980 editorial[25] rekindled an old interest in high dosage vitamin A treatment of benign breast disease (BBD) with premenstrual mastalgia. Nevertheless, the encouraging results obtained in 1984 both with regard to complete or partial responses of BBD and pain reduction were still associated with toxic effects, because of the high vitamin A dosage (150,000 IU/day for 3 months) required to achieve these clinical results.[26] Hence, it was posited in the Pavia Tumor Center that mastalgia might possibly be treated with BC as a vitamin A-precursor and as a *per se* antioxidant agent devoid of any toxicity. This approach, however, proved to be unsuccessful. But, when BC oral supplementation at low dosage (20 mg/day) was associated with intermittent retinol (palmitate or acetate ester) administration at very high dosages (300,000 IU/day) for seven days just before the beginning of the menstrual period, the same positive responses as mentioned above were detected soon after the first menstrual cycle in women aged 21-41 (average 35 yr.), suffering from cyclical mastalgia. Remarkably, no toxic side effects were detected, even after prolonged treatment (22) with a clear cut synergism. This treatment had no effect in premenopausal non-cyclical mastalgia (women aged 41-50).

To explain the mechanism of action of BC-Vitamin A synergism it is suggested that what is involved is the powerful antioxidant activity of BC in that this is efficient in cutting down all the oxygen radicals produced by the phlogistic component of the syndrome associated with the greater water solubility of retinol permitting it to cross the oedema barrier faster than BC and to exert its possible antiprolactin-oestrogen activity. The synergistic effect may also depend on a competition for a receptor due to the same structure in BC and retinol molecular end points.

5. ANTICLASTOGENIC ACTION IN HUMANS AND INCREASE IN MOUSE LIVER MASTOCYTES BY CARs

In a one year-study, 9 healthy human donors were supplemented with beta-carotene (BC) plus canthaxanthin (CX), to determine the effect of carotenoids on chromosomal damage (micronuclei) induced in the donors' lymphocyte cell cultures by exposure to bleomycin (BLM), an antineoplastic drug that has been shown to produce chromosomal aberrations through the production of free radicals. The data showed that the micronuclei induced by BLM in human lymphocyte cell culture was decreased up to 50% when lymphocytes were from donors supplemented with BC at different doses. Significantly, the above micronuclei induction was inversely correlated with donors' carotenoid blood levels.[27]

In another study, the immunostimulating effect of BC was confirmed by a dramatic increase in the number of mastocytes in the liver imprints from BC treated BALB/c mice. This increase was quantifiable in a 23:1 ratio, respect to controls, thus revealing the important role of mastocytes in modulating host immune response. This may well explain the increase in survival observed in tumour transplanted mice when the animals are BC supplemented.[28]

6. BC SUPPLEMENTATION AS A THERAPEUTIC ADJUVANT IN NON-SURGICALLY TREATABLE LUNG CANCER PATIENTS

On the basis of the above BC biomodulation and Seifter's data on BC immunostimulation and local barrier to malignancy,[7,8] four non-surgically treatable lung cancer patients were admitted from July 1989 to July 1990, to a tentative trial in an effort to increase their expected median survivals by BC supplementation at high dosage (80 mg/day). The recruited patients had the following characteristics: three of them suffered from squamous cell carcinoma T_3 N_1 M_x and one from limited type microcytoma; none of them could undergo chemotherapy because of their advanced age and/or concomitant chronic pathologies, nevertheless, they performed well on the Karnowsky Index (K.I.) with a score of 100 or almost; two of them underwent telecobalt therapy. Their expected median survivals ranged from 8 to 12 months. They all complied with the prescription of two gelatin pearls of BC 20 mg each after the two main daily meals. Significantly, the first year follow-up showed a stable disease (SD) for all patients due to a tumor mass stationary status as monitored, in a blind manner, by both chest X-ray and K.I. performance. The X-ray showed rounded opacities sharply delimited from the surrounding tissues. In one case, the squamous cancer opacity in stationary status underwent an apparent colliquation in 2 years, step by step. The patient died from "atypical pneumonia" at the lobe with cancer with no diffusion of the latter. The overall survivals in all the above cases resulted to be increased from 1.5 to 3 times more than their expected median survivals, with a sustained high K.I. performance over a long period of time. The significance of these data apparently depended on the strict admission criteria adopted including no chemotherapy and especially high K.I. performance. The high dosage BC efficacy inducing an increase in overall survivals should in all probability be attributed to both antioxidant and retinoid potential activities of BC, displaying immunostimulation, antiproliferation and differentiation effects, thus accounting for the build-up of biological barriers against malignancy.[29]

ACKNOWLEDGEMENTS

Research partially supported by the Ministero della Sanità, Roma, Dir. Gen. Serv. Med. Soc., Div. IV, (Contract N. 500/4/RSC/57.3/T/1879 - 1989). English text revised by Dr. A.P. Baldry, Supply Professor of Medical English, Univ. of Pavia.

KEYWORDS: carotenoids / antioxidants / retinol / anticarcinogenesis / chemoprevention / human interventions / mastalgia.

REFERENCES

1. A.C. Dorogokupla, E.G. Troitzkaia, L.K. Adilgereieva, S.F. Postolnikov and Z.P. Chekrigina, Effect of carotene on the development of induced tumors, Zdravoor. Kazak., 1973, 10, 32-34.
2. J.H. Epstein, Effects of β-carotene on ultraviolet induced cancer formation in the hairless mouse skin, Photochem. Photobiol., 1977, 25, 211-213.
3. L. Santamaria, A. Bianchi, A. Arnaboldi and L. Andreoni, Prevention of the benzo(a)pyrene photocarcinogenic effect by beta-carotene and canthaxanthine. Preliminary study, Boll. Chim. Farmaceutico, 1980, 119, 745-748.
4. L. Santamaria, G.G. Giordano, M. Alfisi and F. Cascione, Effects of light on 3,4-benzpyrene carcinogenesis, Nature, 1966, 210, 824-825.
5. L. Santamaria, A. Bianchi, A. Arnaboldi, L. Andreoni and P. Bermond, Dietary carotenoids block photocarcinogenic enhancement by benzo(a)pyrene and inhibit its carcinogenesis in the dark, Experientia, 1983, 39, 1043-1045.
6. M.M. Mathews-Roth, Carotenoid pigments as antitumor agents. In J.D. Nelson and C. Grassi, Eds. Current Chemotherapy and Infection Disease, Washington, DC, Am. Soc. Microbiol., 1980, pp. 1503-1505.
7. E. Seifter, G. Rettura, F. Stratford and S.M. Levenson, CH3BA tumor prevention and treatment with beta-carotene, Fed. Proc., 1981, 40, 652-656.
8. E. Seifter, G. Rettura, J. Padawer and S.M. Levenson, Moloney murine sarcoma virus tumors in CBA/J mice: chemopreventive and chemotherapeutic action of supplemental beta-carotene, J.N.C.I.,

1982, 68(5), 835-840.

9. L. Santamaria, A. Bianchi, L. Andreoni, G. Santagati, A. Arnaboldi and P. Bermond, 8-Methoxypsoralen photocarcinogenesis and its prevention by dietary carotenoids. Preliminary results, Med. Biol. Environn., 1984, 12, 533-537.
10. L. Santamaria, A. Bianchi, A. Arnaboldi, L. Andreoni, G. Santagati, C. Ravetto, L. Bianchi, R. Pizzala and P. Bermond, Supplemental carotenoids prevent skin cancer by benzo(a)pyrene, breast cancer by PUVA, and gastric cancer by MNNG. Relevance in human chemoprevention. In: F.L. Meyskens and K.N. Prasad (Eds.) Vitamins and Cancer-Human Cancer Prevention by Vitamins and Micronutrients, Clifton, NY, The Humana Press, 1985, pp.139-159.
11. B.S. Alan, S.Q. Alam, J.C. Weir Jr. and W.A. Gibson, Chemopreventive effects of beta-carotene and 13-cis-retinoic acid on salivary gland tumors, Nutr. Cancer, 1984, 6, 4-12.
12. B.S. Alam, S.Q. Alam. The effect of different levels of dietary beta-carotene on DMBA-induced salivary gland tumors, Nutr. Cancer, 1987, 9, 93-101.
13. B.S. Alam, S.Q. Alam, J.C. Weir Jr., Effects of excess vitamin A and canthaxanthin on salivary gland tumors, Nutr. Cancer, 1988, 11, 233-241.
14. A.S. Rai and M. Katz, Beta-carotene as an inhibitor of benzo(a)pyrene and mitomycin C induced chromosomal breaks in the bone marrow of mice, Can. J. Genet. Cytol., 1985, 27, 598-602.
15. D. Suda, J. Schwartz and G. Shklar, Inhibition of experimental oral carcinogenesis by topical beta-carotene, Carcinogenesis, 1986, 7, 711-715.
16. J. Schwartz, D. Suda and G. Light, Beta-carotene is associated with the regression of hamster buccal pouch carcinoma and the induction of tumor necrosis factor in macrophages, Biochem. Biophy. Res. Commun., 1986, 136, 1130-1135.
17. D. Suda, J. Schwartz and G. Shklar, GGT reduction in beta-carotene inhibition of hamster buccal pouch carcinogenesis, Eur. J. Cancer Clin. Oncol., 1987, 23, 43-46.
18. J. Schwartz and G. Shklar, Regression of experimental hamster cancer by beta-carotene and algae extracts, J. Oral. Maxillofac. Surg., 1987, 45, 510-515.
19. N.J. Temple and T.K. Basu, Protective effect of beta-carotene against colon tumors in mice, J.N.C.I., 1987, 78(6), 1211-1214.
20. M.M. Mathews-Roth, N. Lausen, G. Drouin, A. Richter and N.I. Krinsky, Effects of carotenoid administration on bladder cancer prevention, Oncology, 1991, 48, 177-179.
21. L. Santamaria, L. Bianchi, A. Bianchi, R. Pizzala, G. Santagati and P. Bermond, Photomutagenicity by 8-Methoxypsoralen with and without singlet oxygen involvement and its prevention by beta-carotene.

Relevance to the mechanism of 8-MOP photocarcinogenesis and to PUVA application, Med. Biol. Environn., 1984, 12(1), 541-549.

22. L. Santamaria and A. Bianchi Santamaria, Cancer chemoprevention by supplemental carotenoids and synergism with retinol in mastodynia treatment, Med. Oncol. Tumor Pharmacother, 1990, 7(3-3), 153-167.
23. M.B. Sporn, N.M. Dunlop, D.L. Newton and J.M. Smith, Prevention of chemical carcinogenesis by vitamin A and its synthetic analogs (retinoids), Fed. Proc., 1976, 35, 1332-1338.
24. L. Santamaria, L. Benazzo, M. Benazzo and A. Bianchi, First clinical case report (1980-88) of cancer chemoprevention with beta-carotene plus canthaxanthin supplemented to patients after radical treatment, Med. Biol. Environn., 1988, 16, 945-950.
25. Editorial. Vitamin A, retinol, carotene and cancer prevention, Brit. Med. J., 1980, 281, 957-958.
26. P.R. Band, M. Deschamps, M. Falardeau, J. Ladouceur and J. Cote, Treatment of benign breast disease with vitamin A, Preventive Medicine, 1984, 13, 549-554.
27. L. Bianchi, A. Bianchi, F. Tateo, R. Pizzala, L. Stivala and L. Santamaria, Reduction of chromosomal damage by bleomycin in lymphocytes from subjects supplemented with carotenoids, Relevance in bleomycin tumour chemotherapy, Preliminary results, Boll. Chim. Farmaceutico, 1990, 129(12), 83s, 87s.
28. A. Bianchi, G. Roveta, R. Rizzi, F. Re, R. Pizzala *et al.*, Increase in mouse liver mastocyte frequency induced by beta-carotene, Pharmacol., 1990, 2, 22s.
29. M. Dell'Orti, A. Bianchi Santamaria and L. Santamaria, Survival increase by beta-carotene supplementation in non-surgically treatable lung cancer, A preliminary study, Med. Biol. Environ., 1992, 30(2), 3515-355.

WORKSHOP REPORT: ROLE OF ANTI-OXIDANTS IN CANCER PROTECTION

D.G. Lindsay

Ministry of Agriculture, Fisheries and Food
Nobel House
17 Smith Square
London
SW1P 3JR

The role of anti-oxidants in minimising free-radical damage is under very active investigation, particularly in relation to the initiation of those degenerative diseases where free-radical mechanisms have been implicated, both in the initiation of any lesion, and in the response of the organism to tissue damage.

Free-radicals are known to play an important role in the initiation and progression of malignant disease both as a result of radiation damage, and as a consequence of the exposure to specific chemical carcinogens which produce free-radicals either directly or indirectly, or through the inhibition of processes leading to their de-activation. Nonetheless, even though radiation carcinogenesis exerts its effects as a result of free-radical damage, the specific processes through which this occurs are still far from understood. However, they are likely to differ fundamentally from chemically-induced free-radical formation, since the energy resulting from the radiation could easily penetrate through the nuclear membrane to directly affect DNA.

Free-radical damage to nuclear DNA can be detected in humans. Hydroxylated nucleosides are formed in normal cells, and in individuals not subjected to any known sources of radiation damage, but nothing is understood about the mechanisms which limit the extent of this damage, and whether they are predominately genetically determined or are influenced by the diet. Mixed function oxidases and other metallo-enzymes are present in the nucleus. These could give rise to the formation of free-radicals if the normal control processes are effected. The nuclear DNA could be more susceptible to damage if the cell is undergoing rapid proliferation. In chemically-induced free-radical damage is it conceivable that damage to the lipid membranes and the protein transmembrane receptors, which are involved in the regulation of cell division and differentiation, could be affected without affecting DNA directly. It is also possible that free-radicals lead to the activation of key anti-oxidant enzyme systems, such as glutathione peroxidase or superoxidase dismutase, thereby reducing the capacity of the cell to respond to the burst of oxygen radicals produced in the mitochondria and exported to the cytoplasm. However, in this case it is more likely that this would lead to cell death, rather than cell proliferation.

There is no doubt that oxidative metabolism leads to free-radical formation and that the diet must contribute to this formation. Nonetheless, on present evidence it is impossible to know whether specific factors in the diet are important in initiating free-radical damage, or whether energy intake in general is the most significant factor. At present, the anti-oxidant vitamins are being studied intensively since they are known to protect against free-radical damage. However, it remains to be proved that the current levels of intake of those vitamins are not optimal in minimising this damage. A major obstacle to determining their role is the fact that there is no consensus as to the validity and reproducibility of the present techniques, which are being used to measure oxidative stress.

Since oxygen free-radicals are also implicated in the processes leading to degenerative disease and ageing, it should be possible to demonstrate whether the anti-oxidant vitamins are capable of leading to a greater life-span in experimental animals and what the optimal levels are which achieve this. At present, there are no animal studies which indicate any such protective effects.

Further research is required both to refine the existing methods for measuring oxidative status in relation to specific cell functions, and to study the effects which specific dietary factors may play in inhibiting the rate of oxygen radical formation *in vivo*.

PART 4 TUMOUR INITIATION: THE SIGNIFICANCE OF ENDOGENOUS BIOTRANSFORMATION ENZYMES AND THEIR MODULATION BY DIET

MODULATION OF BIOTRANSFORMATION ENZYMES BY NON-NUTRITIVE DIETARY FACTORS

Peter J. van Bladeren

Department of Biological Toxicology, TNO-Toxicology and Nutrition Institute, Zeist, The Netherlands;
Department of Toxicology, Agricultural University, Wageningen, The Netherlands

1 INTRODUCTION

Organisms are exposed to a large number of xenobiotics (compounds foreign to the body), such as drugs, pesticides, natural food constituents etc. To deal with these usually lipophilic substances, a range of biotransformation enzyme systems are available. These are divided in phase 1 and phase 2 enzymes: In phase 1 a xenobiotic undergoes a transformation, by oxidation, reduction or hydrolysis. In phase 2 the xenobiotic or its metabolite is conjugated to an endogenous molecule. The net result is a much more hydrophilic derivative which can be excreted in urine, or via the bile in the faeces. In phase 1, oxidation is the dominant reaction, catalyzed by the cytochrome P450 mixed-function oxidase system. Phase 2 can be divided into conjugations of electrophiles, catalyzed by e.g. the glutathione S-transferases and epoxide hydrolase, and conjugations of nucleophiles, catalyzed by sulphotransferases and glucuronyl transferases (see table 1).
In addition to the well-known role in detoxication and sometimes activation of xenobiotics, most of the drug-metabolizing enzymes are involved in the biosynthesis or breakdown of endogenous compounds. For instance, several P450 isoenzymes catalyze the oxidation of steroid hormones ([1]), as well as the formation of epoxides from arachidonic acid, compounds with a distinct physiological effect. The glutathione S-transferases play a role in the formation of prostaglandin isomers from the endoperoxide prostaglandin H2 ([2]), and glucuronidation and sulphation of steroid hormones is a prerequisite for the biliary excretion of these hormones.
Most of the enzymes discussed above do not exist as single species, but occur as multigene or supergene families of enzymes (see table 1). When multigene families exist, the individual isoenzymes differ in their catalytic as well as their regulatory properties. In spite of the fact that drug metabolizing enzymes are usually described as having "broad" substrate selectivities, striking differences are known between isoenzymes.

Table 1 Enzymes involved in metabolism of xenobiotics ([3])

Enzyme systems	No of genes	Reactions
cytochrome P450s	>30	oxidation at carbon, nitrogen and sulphur
cytochrome P450 reductase	1	one electron reduction
quinone reductase	1	red. of quinones
glutathione S-transferases	>10	GSH conjugation of electrophiles
epoxide hydrolase	1	hydration of epoxides
UDP-glucuronyl transferases	> 5	conjugation of gluc. acid to -OH, -NH
sulphotransferases	?	conjugation of SO4 to -OH, -NH
N,O-acetyl transferases	> 2	acetyl transfer to -NH, -OH

In fact for most of them substrates are known that are quite specific ([2]).
Thus, factors that cause differences in the "isoenzyme pattern" of an individual give rise to differences in the way a given xenobiotic will be metabolized, and can markedly influence the individual susceptibility to adverse drug reactions, drug-induced diseases and chemically -induced cancers ([1,3]).
In principle, differences in biotransformation enzyme levels between individuals can be of genetic or environmental origin. In the latter case, three modes of action can be envisaged: i) inhibition, ii) induction and iii) activation. The first two mechanisms will be discussed below for two key enzyme systems in biotransformation, cytochrome P450 and the glutathione S-transferases, together with the relevant genetic polymorphisms.
As will be shown, both in inhibition as well as induction, nutrition plays an important role. The effects of macronutrients,although sometimes quite large, are usually not very selective. The same holds true for most micronutrients. Striking effects on activity as well as isoenzyme patterns of drug-metabolizing enzymes are best-known for non-nutritive dietary constituents ([4]).

2 ACTIVATION AND DETOXICATION

Almost all of the xenobiotics to which man is exposed, including the carcinogens need metabolic activation. The reactive intermediates that are formed during metabolism are responsible for binding to cellular macromolecules such as DNA. In general, other biotransformation enzymes can detoxify these metabolites. Thus, the concentration of the ultimate carcinogen, or toxicant in general, is the result of a delicate balance between the rate of activation and the rate of detoxication. Although the process of carcinogenicity is much more complex, inter-individual differences in susceptibility are certainly also a result of interindividual differences in this balance between metabolic activation and detoxication. As examples of the complexities that may arise from this situation, two classes of compounds will be discussed, ethylene dibromide and the halogenated benzenes.

Ethylene dibromide

Although ethylene dibromide (EDB) has not definitively been shown to be a human carcinogen, the evidence from animal experiments for its tumorigenicity is quite clear ([5]). Biotransformation of DBE involves the generation of two highly reactive intermediates (fig 1): oxidation by cytochrome P450 to bromoacetaldehyde and glutathione conjugation to a reactive episulphoniumion ([5]). The first reactive intermediate binds primarily to proteins, and the second to DNA as well as protein. The carcinogenic as well as the mutagenic effect of EDB has conclusively been shown to be the result of the second reactive intermediate, resulting from the glutathione pathway. Isoenzyme selectivity for both primary reactions has been studied extensively. The alpha class glutathione S-transferases are responsible for the conjugation of EDB both in rats and man. The oxidative pathway is catalyzed by cytochrome P4502E1, an isoenzyme responsible for the conversion of many low molecular weight cancer suspects ([6]). For both of these enzymes enormous differences in levels between individuals have been found, which may be due to genetic differences, but are certainly also influenced by induction. One might expect individuals with an increased relative amount of glutathione S-transferases to be at increased risk.

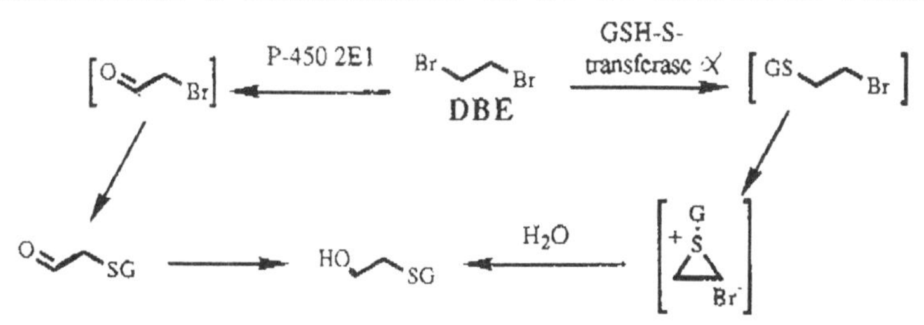

Figure 1 The first steps in the biotransformation of ethylene dibromide.

Halogenated benzenes

In figure 2 the general scheme for the biotransforma-tion of halogenated benzenes is given ([7]). Bioactivation has long been thought to be the result of oxidation to an epoxide. However, recent studies have shown that the covalent binding to cellular macromolecules is not the result of the first oxidative step, but of the second, the formation of a quinone or hydroquinone from the initially formed phenol. The quinone in turn can be detoxified by glutathione conjugation. However, although glutathione protects the liver against toxicity due to these quinones, the conjugates are transported to the kidney and are there activated to new reactive intermediates ([5]). Thus, increasing the relative amount of glutathione S-transferases in this case would not really protect the organism, but merely change the target organ of the active metabolites.

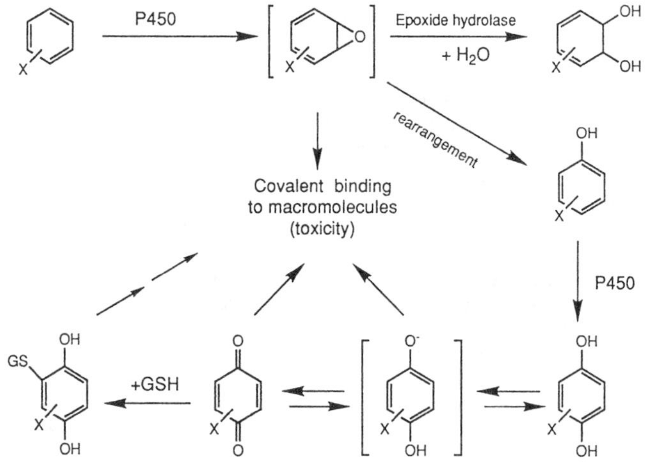

Figure 2 The formation of reactive intermediates during the metabolism of halogenated benzenes ([7]).

3 CYTOCHROME P450

The cytochrome P450 enzymes are a group of hemoproteins, whose Fe(2+)-carbon monoxide complexes show an absorption spectrum with a maximum near 450 nm. These enzymes are monooxygenases, although less usual oxygen transfer reactions also occur. The mechanisms underlying their reactions have been intensively studied and are for the most part known ([8]). Cytochrome P450 plays without doubt the main role in the metabolism of numerous classes of compounds, including drugs, carcinogens, pesticides, as well as natural products. Recently, the importance of P450 in the metabolism of endogenous compounds is also becoming clear: important physiological substrates include steroids, prostanoids, fat-soluble vitamins and fatty acids ([1,2,8]).
The cytochrome P450 enzymes can be grouped into gene families, based on either primary sequences or cDNA work ([3]). Substrate selectivities for the most important and/or interesting isoenzymes are given in table 2. For some substrates, the oxidation can be catalyzed by a number of different P450 forms, while other substrates,

e.g. some steroids are highly specific for one form. In man, the activation of carcinogens appears to be due to only a small number of P450's. P4501A1 activates polycyclic aromatic hydrocarbons; P4501A2 arylamines; P4502E1 activates a variety of low molecular weight cancer suspects, such as urethane, vinyl chloride and ethylene dibromide; while finally the almost "universal" P4503A4 activates aflatoxins, polycyclic hydrocarbon dihydrodiols and polyhalogenated benzenes ([6]).

Genetic variation

Although genetically based differences in P4501A1 have been postulated in the past, the main isozyme known for genetic polymorphism is P4502D6, for which debrisoquine and many related amines are the substrates. The absence of this P450 form has been implicated in an increased risk for bladder cancer as well as for bronchogenic carcinoma ([9]).
Furthermore, a deficiency of P45021A2 is known. However, this enzyme has only a few, albeit very important steroids as substrates, and deficiency results in a serious disease ([10]).

Induction

Human P450's appear to be much more affected by induction than by mutations that cause genetic polymorphisms. Induction levels can be an order of magnitude or more. Studies in animals have indicated that altered levels of protein can have different causes, such as transcriptional activation, mRNA or protein stabilization, and even selective translational enhancement ([1,3]). Numerous compounds and mixtures such as cigarette smoke are known to induce a or (more usually) several forms of P450. For the most important human enzymes, the inducers are given in table 2. The mechanism of induction has been studied most thoroughly for P4501A1, which occurs through the Ah receptor and has been reviewed extensively ([11]). For the sofar much less accessible case of induction of P4502B6 and related forms by phenobarbital, progress is also being made ([12]).
The best studied examples of dietary constituents inducing P450 are the glucobrassicin products, indole-3-carbinol, indole-3-acetonitrile and indole-3-carboxyaldehyde. They induce both hepatic and intestinal P450 in rats. Indole-3-carbinol is the most potent of the three, but treatment with acid such as occurs in the stomach, gives rise to much more potent dimer and trimer condensation products. These would be expected to have a much higher affinity for the Ah receptor. In line with that theory, a much higher induction of P4501A1 was observed ([13]).

Table 2 Inducers, inhibition and substrates for human P450 enzymes ([1-3])

Human P450 enzymes	Inducers	Inhibitors	Substrates
P4501A1	cigarette smoking	7,8-benzoflavone, ellipticine	polycyclic aromatic hydrocarbons
P4501A2	cruciferous vegetables	7,8-benzoflavone	arylamines
P4502C8	rifampicin	sulphaphenazole, barbiturates	hexobarbital
P4502D6	-	quinidine, alkaloids	debrisoquine and related amines
P4502E1	ethanol	disulfiram	ethanol, N-nitroso dialkylamines vinylchloride, ethylene dibromide
P4503A4	dexamethasone, troleandomycin	gestodene, naringenin	aflatoxins, halogenated benzenes

Inhibition

Enzyme inhibition, both competitive and non-competitive is well-known to occur for P450. An interesting example of the former is naringenin, a flavonoid from grapefruit juice, which was found to inhibit the P4503A4 mediated oxidation of nifedipine ([1,14]). In addition inhibitory effects have been noted for numerous flavonoids. Examples of the non-competitive inhibition are known to occur with synthetic compounds, such as troleandomycin, from which a nitroso-derivative is formed that binds extremely tightly to the ferrous heme ([1]), but compounds are also known that actually form a covalent bond with the apoprotein (chloramphenicol) or the porphyrin. Diallyl disulfide a component of garlic oil was shown to inhibit P4502E1, following a typical suicide inhibition pattern ([14]) and the same is known for phenethyl isothiocyanate ([14]). Of course initial inhibition might lead to subsequent induction, and indeed diallyl disulfide has been shown to induce P3402B1 ([14]).

4 GLUTATHIONE S-TRANSFERASES

The cytosolic GST isoenzymes all consist of two subunits, with a molecular weight between 24 and 28.000. The isoenzymes described in rat, man and mouse can be divided into four classes, alpha, mu, pi and theta, based on similar structural and catalytic properties of their subunits ([15]). Amino acid sequence homology and immunological cross-reactivity indicate considerable similary between isoenzymes from one class but from different species, allowing relatively easy extrapolation of results from one species to another. In the rat, more than 10 subunits have been characterized, which are designated by arabic numerals ([16]). From these subunits 8 homodimers and 4 heterodimers are formed, named according to their respective subunit composition. Although substrate selectivities of the GST isoenzymes are generally described as broad and overlapping, major differences between the alpha, mu and pi classes exist: some substrates are specific enough to be used for the classification of the isoenzymes ([17]). Class alpha isoenzymes generally exhibit high peroxidase activity, class pi isoenzymes are highly active towards ethacrynic acid while trans-stilbene oxide is used for the classification of class μ isoenzymes (both μ and ψ exhibit a similar activity towards this model substrate ([18]). In addition, the human μ isoenzymes exhibit by far the highest rates of conversion of polycyclic aromatic hydrocarbon epoxides and diolepoxides ([19]).

Genetic variation

For class μ isoenzymes a clear polymorphism has been observed in humans: isoenzyme μ was found to be expres-

sed in only 60% of the samples analysed ([20]). It is clear that in addition to the phenotype 1-0 which is characterized by an absence of near-neutral enzymes, at least three other phenotypes exist : 1-1, 1-2 and 1 2-1. The first one expresses ψ, the second μ and the third both isoenzymes plus a heterodimer. The results are in agreement with [21], who used trans-stilbene oxide, a model substate only conjugated via μ and ψ, to show that cytosolic GST activity in both liver and mononuclear lymphocytes falls into three groups with resp. low, high and very high activity. The group with "very high" activity may thus express both transferases.
However, documented examples of increased toxicity as a result of modification of GST levels are. In a study on the excretion of the mercapturate derived from 1,3-dichloropropene in exposed workers, no difference was observed between mu-positive and mu-negative subjects ([22]). Although the mu enzyme had by far the highest Vmax, obviously the lower activity of the other isozymes still allowed them to cope. In contrast to this finding, a survey of a large number of smokers clearly showed a higher amount of sister-chromatid-exchanges in the lymphocytes of mu-negative compared to mu-positive volunteers ([23]), indicating that these people are less well protected against DNA damage.
Considerable polymorphism has been observed for the human liver α class isoenzymes. The ratio of B_1 and B_2 subunits, as determined by HPLC, was found to range from 0.5 to over 10 ([18]). However, a division into two groups, with average ratios of 1.6±0.3 and 3.8±0.6 could be made, suggesting an α class polymorphism.

Induction

It has long been known that GST activity towards a number of different substrates can be induced by several agents. Most studies have concentrated on rat liver GST, induced by phenobarbital and 3-methylcholanthrene on the one hand, and a number of "anticarcinogenic" naturally occurring compounds on the other hand. Only recently the induction of individual isoenzymes has been studied (e.g. [24]). In that study it was shown that the changes in the glutathione S-transferase isoenzyme pattern induced by Brussels sprouts in rat liver and intestine was very similar to that caused by administration of allyl isothiocyanate, and not to that resulting from goitrin.
[25] and [26] have shown differential increases in mRNA levels coding for subunits 1 (5-10 fold) and subunits 3 and 4 (5-6 fold) by phenobarbital and 3-methyl-cholanthrene. However, on a protein level, induction is considerably smaller, and displays a different subunit selectivity, indicating that differences in transla-tional efficiency and/or turnover rates between mRNA's coding for individual subunits may exist <u>in vivo</u> ([27]). Recently a theory on phase II enzyme induction (mainly

NADH quinone-reductase and GST) was expounded by Talalay and coworkers ([28]). It was suggested that the common factor in inducing agents for GST is the existence or development during biotransformation of a Michael acceptor. In addition, the "classic" inducers such as TCDD could also work via a different, receptor mediated, mechanism. No mention of isoenzyme selectivity is made in this theory. However, recently socalled Anti-oxidant as well as Xenobiotic Responsive Elements have been recognized in the DNA-sequences ([20,3]).

Inhibition

A large variety of inhibitors of the GST are known. Some of these are strong, and/or selective enough to be used to characterize individual isoenzymes: triphenyl-tinchloride, bromosulphophthalein, cibacron blue and hematin thus form a panel useful for the classification of GST isoenzymes ([17]). Others include drugs from a variety of classes, metal compounds, and a considerable amount of naturally occurring compounds.
However most of the studies described so far have been performed on either cytosol or mixtures of affinity-purified isoenzymes and only a few isolated cases are known where an actual <u>in vivo</u> effect was observed. Because of the potential modulation of biotransformation pathways <u>in vivo</u>, but also because inhibition of glutathione S-transferases might have potential therapeutic application in the treatment of (multi) drug resistant cancer cells this subject is an important one. Two classes of inhibitors can be distinguished, reversible inhibitors, comprising substrates and analogs of substrates, as well as socalled non-substrate ligands (mainly of importance for α class subunits) and irreversible inhibitors, which act by covalent binding to the enzymes.
By far the largest range of competitive inhibitors of GST is found in the compounds that bind to the electrophilic substrate site, the "second substrate analogs". However, the distinction between substrates and inhibitors in this case is not straightforward. In fact, all substrates, due to their binding capacity, will act as competitive inhibitors for other substrates. A good example in this respect is ethacrynic acid, both used as an inhibitor of GST ([29]) and as a substrate with selectivity towards certain mu class isoenzymes ([17]). Also, the glutathione conjugate of this compound is a strong competitive inhibitor of GST isoenzymes ([30]).
A large number of phenols have been shown to effectively inhibit glutathione S-transferases in a competitive manner. Among these phenols are many naturally occurring compounds, such as the plant phenols ellagic acid, caffeic acid, quercitin, chlorogenic acid and ferrulic acid, all of which show IC50 values between 0.4 and 100 µM towards the human anionic forms, and substantially higher IC50 values towards human cationic forms ([31,32]).

Rat glutathione S-transferase isoenzymes appear to be much more sensitive towards these compounds than the human forms ([32]). A large number of other synthetic and naturally occurring phenols were able to inhibit house fly GST in a similar manner ([33]).
A special kind of inhibition of the GST is caused by the "non-substrate ligands", and should be mentioned here, although thus far no dietary constituents have been shown to display activity similar to the best studied examples, heme, bilirubin and several bile acids. The glutathione S-transferases are rather selective in their ability to bind these non-substrate ligands: although all isoenzymes appear to bind these compounds to some extent, in general only the alpha class isoenzymes containing subunit 1 have a low (<1μM) binding constant. The binding usually coincides with loss of catalytic activity, although it has been established that this binding occurs at a site distinct to the binding sites of glutathione and the electrophilic second substrate ([34]).
Although covalent binding to Glutathione S-transferases has been described as a useful step in the detoxification of electrophiles, only a few systematic studies have been performed on the consequences and mechanism of the interaction of covalently binding compounds with GST Several quinones have long been known to inhibit glutathione S-transferases ([35,36,37]). Among these are several naturally occurring compounds such as juglone and vitamin K, as well as synthetic ones such as tetrachloro-1,2- and 1,4-benzoquinones. The nature of the inactivation was elucidated only recently.
Quinones as a rule react efficiently with sulfhydryl groups, in one of two ways: arylation of the thiol group, or oxidation of two thiols to a disulfide. To what extent these two pathways are followed depends on the quinone. Certainly the reaction of a series of quinones with (presumably) a thiol group in the enzyme led to inhibition ranging from 100 to 75% ([38]). A special case is tetrachloro 1,4-benzoquinone (TCBQ), which like many other quinones, forms conjugates with glutathione and reacts efficiently with proteins ([39]). However, the reaction pathway is substitution of a chloride atom by sulfur, leaving the quinone structure intact. Instead of the more usual case, where from the quinone a hydroquinone is formed which is no longer reactive. The initial glutathione conjugate of TCBQ (TCBQ-GSH) is thus a reactive glutathione derivative, capable of alkylating more thiols. In fact, in the presence of an excess of glutathione ultimately a tetra-GSH-conjugate is formed ([39]). In fact, the reactive glutathione conjugate derived from TCBQ might be targeted to the active site of the enzyme: the combination of a reactive group and a substrate moiety could lead to a preferential covalent inhibition of the glutathione S-transferases.

5 CONCLUSION

Each individual has its own isoenzyme pattern for the various drug metabolizing enzymes, as was demonstrated above for P450 and the glutathione S-transferases. The multiplicity of these enzymes results in differential responses to dietary constituents. A substance may increase the level of a certain P450, and decrease the level of another. The complexity of the problem is such that it is premature to call a compound an anticarcinogen, since although its administration may inhibit the tumorigenicity of one compound, the effects of another may be exacerbated.

A sofar neglected area is that of modulation of the metabolism of endogenous compounds. Changes in the biotransformation enzymes might very well have subtle effects on the levels of various messenger molecules which are metabolized by those same enzymes.

Several approaches for future studies on the effects of dietary constituents are indicated:

i) Further studies on the mechanisms of induction and inhibition of biotransformation enzymes.

ii) Careful studies using human volunteers, where the effects can be studied in isolation as much as possible. A considerable number of non-invasive assays to estimate the amount of a particular enzyme in an individual are already available. However, for many relevant drug-metabolizing enzymes such tools are still lacking, and there is no doubt that considerable progress needs to be made in that area, based on classical assays using model-drugs as well as modern approaches using DNA-technology.

iii) Studies of the disposition and kinetics of the dietary constituents themselves. In these latter studies, the organ selectivity of the effects, as well as the different responses after an acute high dose versus a chronic low dose would be primary goals, to assess the day to day relevance of e.g. inducing agents in food for the human situation. In that respect the recent developments in computer PBPK-modelling are interesting. With the aid of such a system *in vitro* data may be used to extrapolate and predict *in vivo* kinetics and effects.

REFERENCES

1. F.P. Guengerich, *Faseb J.*, 1992, *6*, 745.
2. M. Ujihara, S. Tsuchida, K. Satoh, H. Sato and Y. Urade, *Arch.Biochim.Biophys.*, 1988, *264*, 428.
3. C.R. Wolfe, *Cancer Surveys*, 1990, *9*, 437.
4. I.R. Rowland (ed), Nutrition, Toxicity and Cancer, CRC Press Inc. Boca Raton, 1991.
5. T.J. Monks, M.W. Anders, W. Dekant, J.L. Stevens, S.S. Lau and P.J. van Bladeren, *Tox.Appl.Pharmacol.*, 1990, *106*, 1.
6. F.P. Guengerich, *Life Sciences*, 1992, *50*, 1471.
7. C. den Besten, J.R.M. Vet, H.T. Besselink, G.S. Kiel, B.J.M. van Berkel, R.B. Beems and P.J. van Bladeren, *Tox.Appl.Pharmacol.*, 1991, *111*, 69.

8. F.P. Guengerich, Chem.Res.Toxicol., 1991, 4, 391.
9. J.R. Idle, Mut.Res., 1991, 247, 259.
10. Y. Higashi, T. Hiromasa, A. Tanae, T. Miki, J. Makura, T. Kondo, T. Ohura, E. Ogawa, K. Nakayama and Y. Fujii-Kuriyama, J.Biochem. 1991, 109, 638.
11. D.W. Hebert and F.J. Gonzalez, Annu.Rev.Biochem., 1987, 56, 945.
12. D.J. Waxman and L. Azaroff, Biochem.J., 1992, 281, 577.
13. H.M. Wortelboer, Ph.D. Thesis, Utrecht, 1990.
14. C.S. Yang, J.F. Brady and J. Hong, Faseb J., 1992, 6, 737.
15. B. Mannervik and U.H. Danielson, C.R.C. Crit.Rev.Biochem., 1988, 23, 283.
16. W.B. Jacoby, B. Ketterer and B. Mannervik, Biochem.Pharmacol., 1984, 33, 2539.
17. B. Mannervik, Adv. Enzymol., 1985, 57, 357.
18. B. van Ommen, J.J.P. Bogaards, W.H.M. Peters, B. Blaauboer and P.J. van Bladeren, Biochem.J., 1990, 269, 609.
19. M. Warholm, C. Guthenberg and B. Mannervik, Biochemistry, 1983, 22, 3610.
20. P. Board, M. Coggan, P. Johnston, V. Ross, T. Suzuki and G. Webb, Pharmacol.Ther., 1990, 48, 357.
21. J. Seidegard and R.W. Pero, Hum. Genetics., 1985, 69, 66.
22. R.M.E. Vos, R.T.H. van Welie, W.M. Peters, C.T.A. Evelo, J.J.P. Bogaards, N.P.E. Vermeulen and P.J. van Bladeren, Arch. Toxicol., 1991, 65, 95.
23. G. van Poppel, N. de Vogel, P.J. van Bladeren and F.J. Kok, Cancer Res., submitted.
24. J.J.P. Bogaards, B. van Ommen and P.J. van Bladeren, J.Chromatogr., 1989, 474, 430.
25. C.B. Pickett, C.A. Telakowski-Hopkins, G.J.F. Ding, L. Argenbright and A.Y.H. Lu, J.Biol.Chem., 1984, 259, 5182.
26. G.J.F. Ding, V.D.H. Ding, J.A. Rodkey, C.D. Bennett, A.Y.H. Lu and C.B. Pickett, J.Biol.Chem., 1986, 261, 7952.
27. R.M.E. Vos, M.C. Snoek, W.J.H. van Berkel, F. Muller and P.J. van Bladeren, Biochem.Pharmacol., 1988, 37, 1077.
28. H.J. Prohaska and P. Talalay, Cancer Res., 1988, 48, 4776.
29. J.T. Ahokas, F.A. Nicholls, P.J. Ravenscroft and B.T. Emmerson, Biochem.Pharmacol. 1985, 34, 2157.
30. J.H.T.M. Ploemen, B. van Ommen and P.J. van Bladeren, Biochem.Pharmacol., 1990, 40, 1631.
31. M. Das, D.R. Bickers and H. Mukhtar, Biochem.Biophys.Res. Commun., 1984, 120, 427.
32. M. Das, S.V. Singh, H. Mukhtar and Y.C. Awasthi, Biochem. Biophys.Res.Commun., 1986, 141, 1170.
33. N. Motoyama, A.P. Kulkarni, E. Hodgson and W.C. Dauterman, Pestic.Biochem.Physiol., 1978, 9, 255.
34. D.A. Vessey and T.D. Boyer, Toxicol.Appl.Pharmacol., 1984, 73, 492.
35. A.P. Kulkarni, N. Motoyama, W.C. Dauterman and E. Hodgson, Bull.Environm.Contam.Toxicol., 1978, 20, 227.
36. P.J. Dierickx, Res.Commun.Chem.Pathol.Pharmacol., 1983, 41, 517.
37. P.J. Dierickx, Pharmacol.Res.Commun., 1983a, 15, 581.
38. R.M.E. Vos, B. van Ommen, M.S.J. Hoekstein, J.H.M. de Goede, and P.J. van Bladeren, Chem.-Biol.Interact., 1989a, 71, 381.
39. B. van Ommen, C. den Besten, A.L.M. Rutten, J.H.T.M. Ploemen, R.M.E. Vos, F. Muller and P.J. van Bladeren, J.Biol.Chem., 1988, 263, 12939.

EFFECT OF COOKING AND OF VEGETABLES AND FRUIT ON 1,2-DIMETHYLHYDRAZINE-INDUCED COLON CARCINOGENESIS IN RATS

G. M. Alink, H. A. Kuiper,* V. M. H. Hollanders** and J. H. Koeman

Department of Toxicology
Agricultural University Wageningen
The Netherlands

**TNO Toxicology and Nutrition Institute
Zeist, The Netherlands

*Department of Toxicology
State Institute for Quality Control of Agricultural Products (RIKILT-DLO)
Wageningen, The Netherlands

1 INTRODUCTION

Epidemiological studies have shown that diet is a major factor in the etiology of colon cancer.[1,2]
As processed meat contains heterocyclic amines which have been shown to induce colon cancer in experimental animals,[3] a possible role of heterocyclic compounds in the etiology of colon cancer may be assumed. The protective role as shown by vegetables is mostly attributed to vitamin A and fibre.[4] In addition glucosinolates in cruciferous vegetables may protect against colon cancer.[5] Although colon cancer seems a multifactorial disease, only a few animal experimental studies have been performed on the influence of combined food items on colon cancer. So far no attention has been paid to the effect of non-nutrients (except glucosinolates) and baking and frying of food items on colon carcinogenesis.

The colon carcinogen 1,2-dimethylhydrazine (DMH) is frequently used to study colon carcinogenesis in animal models.[6] The purpose of the present study was to examine the modulating effect of heat processing and of vegetables and fruit in human diets and of vegetables and fruit in animal diets on the DMH-induced colon carcinogenesis in rats.

2 MATERIALS AND METHODS

Animals

Two hundred and sixteen 4-week-old male Wistar rats (CPB: WU) were obtained from Harlan, Zeist, The Netherlands. The study was carried out at the Centre for Small Laboratory Animals (CKP) of the Agricultural University. During 4 weeks of adaptation to the experimental diets and after DMH-treatment, rats were housed in stainless-steel cages with wire-mesh bases in a room with air conditioning (21 ± 1°C), controlled humidity (55 ± 10%) and artificial lighting (12-hr light/12-hr dark). Food and drinking-water were provided *ad libitum*. During the DMH-treatment and two weeks afterwards the rats stayed in cages placed in an animal isolator maintained under negative pressure. For dietary group B, 36 animals and for each of the other dietary groups 45 animals were used.

Diets

Five types of diets with a similar composition as those previously described (Tables 1 and 2) have been investigated.[8]

Diet A (animal diet). This was the control diet and consisted of a commercial semi-synthetic diet.

Diet B (animal diet). This was a modification of diet A in which part of the macro- and micronutrients were replaced by a vegetable and fruit mixture prepared according to mean consumption figures in The Netherlands.[7]

Diet C (human diet). This was composed of meat, bread and eggs at levels calculated according to mean levels of consumption in The Netherlands,[7] without processing (baking or frying).

Diet D (human diet). This consisted of the same food items as diet C but they were processed under usual household conditions.

Diet E (human diet). This represented a complete human diet, including vegetables and fruit.

The macronutrient composition differed between animal and human diets, but were the same for each type of diet. The animal diets (A and B) contained 21.6 energy (E) % fat, 26.0 E % protein, 52.4 E % carbohydrate and 10.7 % (w/w) fibre. The human diets (C, D and E) contained 40.6 % fat, 13.2 E % protein, 46.2 E % carbohydrate and 5 % (w/w) fibre. The micronutrient composition was the same in all diets and was based on diet A. Details on preparation of the diets have been presented in a previous paper.[8]

Experimental design

The rats were fed the diets for a period of eight months starting from the beginning of the experiment, at the age of 4 weeks. Food intake per cage and body weights of individual rats were recorded weekly during the entire experimental period. Starting at 8 weeks of age, all animals were injected once weekly for 10 weeks, 50 mg DMH per kg body weight, subcutaneously (in the neck). DMH was dissolved in a 1.5 % solution of EDTA in 0.9 % NaCl, which was adjusted to pH 6.5. Rats were injected 1 ml/kg b.w. of the DMH solution.

At the end of the experiment all animals were killed by decapitation and subjected to detailed gross examination. The colon was removed, rinsed with cold phosphate buffered saline and examined for the presence of tumors and lesions suspected of being a tumor. The number of tumors, their size and gross appearance were recorded. Each tumor and tumor-like lesion was fixed in 10 % buffered formalin. These tissues were processed and embedded in a paraffin wax. Five μm thick sections were made and stained with hematoxylin and eosin. The proliferative epithelial lesions in the colon were classified as sessile or polypoid adenomas and adenocarcinomas.

Statistical analysis

Data on the tumor status of the animals and the number of carcinomas per carcinoma-bearing animal were analyzed with a generalized linear model using a Poisson error distribution. A logarithmic link function has been used, implying that effects are additive on the logarithmic scale. Additionally, tumor incidences were analyzed using the Fisher exact probability test. P values of ≤ 0.05 were considered significant.

3 RESULTS

Food intake and body weight

Food intake of rats consuming animal diets (A and B) was higher than of rats maintained on the human diet (C, D and E). This is in accordance with previous findings and may be attributed to the difference in calorific density and subsequent calorific adaptation.[8] After 8 months no significant difference was observed in body weight between animal and human diet groups.

Colon tumor incidence

Table 3 summarizes the incidences of colon tumors in rats fed the five different diets. Tumors were mainly classified as adenomas and adenocarcinomas. The highest number of adenomas was observed in the group fed the animal diet (A), while in the group fed the animal diet with vegetables and fruit added (B) significantly less adenomas were found ($P < 0.01$). No significant differences were observed between the combined human (C, D, E) and combined animal diet groups (A, B), neither was there a significant difference between the human diet groups in the number of adenomas. However, the overall incidence of carcinomas was significantly higher in the combined human diet groups than in the combined animal diet groups ($P < 0.05$). In the pairwise comparison of human diets the incidence of carcinomas was a factor 1.43 higher in rats fed the human diet including vegetables and fruit (E) in comparison with rats consuming the corresponding diet without vegetables and fruit (D) ($P < 0.05$). No significant differences were observed in the incidences of colon carcinomas between group C and D, and between group A and B.

4 DISCUSSION

The present study was designed to evaluate the effects of heating of human diets and the presence of vegetables and fruit separately and in combination on DMH-induced colon carcinogenesis in rats. In contrast to previous experiments[8] where no effect was found of vegetables and fruit on the spontaneous tumor incidence in human nor in animal diet groups, in the present study vegetables and fruit had a marked effect on DMH-induced tumors, which was inhibitive for the animal diets but enhancing for the human diets. Like in

Table 1. Composition of the diets

Components	Levels (% dry weight) in diet: A	B	C	D	E
Meat, bread, eggs (raw)	—	—	55.1	—	—
Meat, bread, eggs (fried or baked)	—	—	—	55.5	51.5
Vegetables and fruit	—	19.5	—	—	19.5
Semi-synthetic products					
Muracon SSP Tox	100	80.5	—	—	—
Lard	—	—	4.2	4.8	5.8
Potato flour	—	—	15.4	15.5	—
Sugar	—	—	19.1	18.9	22.6
Bran	—	—	5.7	4.8	0.6
Pectin	—	—	0.5	0.5	—

Table 2. Composition of the product groups

Product group . . .	Meat, bread and eggs: Component	Level (% by wet weight)	Vegetables and fruit: Component	Level (% by wet weight)
	Eggs	7.0	Potato	35.1
	White bread	19.4	Banana	3.0
	Wheaten bread	17.1	Orange	9.0
	Whole bread	2.3	Apple	19.1
	Margarine	9.7	Salad	3.75
	Minced meat	9.9	Pepper	1.25
	Chicken	5.0	Tomato	3.75
	Pork liver	2.8	Cucumber	3.75
	Beef steak	3.5	Cauliflower	3.75
	Steak tartare	4.0	Spinach	2.5
	Fricandeau	7.5	Leek	2.5
	Pork steak	9.9	Red cabbage	2.5
	Bacon	2.0	White cabbage	2.5
			Sauerkraut	2.5
			Carrot	1.25
			Brussels sprouts	1.25
			Beet	2.5

<u>Table 3</u> Summary of colonic neoplastic changes

Dietary group	Total number of: Polypoid adenomas	Adeno-carcinomas
A	68 (27)	67 (31)
B	19 (14)**	42 (22)
C	31 (20)	70 (28)
D	45 (20)	72 (34)
E	42 (23)	100 (35)*

In brackets number of rats bearing adenomas or carcinomas.
* compared to D $p < 0.05$
**compared to A $p < 0.01$

previous experiments[8] heating had no significant effect on the tumor incidence.

Our study suggests that the cancermodulating effect of vegetables and fruit may depend on the fat content of the diet. As far as we know this is the first animal study in which an increase of chemically induced colon carcinogenesis due to the introduction of vegetables and fruit in a human diet is found. As the animal diets and the human diets were balanced for macro- and micronutrients and fibre, the modulating effects must be ascribed to non-nutrients other than fibre. Which components in vegetables or fruit in human diets are responsible for the observed effects on tumor incidence is unknown. One may speculate that interaction between compounds present in vegetables and fat could result in modification of metabolic pathways. For example by interference with the natural metabolic activity in the colon. The influence of human diets on metabolic activation of carcinogens was shown in a previous study.[9] In this study it was found that liver homogenate obtained from rats fed a complete human diet (baked and fried plus vegetables and fruit) had a higher bioactivation capacity towards dimethylnitrosamine than the human diet without vegetables and fruit.

As in our study fat content and heat processing were main variables between the animal and human diets containing vegetables and fruit, the data suggest that one of these factors or both influence the tumor modulating effect of non-nutrient substances in vegetables and fruit. If this hypothesis is correct the conclusion would be that vegetables and fruit only exert a protective effect in diets with a low fat content. Further experimentation is needed to conclude whether or not the supposed interactive effects between fat and vegetables and fruit may have health implications for the Western diet.

REFERENCES

1. R. Doll and R. Peto, J.Natl.Cancer Inst., 1981, 66, 1192.
2. W.R. Bruce, Cancer Res., 1987, 47, 4237.
3. T. Sugimura, Environ.Health Perspect., 1986, 67, 5.
4. L.W. Wattenberg, Cancer Res., 1983, 43, 2448.
5. S. Graham, S. Dayal, M. Swanson, A. Mittelman and G. Wilkinson, J.Natl.Cancer Inst., 1978, 61, 709.
6. H.P. Glauert and J.A. Weeks, Toxic.Letters, 1989, 48, 283.
7. H.J.K. van den Berg, Report of the Ministry of Agriculture and Fisheries, The Netherlands, 1981.
8. G.M. Alink, H.A. Kuiper, R.B. Beems and J.H. Koeman, Fd.Chem. Toxic., 1989, 27, 427.
9. G.M. Alink, P.L.M. Reijven, S.R. Sijtsma, W.M.F. Jongen, R.J. Topp, H.A. Kuiper and J.H. Koeman, Fd.Chem.Toxic., 1988, 26, 883.

STUDIES OF ANTIMUTAGENIC FACTORS IN FOOD

G. Bronzetti, E. Morichetti, C. Salvadori* and C. Della Croce
Istituto di Mutagenesi e Differenziamento, CNR, Via Svezia 10 - 56123 - Pisa, Italy.
*Parmalat S.p.A., Via O. Grassi 26 - 43044 - Parma, Italy.

INTRODUCTION

The role of the diet in the etiology of cancer received increasing attention in these last years. It is known that human diet is a complex mixture containing both mutagenic and antimutagenic factors. For this reason it is important to identify both these agents to minimize the human hazard.

Many antimutagens have been discovered by the use of short term assays that are considered a tool for elucidating mechanisms and specificity of dietary factors.

Since it is very difficult to eliminate man's exposure to mutagenic agent it could be very important to increase the use of antimutagenic agents in the diet.

In the present study we have chosen chlorophyllin, spermine and fermented milk as hypotetic antimutagens for their importance as natural substances contained in the diet. Their antimutagenic activity was evaluated in the D7 strain of *S.cerevisiae* using standard mutagens.

Sodium-copper-chlorophyllin:

Chlorophyllin (Chl) is a derivative of chlorophyll (1), a known food additive (E141) used as colouring matter and also employed as remedy for acceleration of wound healing (2,3); it is an antioxidant, protects against peroxidative damages and acts as a membrane stabilizer (4). It was reported that it decreases the genetic effects induced in *S.cerevisiae and S.typhimurium* by environmental and dietary complex mixtures (5) and it inhibited the mutagenicity induced by aflatoxin B1 (6).

To evaluate the influence of chl on genetic effects induced by some chemical (styrene oxide, ethidium bromide and sodium chromate) and physical (X-rays) agents, yeast cells were treated in the presence of different concentrations of chl.

Spermine:

Spermine (Spe) is a polyamine present in food from plants, in fresh and cured meat, in many biological materials and it is implicated in a variety of biological reactions; it decreases the induced mutation in various bacterial systems (7,8,9,10). In cultured human lymphocytes exposed to X-rays it reduced the chromosomal aberrations and in Chinese hamster ovary cells it decreased the level of sister chromatid exchanges induced by psoralen and UV-rays (11,12).

To evaluate a possible effect of spe in the prevention of EMS and MMS induced effects, cells were pretreated for an hour in the presence of different concentrations of spe and then incubated with EMS or MMS for two hours in phosphate buffer. To analyze the spe influence on UV-induced repair, after the exposure to UV-rays, cells were postincubated in liquid growth medium in the dark.

Fermented milk:

It is known that consumption of milk decreased the incidence of some induced cancers (13-17). In rats dietary supplementation with viable *Lactobacillus acidophilus* significantly lowered the activity of fecal bacterial enzymes (azoreductase, β-glucuronidase and nitroreductase) that play an important role in the conversion of chemical procarcinogens to carcinogens (18,19).

In this work we have assayed a commercial fermented milk (Kyr from Parmalat) prepared from a stock yogurt culture (containing only *Lactobacillus bulgaricus and Streptococcus thermophilus*) by adding fermented milk obtained using *Lactobacillus acidophilus and Bifidobacterium bifidum.* We have tested five Kyr-samples obtained by different productions.

To evaluate the antimutagenic effect yeast cells were treated with EMS and MMS in the presence of fermented milk samples.

MATERIALS AND METHODS

Yeast strain:

D7 strain of *Saccharomyces cerevisiae*, obtained from F.K. Zimmermann was used (20).

Experimental procedures:

Chemical treatment and X-irradiation were performed as reported by Bronzetti et al. (21); UV-irradiation was performed as reported by Galli et al. (22).

RESULTS AND DISCUSSION

It is important to note that none of the hypothetic antimutagens used influence the spontaneous revertant and convertant frequencies in our experimental conditions.

Our results showed that chl possess antimutagenic activity toward styrene oxide , ethidium bromide, sodium chromate and X-rays as reported by Bronzetti et al. (23).

Spe reduced the mitotic gene conversion frequency, but mainly the point reverse mutation frequency induced by UV-rays (table 1c). Spe had no effect on survival percentage in MMS and EMS treated cells. In addition significant dose dependent decrease of mitotic gene conversion and particularly of point reverse mutation was observed in the presence of spe in MMS and EMS treated cells(table 1a,b).

The results obtained by treating cells with alkylating agents indicated that spe is a desmutagenic agent; probably it binds to DNA preventing the reaction with alkylating groups. We can hypothesize that spe acts preventing only in part DNA damage but it does not interfere with cellular functions.

The significant decrease of UV-induced genetic activity, when cells were postincubated with spe, confirms an activity of polyamines in repair of pyrimidine dimers .

Table 1b shows that all samples significantly decreased genetic activity induced by EMS. Sample 4 is the only sample that decreased both gene conversion and point reverse mutation.

The same samples did not influence the genetic activity induced by MMS (data not shown).

Literature data showed that dietary supplementation with Bifidobacterium bifidum and Lactobacillus acidophilus decreased the incidence of some kinds of cancer.

Results obtained with samples of fermented milk are very interesting because all commmon yogurt contained only two kinds of bacteria (Lactobacillus acidophilus and Streptococcus thermophilus)
To estabilish which bacteria species are responsible for the antimutagenic activity, experiments with samples containing only one kind of microorganism are in progress.

It would be interesting to investigate why these samples determine different antimutagenic activity. For this purpose different experimental conditions and different mutagens will be employed.

TABLE 1. EFFECT OF SPERMINE (Sp) ON GENE CONVERSION AND POINT REVERSE MUTATION INDUCED BY MMS (a) EMS (b) AND UV-RAYS (c) AND OF FERMENTED MILK (S) INDUCED BY EMS (b).
DATA REPRESENT MEAN OF 4 INDEPENDENT EXPERIMENTS ± SD.

(a)

	Surv.(%)	Conv./10^5surv.	Rev./10^6surv.
Control	100	1.3±0.2	0.2±0.01
MMS 7mM	77.2±6.3	185.1±27.2	102.5±11.5
MMS+Sp. 8mM	63.4±4.2	113.4±28.7*	54.8±5.5*

(b)

	Surv.(%)	Conv./10^5surv.	Rev./10^6surv.
Control	100	1.3±0.2	0.2±0.01
EMS 110mM	58.3±3.1	178.1±8.11	730.4±66.6
EMS+Sp. 8mM	57.3±9.2	88.8±9.7*	320.2±14.0*
EMS+S1(100µl)	51.0±8.1	85.2±11.3*	714.9±96.3
EMS+S2(100µl)	43.6±8.1	157.7±29.8	662.1±40.5
EMS+S3(100µl)	30.3±2.0	59.5±8.7*	751.2±71.5
EMS+S4(100µl)	59.0±6.3	65.9±17.8*	460.9±60.7*
EMS+S5(100µl)	78.0±15.2	133.3±42.4	418.5±41.1*

(c)

	Surv.(%)	Conv./10^5surv.	Rev./10^6surv.
Time: 0h			
Control	100	1.3 0.2	0.2 0.01
UV (200J/m^2)	24.6±6.7	826.8±172.1	1016.1±161.7
Time: 2h			
Control	100	1.3±0.2	0.3±0.1
UV (200J/m^2)	25.1±8.1	1080.2±152.3	885.5±66.7
UV+Sp. 4mM	37.6±13.2	768.1±79.6*	577.4±41.4*
UV+Sp. 8mM	28.6±15.1	811.9±93.5*	340.8±79.3*

*$P<0.05$.

REFERENCES

1. J.C. Kephart, Econ. Bot., 1955, 9, 3.
2. K. Imai, T. Aimoto, M. Sato, K. Watanabe, R. Kimura and T. Murata, Chem. Pharm. Bull., 1986, 34, 4287.
3. M. Sato, K.Konagai, R. Kimura and T. Murata, Chem. Pharm. Bull., 1983, 31, 3665.
4. M. Sato, R.Imai, R. Kimura and T. Murata, Chem. Pharm. Bull., 1984, 32, 716.
5. T. Man Ong, W.Z. Whong, J. Stewart, and H.E. Brockman, Mutat. Res., 1986, 173, 111.
6. E. Robin, "Antimutagenesis and Anticarcinogenesis Mechanisms" Plenum Press, New York, 1986, Vol. 39, 575.
7. C.H. Clarke and D.M. Shankel, Bacteriol. Rev.,1975, 39, 33.
8. P.E. Hartman "Chemical mutagens", 1982, Vol. 7, 211.
9. C.H.Clarke, D.M. Shankel, Mutat Res.,1988, 202, 19.
10. J.A. Prendergast, O.P. Kamra,A. T. Nasim, Mutat. Res., 1984, 125, 205.
11. P.E. Hartman, and D.M. Shankel, Environ. Mol. Mutag., 1990, 15, 145.
12. R. Cozzi, P. Perticone, R. Bona, and S. Polani, Environ. Mol. Mutag., 1991, 18, 207.
13. K. Yano, J. Agric. Food Chem, 1979, 27, 456.
14. A.D. Ayebo, I.A. Angelo and K.M. Shahani, Milchwissenschaft, 1980, 35, 730.
15. I. Bogdanov, P. Popkhristov, and L. Marinov, Abstract of VIII International Cancer Congress, Moscow, 1962, 364.
16. B.A. Friend, R.E. Farmer and K.M. Shahani, Milchwissenschaft, 1982, 37, 708.
17. B.R Goldin, L. Swenson, J. Dwyer and S.L. Gorbach, J. Natl. Cancer Inst., 1980, 64, 255.
18. B.R. Goldin, S.L. Gorbach. Cancer., 1977, 40, 2421.
19. B.R. Goldin and S.L. Gorbach, J. Natl. Cancer Inst., 1976, 57, 371.
20. F.K. Zimmermann, R. Kern and H. Rasemberger,Mutat. Res., 1975, 28, 381.
21. G. Bronzetti, A. Galli and C. Della Croce, "Antimutagenesis and Anticarcinogenesis Mechanisms", Plenum Press, New York, 1990, Vol 52, 463.
22. A. Galli, C. Della Croce, S. Minnucci, R. Fiorio and G. Bronzetti, Mutat. Res., 1992, 282, 55.
23. G. Bronzetti, A. Galli and C. Della Croce, Environ. Health Perspectives, 1992, (in press).

DOES THE TYPE OF FAT INFLUENCE INTESTINAL AND HEPATIC MICROSOMAL METABOLISM?

R. Chinery[1], R. A. Goodlad[1], N. A. Wright[1], J. T. Borlak[2*]

1 Imperial Cancer Research Fund, Histopathology Unit,
35-43 Lincoln's Inn Fields, London WC2A 3PN
2 Marion Merrell Dow Research Institute, Department of Clinical Biochemistry and Metabolism, 16 Rue d'Ankara, 67009 Strasbourg, France
* To whom correspondence should be sent

1 INTRODUCTION

Cytochrome P450 isoenzymes are located on the endoplasmic reticulum membranes of mammalian cells.[1] More than 71 P450 genes are known and some of their chromosomal locations have been reported.[2] These mono-oxygenases display discrete, but overlapping substrate specificities and exist in multiple forms. They require NADPH cytochrome P450 reductase for sequential electron transfer to heamoprotein pigments termed cytochrome P450. These cytochromes catalyse via redox-reactions the insertion of a single oxygen atom into endogenous and foreign compounds thereby rendering them more polar to facilitate their excretion. Specific cytochrome P450 isoenzymes are induceable by chemical agents commonly found in the environment, such as polychlorinated biphenyls, TCDD, etc.[3] In addition, there is strong evidence for a pivotal role of certain cytochrome P450s (i.e. CYP1A1, CYP2E1, see reference 2 for nomenclature) in the metabolic activation of procarcinogens.[4]

The distribution and regulation of drug metabolising enzymes in mammalian tissues is not uniform.[5] For instance, treatment of rats with phenobarbital resulted in the induction of CYP2B1 in liver and small intestine, but the expression of this protein was absent in the colon. For comparison, treatment with beta-naphthaflavone resulted in the concurrent induction of CYP4501A1 in colonic epithelium and hepatic tissue, as shown in Western blot experiments.[6] Although several authors reported the existence of a mono-oxygenase system in the colon,[7,8] it remains controversial to what extent colon tumourigenesis can be attributed to the biotransformation of procarcinogens by cytochrome P450 isoenzymes. Moreover, some epidemiological studies have shown a correlation between dietary fat and risk of cancer,[9] but it appears that only certain fatty acids promote tumourigenesis in animals when treated with chemical carcinogenesis.

Therefore, the objective of the present study was to assess cytochrome P450 catalysed reactions in groups of rats that received a diet either low or high in saturated or unsaturated fats. Microsomes of duodenum, proximal and distal ileum, and colon, as well as hepatic tissue were isolated and the metabolism of marker substrates was studied. The results should provide further information on the role of dietary fat in the regulation of P450 isoenzymes in liver and gut and to what extent types of fat may or may not modulate the expression of procarcinogen metabolising P450 isoenzymes.

2 METHODS

Materials. All chemicals were purchased from Sigma Chemical Company (St Louis, M.O., U.S.A.).

Animal diets. The animal diets were prepared by Special Diet Services (SDS) Limited, Wiltham, Essex. Four dietary regimes were prepared containing either 5% or 30% w/w lard and 5% or 30% sunflower margarine, respectively. The fatty acid composition of each fat type (SAT and UNSAT) respectively were: 16:0 24.85 *versus* 8.3; 18:0 11.52 *versus* 7.95; 18:1 45.2 *versus* 31.63; 18:2 10.3 *versus* 50.45; 18:3 0.6 *versus* 0.32; and 20:0 0.14 *versus* 0.41. dl-α-Tocopherol was added to all diets, producing a final concentration of 5.7 IU vitamin E/100g in the diet.

The diets were stored at 4°C in airtight containers to minimise lipid peroxidation. The digestible energy values (MJ/kg) of each diet was: 5%SAT 12.09; 5%UNSAT 11.93; 30% SAT 18.01; 30% UNSAT 17.03.

Animals and Treatment Groups. Male Wistar rats (220-240g) were bred at Clare Hall, South Mimms. After a period of acclimatisation, the rats were randomly divided into four dietary groups of 18 animals each. Animals were housed four to a cage with diets and water being given *ad libitum*. Each rat was examined daily and weighed twice weekly. There was no significant difference in body weight gain or dietary intake between groups.

Preparation of Subcellular Fractions and Assessment of Microsomal and Cytosolic Enzyme Activities. All animals were sacrificed by cervical dislocation. Liver microsomes were prepared, stored, and utilised as described.[10] Intestinal and colonic microsomes are prepared as above, with the following modifications. The entire small intestine and colon was removed and washed 2-3 times by forcing ice-cold sucrose (0.25M) through the lumen until the gastrointestinal tract was visibly free from excreta. The duodenum, proximal and distal ileum, and colon were dissected, and specimens were examined histologically using

Mayer's haematoxylin and eosin. Samples were pooled and each pool contained six animals. The resultant pools were homogenised in 3 volumes of ice-cold potassium phosphate buffer (0.1M, pH 7.4) containing sucrose (0.25M), 20% glycerol (v/v), trypsin inhibitor (5mg/ml), and heparin (5U/ml), and centrifuged as for the preparation of hepatic membranes. The microsomal fractions were resuspended in ice-cold buffer containing 0.25M sucrose, 20mM Tris buffer and 5mM EDTA (pH 7.4), and stored at -80°C until assayed.

Protein concentrations were determined using bovine serum albumin as standards.[11] Cytochrome b_5 and cytochrome c-(P450)-reductase were determined as previously described.[12] Cytochrome P450 was measured by the method of Omura and Sato.[13] Glutathione-S-transferase activity was assayed using 1-chloro-2,4-dinitro benzene as the substrate.[12]

The N-demethylation of aminopyrine was assayed by the methods of Cochin and Axelrod[14] and Nash.[15] Aniline hydroxylase was measured as detailed by Schenkman *et al.*[16] The metabolism of 7-ethoxyresorufin was measured fluorometrically using the method of Burke and Mayer.[17]

3 RESULTS

Microsomal cytochrome P450, cytochrome b_5 and P450 reductase: There was little evidence to suggest significant differences in hepatic cytochrome P450 and cytochrome b_5 concentrations amongst the various dietary regimes. Similar results were obtained when the activities of P450 reductase were assessed.
Comparable results were obtained with microsomes isolated from the duodenum, but microsomes isolated from the ileum and colon expressed higher NADPH-cytochrome-c-(P450) reductase activity, as well as cytochrome P450 and cytochrome b_5 in response to either a 5% or 30% UNSAT diet.

Enzyme activities of marker substrates for CYP1A1 and CYP1A2: Tables 1 to 5 summarise the results with EROD and aniline as substrates. It is well established that EROD is the preferred substrate for CYP1A1 whereas aniline is preferentially metabolised by CYP1A2. The data gives some support for higher hepatic EROD activities when a saturated fat diet (5% or 30%) was given, but, when the 4-hydroxylation of aniline was measured, this difference became marginal. With the exception of EROD activities determined for the duodenum and distal ileum (UNSAT in the diet) there was little evidence for a dose and fat related change in the expression of CYP1A1. Comparable results were obtained with aniline as substrates. It is noteworthy, that the 4-hydroxylation of aniline was measurable at highest rates with microsomes isolated from the colon.

Metabolism of aminopyrine, a marker substrate of phenobarbital inducible P450 isoenzymes. Tables 1 to 5 summarise the results with aminopyrine as the substrate. Hepatic microsomes of rats fed the UNSAT (5% or 30%) diets expressed marginally less aminopyrine-N-demethylase activity. Highest activities were found with microsomes isolated from the duodenum (30% SAT diet group), but there was no obvious trend in the metabolism of this substrate amongst the various treatment groups. For instance, a 30% SAT diet produced maximal rates of metabolism with microsomes isolated from the proximal small intestine, whereas a 5% UNSAT diet resulted in maximal activities with microsomes isolated from the distal ileum. Noticeably, no activity was found with microsomes isolated from the colon.

Activity of glutathione-S-transferase (GST) There was significant evidence for higher rates of hepatic GST activities in response to the 30% UNSAT diet. Similar results were obtained with cytosolic preparations of the proximal ileum, but there were no effects of diet in the distal ileum and the colon, when the various treatment groups were compared. GST activities in the duodenum were as high as those found in the hepatic samples (see tables 1 to 5).

4 DISCUSSION

The present study provides evidence for the metabolism of marker substrates by microsomes isolated from duodenum, proximal and distal ileum as well as the colon.

Evidence for CYP1A1 expression in the colon and small intestine was demonstrated in a recent report, employing Western immunoblotting techniques.[5] It was found that treatment of male rats with beta-naphthoflavone was essential to induce this protein. Comparable results were obtained, when the expression of CYP2B1 was assessed. However, phenobarbital treatment did not result in the expression of CYP2B1 in the colon, which contrasts with its expression in the small intestine. A similar result was obtained in the present study, as aminopyrine, was not metabolised by colonic microsomes. Therefore, the results of the present study and those reported by Rosenberg (1991) are in agreement.

A comparison of liver and gut enzyme activities (see tables 1-5) provides little evidence for diet consistently affecting the metabolism of EROD, aniline, aminopyrine and GST, but hepatic cytochrome P450 and b_5 concentrations were significantly higher, when compared with the various gut sections. It is also evident that the diets used in this study did not greatly alter the

Table 1. Hepatic P450 components and microsomal metabolism of marker substrates.

	5%SAT	5%UNSAT	30%SAT	30%UNSAT
Cytochrome P450[a]	0.89±0.12	0.95±0.11	0.92±0.03	0.63±0.10
Cytochrome b_5[a]	0.42±0.06	0.41±0.03	0.38±0.01	0.30±0.05
P450 reductase[b]	30.50±3.95	29.26±1.29	32.39±2.95	38.66±4.48
EROD[c]	91.57±7.49	63.70±11.30	85.14±7.52	66.49±7.34
Aniline-4-hydroxylase[b]	0.07±0.00	0.06±0.00	0.09±0.00	0.06±0.00
Aminopyrine-N-demethylase[b]	10.74±0.77	8.24±0.60	11.31±1.10	7.58±1.13
Glutathione-S-transferase[b]	19.27±2.10	23.66±1.77	32.65±2.06	22.19±1.12

Values are mean ± SEM, n=5. EROD: Ethoxyresorufin-O-deethylase; SAT: saturated fat; UNSAT: unsaturated fat; [a]: nmol/mg protein; [b]: nmol/min/mg protein; [c]: pmol/min/mg protein.

Table 2. Components of the P450 mono-oxygenases and microsomal metabolism of marker substrates in the duodenum.

	5%SAT	**5%UNSAT**	**30%SAT**	**30%UNSAT**
Cytochrome P450[a]	43.97±6.95 1088.7±91.7	40.50±10.00 1134.0±109.0	62.80±14.10 611.0±113.0	36.85±9.25 424.6±77.90
Cytochrome b_5[a]	27.43±5.78 665.0±74.5	40.00±1.00 869.2±36.9	35.67±3.18 361.1±49.5	36.85±8.25 424.6±67.0
P450 reductase[b]	13.20±0.29 292.30±32.60	12.19±1.15 243.30±23.00	14.31±2.08 142.30±15.80	14.62±0.33 170.50±7.50
EROD[c]	58.50±2.80 856.40±70.49	31.60±2.38 752.40±5.34	53.20±3.00 504.70±12.2	35.28±7.05 682.23±31.89
Aniline-4-hydroxylase[b]	0.03±0.01 0.77±0.01	0.04±0.04 0.90±0.02	0.05±0.01 0.50±0.01	0.05±0.00 0.58±0.01
Aminopyrine-N-demethylase[b]	4.80±0.16 86.80±2.67	7.27±1.29 101.10±2.61	9.57±0.24 91.10±4.67	7.94±1.98 92.10±1.37
Glutathione-S-transferase[b]	42.91±3.88	41.70±2.38	40.56±2.71	43.10±15.8

Values are expressed as mean ± SEM, n=6 animals per pool. [a]: pmol/mg protein; [b]: nmol/min/mg protein(upper) or g tissue (lower); [c]: pmol/min/mg protein (upper) or g tissue (lower).

Table 3. Components of the P450 mono-oxygenases and microsomal metabolism of marker substrates in the proximal ileum.

	5%SAT	5%UNSAT	30%SAT	30%UNSAT
Cytochrome P450[a]	11.97±1.53 246.3±1.9	10.90±1.04 106.3±9.5	11.17±0.37 87.4±3.7	28.50±1.00 229.5±9.5
Cytochrome b_5[a]	19.15±2.45 394.1±3.1	17.44±1.65 170.0±15.2	17.83±0.59 139.9±5.91	22.80±0.80 183.6±7.6
P450 reductase[b]	12.89±1.14 270.30±28.30	14.18±1.81 138.70±19.20	13.26±0.61 99.33±4.41	17.97±0.34 147.00±1.00
EROD[c]	43.85±4.55 377.00±28.10	36.96±3.77 357.80±13.30	48.15±3.69 375.80±23.00	48.30±19.30 554.21±6.64
Aniline-4-hydroxylase[b]	0.03±0.00 0.53±0.01	0.04±0.00 0.42±0.01	0.05±0.00 0.35±0.00	0.03±0.01 0.39±0.00
Aminopyrine-N-demethylase[b]	5.62±0.16 119.27±14.50	Not determined	7.22±0.28 56.39±0.14	5.32±0.68 43.09±5.51
Glutathione-S-transferase[b]	16.88±1.62	22.95±0.49	16.93±1.58	26.46±5.15

Values are expressed as mean ± SEM, n=6 animals per pool.
[a]: pmol/mg protein; [b]: nmol/min/mg protein(upper) or g tissue (lower); [c]: pmol/min/mg protein (upper) or g tissue (lower).

Table 4. Components of the P450 mono-oxygenases and microsomal metabolism of marker substrates in the distal ileum.

	5%SAT	5%UNSAT	30%SAT	30%UNSAT
Cytochrome P450[a]	32.60±25.40 452.0±13.52	98.70±15.10 1029.0±58.90	78.67±9.40 1040.7±39.9	15.30±0.60 166.45±6.00
Cytochrome b_5[a]	6.87±0.64 77.40±1.40	8.49±1.05 89.00±8.08	12.11±2.40 159.30±20.50	13.20±6.00 143.50±16.00
P450 reductase[b]	5.51±1.13 75.33±7.84	12.48±0.40 115.67±1.16	3.06±0.29 43.67±3.18	12.44±1.16 136.30±20.10
EROD[c]	56.50±10.40 473.82±7.56	26.71±1.04 497.42±9.90	85.50±10.90 744.95±42.60	34.58±6.40 929.63±9.38
Aniline-4-hydroxylase[b]	0.04±0.01 0.49±0.02	0.04±0.01 0.43±0.01	0.04±0.01 0.56±0.02	0.05±0.00 0.51±0.01
Aminopyrine-N-demethylase[b]	4.45±0.92 61.10±4.16	7.48±0.02 69.65±0.10	6.82±0.18 93.26±13.46	5.90±0.35 64.15±0.25
Glutathione-S-transferase[b]	10.45±0.94	11.14±1.11	12.54±2.69	9.29±1.61

Values are expressed as mean ± SEM, n=6 animals per pool.
[a]: pmol/mg protein; [b]: nmol/min/mg protein(upper) or g tissue (lower); [c]: pmol/min/mg protein (upper) or g tissue (lower).

Table 5. Components of the P450 mono-oxygenases and microsomal metabolism of marker substrates in the colon.

	5%SAT	5%UNSAT	30%SAT	30%UNSAT
Cytochrome P450[a]	9.40±0.85 99.27±0.78	14.00±0.20 54.67±0.72	15.10±0.50 90.60±3.00	9.85±1.05 78.70±8.70
Cytochrome b_5[a]	5.09±0.64 51.47±5.49	7.93±1.97 30.90±7.81	32.00±24.00 48.00±2.08	44.00±4.00 35.20±3.20
P450 reductase[b]	6.24±0.60 66.00±1.00	11.81±0.31 46.00±1.15	5.39±0.28 32.33±1.67	8.86±0.80 70.70±6.30
EROD[c]	25.18±1.93 269.10±20.60	35.22±2.79 281.76±10.90	30.53±1.15 183.43±7.09	25.14±0.45 201.11±3.62
Aniline-4-hydroxylase[b]	0.05±0.01 0.49±0.03	0.13±0.00 0.49±0.01	0.09±0.00 0.56±0.00	0.09±0.00 0.72±0.00
Aminopyrine-N-demethylase[b]	Not detectable	Not detectable	Not detectable	Not detectable
Glutathione-S-transferase[b]	12.85±0.61	15.49±0.37	14.41±0.23	15.74±0.48

Values are expressed as mean ± SEM, n=6 animals per pool.
[a]: pmol/mg protein; [b]: nmol/min/mg protein(upper) or g tissue (lower); [c]: pmol/min/mg protein (upper) or g tissue (lower).

concentrations of cytochrome P450 and cytochrome b_5 and enzyme activities attributable to cytochrome P450 isoenzymes. Consequently, there was little experimental evidence to suggest an altered expression of intestinal mono-oxygenases in response to the dietary fats used in this study.

Currently, we are investigating the tissue distribution of cytochrome P450 isoenzymes in Western blot and Northern blot experiments to obtain unambiguous information on the expression of these enzymes at the protein and mRNA level. In the future, we would also like to assess the tumour promoting abilities of certain fatty acids in animals previously treated with a chemical carcinogen to investigate the relationship between the metabolism by intestinal mono-oxygenases, its modulation by dietary fats and the occurrence of malignant tumour growth.

5 REFERENCES

1. E. Hodgson, Drug. Metab. Rev., 1979, 10, 15.
2. D.W. Nebert, D.R. Nelson, M. Adesnik, M.J. Coon, R.W. Estabrook, F.J. Gonzalez, F.P. Guengerich, I.C. Gunsalus, E.F. Johnson, B. Kemper, W. Levin, I.R. Phillips, R. Sato, M.R. Waterman, DNA, 1989, 8, 1.
3. S. Safe, CRC Crit. Rev. Toxicol., 1984, 13, 319.
4. A.H. Conney, Cancer. Res., 1982. 42, 4875.
5. F.J. Gonzalez, Pharmacol. Rev., 1989, 40, 243.
6. D.W. Rosenberg, Arch. Biochem. Biophys., 1991,284, 223.
7. W.F. Fang, H.W. Strobel, Arch. Biochem. Biophys., 1987, 186, 178.
8. R.J. Oshinsky, H.W. Strobel, Mol. Cell. Biochem., 1987, 19, 575.
9. P. Howert, G. Glover, 'Fatty acids in Foods and their Health Implications' Marcel Dekker Inc., New York, USA, 1992.
10. J.T. Borlakoglu, J.D. Edwards-Webb, R.R. Dils, J. Biochem., 1990, 188, 327.
11. O.H. Lowry, N.Y. Rosebrough, A.L. Farr, R.T. Randall, J. Biol. Chem. 1951, 193, 265.
12. G.G. Gibson, P. Skeet, 'Introduction to Drug Metabolism', Chapman and Hall Ltd., London, 1986.
13. R.A. Omura, R. Sato, J. Biol. Chem., 1964, 239, 2370.
14. J. Cochin, J. Axelrod, J. Pharmacol. Exp. Therap., 1959, 125, 105.
15. N.G. Nash, J. Biol. Chem., 1953, 55, 416.
16. J.B. Schenkman, H. Remmer, R.W. Estabrook, Mol. Pharmacol., 1967, 3, 113.
17. M.D. Burke et al., Biochem. Pharmacol., 1985, 34, 3337.

CHEMICAL AND BIOCHEMICAL BASIS FOR BENEFICIAL EFFECTS OF SULFHYDRYL COMPOUNDS ON FOOD SAFETY

Mendel Friedman

Food Safety Research Unit
U.S. Department of Agriculture, Agricultural Research Service
Western Regional Research Center
800 Buchanan Street, Albany, CA 94710 USA

INTRODUCTION

Most naturally occurring food toxicants and many antinutritional compounds possess specific sites that are responsible for their deleterious effects. Therefore, it should be possible to lessen the toxic potential by modifying these sites with site-specific reagents, such as SH-containing amino acids, peptides, and proteins, in a manner that will alter structural integrity and thus preventing them from interacting with receptor sites *in vivo*. The chemical reactivities of negatively charged sulfur anions (RS^-) are much greater than would be expected from their basicities. This greater reactivity presumably results from (a) polarizabilities of outer shell sulfur electrons; and (b) the availability of d-orbitals in the electronic structure of sulfur, permitting d-orbital overlap during the formation of transition states. A related possibility is that sulfur can act as a free-radical trap, whereby free electrons of highly reactive oxygen radicals are transferred or dissipated to the sulfur atoms.[1] I will briefly review some of our approaches to reducing deleterious effects of representative food toxicants, based on the reactivity of the sulfhydryl group with electrophilic centers. These include (a) the double bond of dehydroalanine to prevent lysinoalanine formation; (b) the double bond of furan rings of aflatoxins to suppress mutagenicity; and (c) disulfide bonds of plant protease inhibitors to reduce potential carcinogenicity.

Lysinoalanine (LAL)

Alkali-treated food proteins and synthetic LAL, when fed to rats, induce cytotoxic changes in kidney cells. These changes are characterized by enlargement of the nucleus and cytoplasm, increase in nucleoprotein, and disturbances in DNA synthesis and mitosis. These observations suggest disruption of normal regulatory functions in the *pars recta* cells of the kidneys.[2,3]

Based on a mathematical analysis of the observed equilibria between various functional groups of LAL and metal ions, we hypothesize that LAL exerts its biological effects through chelation to copper and possibly also cobalt in metallothioneins of kidney cells.[4,5]

A postulated mechanism of LAL formation and inhibition by thiols is shown in Figure 1.[6-14] LAL formation can also be reduced by acetylating ϵ-NH_2 groups of lysine before exposing the protein to high pH. However, this decrease in LAL is accompanied by an increase in dehydroalanine residues (Table 1). Since dehydroalanine in dehydroproteins can act as an alkylating agent *in vitro*, a need exists to establish whether it can act as a biological alkylating agent *in vivo*. The role of LAL in metal ion metabolism also merits study.

Table 1 Dehydroalanine content of alkali-treated caseins.[6,14]

PROTEIN	DEHYDROALANINE (g/16 g N)
Casein, untreated	0.00
Casein + alkali	0.33
Acetylated casein, untreated	0.00
Acetylated casein + alkali	1.39

Aflatoxin B_1 (AFB_1)

AFB_1 is a pre-carcinogen that is transformed *in vivo* to an active epoxide which can induce liver cancer by forming DNA-adducts. Prior treatment with a site-specific reagent should modify AFB_1 in a manner that will prevent formation of the epoxide and suppress its mutagenic and carcinogenic activity (Figure 2).[15,16]

A comparison of inactivation of AFB_1 by eleven different thiols showed that several of them effectively suppressed the mutagenicity of AFB_1.

HPLC studies showed that the disappearance of AFB_1 in the presence of N-acetylcysteine was accompanied by the appearance of a single new peak on the chromatogram (Figure 3).

Our observations that many structurally different thiols can suppress the mutagenic activity of AFB_1 suggests that thiols may be useful for inactivating aflatoxins in contaminated foods, as an antidote to treat aflatoxin toxicity, or for prophylaxis to prevent aflatoxin poisoning. In a relevant study, De Flora et al. demonstrated that N-acetylcysteine can prevent urethane-induced lung tumors in mice.[17] Similar studies need to be carried out to find out whether thiols can prevent AFB_1-induced liver cancer.

Soybean Inhibitors of Digestive Enzymes

Feeding rats raw soybeans or pure soybean inhibitors of digestive enzymes, the so-called Kunitz inhibitor of trypsin and the Bowman-Birk inhibitor of trypsin and chymotrypsin, induces hypertrophy, hyperplasia, and hypersecretion of trypsin and chymotrypsin by the pancreas. Raw soy flour diets also potentiate pancreatic carcinogenicity of azaserine and nitrosamines in rats. A so-called biofeedback mechanism has been postulated to explain these consequences of soybean nutrition.[18]

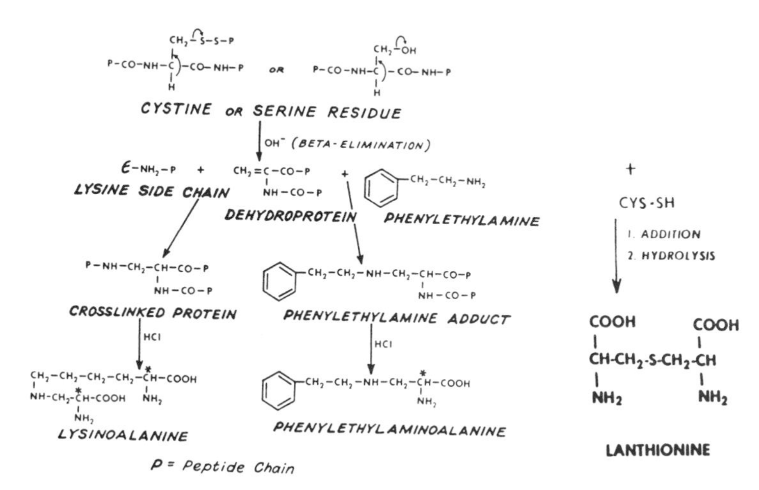

Figure 1 Formation of novel amino acids. Because SH groups react faster with the dehydroprotein than NH_2 groups, thiols suppress LAL formation.

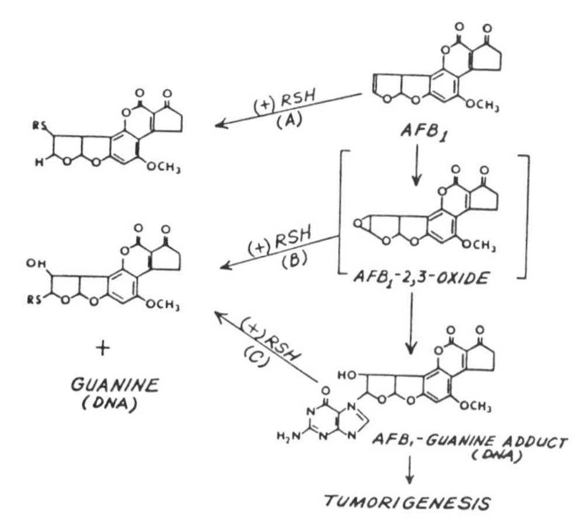

Figure 2 Some possible aflatoxin-thiol interactions: (A) Formation of an inactive thiol adduct; (B) Reaction with epoxide to prevent DNA alkylation; (C) Displacement of aflatoxin-DNA adduct (guanine) adduct blocking tumorigenesis

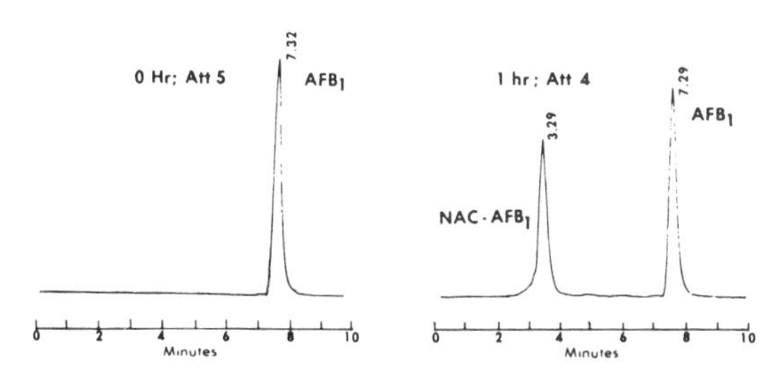

Figure 3 HPLC of AFB_1 and its N-acetylcysteine derivative (NAC-AFB_1)

These considerations suggest a need to find ways to inactivate the inhibitors before soybeans are consumed. Although heat is often used to inactivate inhibitors, such inactivation is often incomplete. The use of high temperature to destroy inhibitors may also destroy lysine and sulfur amino acids and thus damage protein nutritional quality.[19] A key question is whether residual protease inhibitors in heat-treated soybeans endanger human health.[20]

Most inhibitors of trypsin and other proteolytic enzymes contain disulfide bonds, some or all of which are needed to maintain active conformations. In fact, amino acid sequence studies show that the reactive peptide link responsible for the enzyme-inhibiting activity is a cyclic substrate in a loop closed by a disulfide bridge. Since thiols are expected to interact with inhibitor disulfide bonds via sulfhydryl-disulfide interchange and oxidation-reduction reactions, illustrated below, we carried out systematic studies on the abilities of cysteine, N-acetylcysteine, reduced glutathione, and sodium sulfite to synergize heat-inactivation of soybean inhibitors.

Sulfhydryl-disulfide interchange and oxidation pathways. Net effects: network of new disulfide bonds and altered protein configuration

$$\text{R-SH} + \text{In-S-S-In} \rightleftharpoons \text{R-S-S-In} + \text{HS-In}$$
$$\text{R-SH} + \text{Pr-S-S-Pr} \rightleftharpoons \text{R-S-S-Pr} + \text{HS-Pr}$$
$$\text{In-SH} + \text{Pr-S-S-Pr} \rightleftharpoons \text{In-S-S-Pr} + \text{HS-Pr}$$
$$\text{In-SH} + \text{HS-Pr} + \tfrac{1}{2}\,0_2 \longrightarrow \text{In-S-S-Pr} + \text{H}_2\text{0}$$
$$\text{In-SH} + \text{HS-In} + \tfrac{1}{2}\,0_2 \longrightarrow \text{In-S-S-In} + \text{H}_2\text{0}$$

R-SH: Added thiol (Cysteine, N-acetyl-L-cysteine, etc.)
In-S-S-In: Inhibitor (In) disulfide bonds.
Pr-S-S-Pr: Protein (Pr) disulfide bonds.

Our results show that this approach makes it possible to lower the inhibitor content of soybean flour to near zero levels.[21-24] The accompanying improvement in the nutritional quality and safety may result from inactivation of inhibitors and the introduction of new disulfide bonds. This approach should generally be useful for inactivating related disulfide-containing toxic plant proteins such as lectins and ricin, widely distributed in legumes and castor beans, respectively, as well as neurotoxic proteins derived from *Salmonella* and other microorganisms.[56] Efforts to use plant engineering to control the inhibitor content of soybeans[26,27] and the glycoalkaloid content of potatoes[28] should also benefit food safety.

In summary, antioxidant and antitoxic effects of SH-containing amino acids, peptides, and proteins are due to their abilities to act as reducing agents, scavengers of oxygen radicals, strong nucleophiles that can trap electrophilic compounds, precursors of cellular glutathione, and inducers of cellular detoxification.[1,17,30] Future studies should also exploit the practical potential of SH-containing compounds to reduce adverse effects of food processing.[19,30] In general, better understanding of the molecular mechanisms underlying actions of potentially toxic and health-promoting food ingredients should facilitate the development of better and safer diets.

REFERENCES

1. M. Friedman, 'The Chemistry and Biochemistry of the Sulfhydryl Group in Amino Acids, Peptides, and Proteins', Pergamon, Oxford, 1973.
2. J.C. Woodard, 'Protein Nutritional Quality of Foods and Feeds', Marcel Dekker, New York, 1975, p. 595.
3. D.H. Gould and J.T. MacGregor, Adv. Exp. Med. Biol., 1977, 86A, 29.
4. K.N. Pearce and M. Friedman, J. Agric. Food Chem., 1988, 36, 707.
5. M. Friedman and K.N. Pierce, J. Agric. Food Chem., 1989, 37, 123.
6. M. Friedman, M.R. Gumbmann and P.M. Masters, Adv. Exp. Med. Biol., 1984, 177, 367.
7. M. Friedman, ACS Symposium Series, 1982, 206, 231.
8. M. Friedman, J.F. Cavins and J.S. Wall, J. Amer. Chem. Soc., 1965, 87, 3572.
9. J.W. Finley, J.T. Snow, P.H. Johnston and M. Friedman, J. Food Sci., 1978, 43, 619.
10. J.T. Snow, J.W. Finley and M. Friedman, Int. J. Peptide Protein Res., 1976, 7, 461.
11. M. Friedman, C.E. Levin and A.T. Noma, J. Food Sci., 1984, 49, 1282.
12. M. Friedman and A.T. Noma, J. Agric. Food Chem., 1986, 34, 497.
13. R. Liardon, M. Friedman and G. Philippossian, J. Agric. Food Chem., 1991, 39, 531.
14. M.S. Masri and M. Friedman, Biochem. Biophys. Res. Commun., 1982, 104, 321.
15. M. Friedman, C.M. Wehr, J.E. Schade and J.T. MacGregor, Food and Chem. Toxicol., 1982, 20, 887.
16. M. Friedman, Adv. Exp. Med. Biol., 1984, 177, 31.
17. S. De Flora, C. Benicelli, D. Serra, A. Izzotti and C.F. Cesarone, 'Absorption and Utilization of Amino Acids', CRC Press, Boca Raton, FL, 1989, Vol. 3, p. 19.
18. M. Friedman (Editor), 'Nutritional and Toxicological Aspects of Enzyme Inhibitors in Foods', Plenum, New York, 1986.
19. M. Friedman, Annual Review Nutrition , 1992, 12, 119.
20. J. Hathcock, 'Nutritional and Toxicological Consequences of Food Processing', Plenum, New York, 1991, p. 273.
21. M.R. Gumbmann and M. Friedman, J. Nutr. , 1987, 117, 1018.
22. M. Friedman, O.K. Grosjean and J.C. Zahnley, J. Sci. Food Agric., 1982, 33, 165.
23. M. Friedman, M.R. Gumbmann and O.K. Grosjean, J. Nutr. , 1984, 114, 2241.
24. M. Friedman and M.R. Gumbmann, J. Food Sci., 1986, 51, 1239.
25. J.N. Wallace and M. Friedman, Nutr. Rept. Intl., 1985, 32, 748.
26. M. Friedman, D.L. Brandon, A.H. Bates and T. Hymowitz, J. Agric. Food Chem., 1991, 39, 327.
27. J.M. Damagalski, K.P. Kollipara, A.H. Bates, D.L. Brandon, M. Friedman and T. Hymowitz, Crop Sci., 1992, in press.
28. M. Friedman, ACS Symposium Series, 1992, 484, 419.
29. T.K. Smith, Adv. Exp. Med. Biol., 1991, 289, 165.
30. M. Friedman and I. Molnar-Perl, J. Agric. Food Chem., 1990, 38, 1642.

DETERMINATION OF POTENTIALLY ANTICARCINOGENIC FLAVONOIDS IN FOODS AND PRELIMINARY RESULTS ON DAILY INTAKE IN THE NETHERLANDS

M.G.L. Hertog[#]; P.C.H. Hollman[#]; D. Kromhout[*]

[#]DLO-State Institute for Quality Control of Agricultural Products (RIKILT-DLO), Bornsesteeg 45, NL-6708 PD Wageningen, the Netherlands

[*]Department of Epidemiology, National Institute of Public Health and Environmental Protection, Antonie van Leewenhoeklaan 9, NL-3720 MA Bilthoven, the Netherlands

INTRODUCTION

Flavonoids share the common skeleton of diphenylpropanes (C6-C3-C6) (Figure 1) and they occur ubiquitously in plant foods. Average intake of all flavonoids is estimated to be 1 gram/day, of which approximately 160 mg are 4-oxoflavonoids, including flavonols, flavones and flavanones[1]. Flavonoids usually occur in foods as *O*-glycosides with sugars bound to C3. Although flavonoids are generally considered to be non-nutritive agents, interest in flavonoids has arisen because of their potential role in the prevention of cancer. Quercetin and other related flavonoids inhibited carcinogen-induced tumors in rats and in mice[9-12]. Although the mechanism of action is still unclear it is suggested that flavonoids enhance the deactivation of potential carcinogens[13]. Flavonoids are also potent antioxidants and scavengers of free radicals which are possibly involved in cell damage and subsequently tumour development [14-15]. Quercetin was also found to be mutagenic[2-4] and at a level of 2 % in the diet to induce bladder tumours in rats[5]. However, these results could not be confirmed in other animal studies using quercetin levels of up to 10 % of the diet[6-8]. An epidemiological evaluation of flavonoids has not been carried out because reliable quantitative data on the occurrence of flavonoids in foods is lacking. We have therefore developed and validated a Reversed Phase High Performance Liquid Chromatographic (RP-HPLC) method for the determination of the five anticarcinogenic flavonoids quercetin, myricetin, kaempferol, apigenin and luteolin in foods. We then measured the flavonoid content of commonly consumed foods of vegetable origin. We also report some preliminary results on the flavonoid intake and distribution of 5898 subjects in the Netherlands using data of the National Food Consumption Survey 1987-88[16].

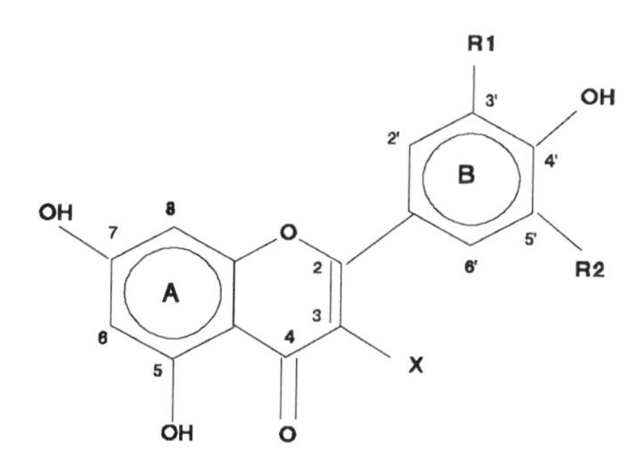

Figure 1. Structure of flavonoids. *Flavonols*: X=OH; Quercetin: R1=OH, R2=H; Kaempferol: R1=H,, R2=H; Myricetin: R1=OH, R2=OH. *Flavones*: X=H; Apigenin: R1=H, R2=H; Luteolin: R1=OH, R2=H

MATERIALS AND METHODS

Method of analysis

A method based on RP-HPLC with UV detection was developed for the quantitative determination of five major flavonoid aglycones viz. quercetin, kaempferol, myricetin, luteolin and apigenin in various vegetables, fruits and beverages, after acid hydrolysis of the parent glycosides. This method was described in detail elsewhere[17]. Briefly, completeness of hydrolysis and extraction were optimized by testing systematically different conditions such as acid concentration, reaction period and methanol concentration in the extraction solution using foods containing various types of flavonoid glycosides. The foods used were lettuce and endive containing flavonol glucuronides, onion, leek and cranberries containing flavonol glucosides and celery containing flavone glucosides. Quantification was carried out by co-chromatography of the pure standards. Identity and peak purity of the flavonoids was confirmed by comparing spectra of the flavonoids in the foods with the spectra of pure standards provided by diode array on-line.

Food analysis

The flavonoid content of 28 vegetables, 12 fruits and 8 beverages commonly consumed in the Netherlands was determined with the method described above. Sampling procedure, analysis and quality control was described in detail before[18]. Briefly, sampling of the foods was carried out in three seasons, spring, summer and winter. Fresh foods were purchased in a supermarket, grocery and street market and subsequently combined to a composite in proportions reflecting the sales. Processed foods were purchased in a supermarket. Three major brands were mixed in equal portions (net weight) to a composite. In addition, six different types of tea (prepared according to Dutch customs), five wines and four fruit juices were analysed. Optimum hydrolysis conditions in foods containing an unknown type of flavonoid glycoside were determined in a three step optimization procedure as described before. Analytical quality control was performe by including control samples with a known amount of flavonoids in every series of analysis during the analysi period. All determinations were carried out in duplicate.

RESULTS AND DISCUSSION

Optimum extraction and hydrolysis conditions were as follows: flavonol glucosides (quercetin, kaempferol, and myricetin) were extracted and hydrolysed during two hours in 50 % aqueous methanol with 1.2 M HCl; flavonol glucuronides (quercetin and kaempferol) were extracted an hydrolysed during two hours in 50 % aqueous methanol with 2.0 M HCl. Flavone glycosides (luteolin and apigenin) wer extracted and hydrolysed during four hours in 50 % aqueou methanol with 2.0 M HCl. Repeatability of the method was good with coefficients of variation ranging from 2.5-3.1 for quercetin, 4.6-5.6 % for kaempferol, 4.6 % for myricetin, 3.3 % for luteolin and 2.8 % for apigenin. CV of the within-laboratory reproducibility was less than tw times the CV of repeatability. Recoveries of the flavonol quercetin, kaempferol and myricetin ranged from 77-110 % and recoveries of the flavones apigenin and luteolin ranged from 99-106 %. A typical HPLC chromatogram of a vegetable extract after hydrolysis is shown in Figure 2.

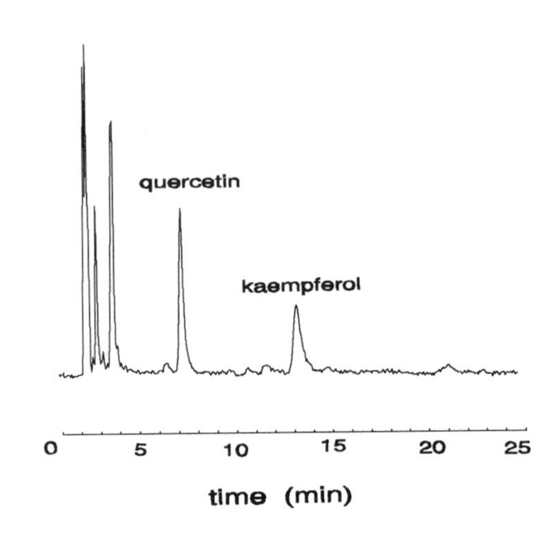

Figure 2. Typical RP-HPLC chromatogram of french bean extract monitored in acetonitrile/phosphatebuffer (25/75, v/v, pH 2.4) (detection: 370 nm).

Table 1 reports the flavonoid content of some selected vegetables, fruits and beverages. The major flavonoid that we found in foods was quercetin followed by kaempferol. Luteolin and apigenin were only found in celery whereas myricetin was found in broad beans, grapes, wine and tea (not shown). The quercetin content of onions (347 mg/kg) and the kaempferol content of kale (211 mg/kg, not shown) was approximately five to ten fold higher than in other vegetables. No flavonoids were found in most brassicas, in mushrooms, chicory, cucumber and in carrots. Most fruits contained only quercetin in levels varying between 6-36 mg/kg. Black tea contained 17-22 mg/L quercetin, 7-16 mg/L kaempferol and 1-4 mg/L myricetin.

Table 1. Mean flavonoid content ± SD (mg/kg fresh weight) of selected vegetables, fruits and beverages.

Food	Quercetin	Kaempferol	Myricetin
Lettuce	14 ± 14	<2	<1
Onion	347 ± 63	<2	<1
Endive	<1	46 ± 42	<1
Broad beans	20	<2	25
Apple¶	36 ± 19	<2	<1
Strawberry	8.6	12	<1
Wine (red)¶✲	11 ± 5	<1	9 ± 3
Apple Juice¶✲	2.8	<1	<0.5

<0.5,<1,<2 below limit of detection
¶ mean ± SD of five varieties
✲ mg/L

A preliminary estimation of the mean flavonoid intake of 5898 subjects in the Netherlands showed that it was almost 20 mg/day. Quercetin contributed to approximately 75 % of the total flavonoid intake, followed by kaempferol which contributed to approximately 16 %. Flavonoid intake was not normally distributed but strongly right-skewed[18].

We conclude that potentially anticarcinogenic flavonoids, especially quercetin, occur in various commonly consumed foods in the Netherlands. They are therefore a common component of the Dutch diet. The quantitative determination of quercetin, kaempferol, myricetin, apigenin and luteolin in various foods makes an accurate estimation of the individual intake of these flavonoids possible. Our data thus provide a base for epidemiological studies investigating the relation between flavonoid intake and cancer risk.

REFERENCES

1. J. Kuhnau. World Rev Nutr Diet 1976, 24, 117
2. L.F. Bjeldanes and G.W. Chang. Science (Washington, D.C.) 1977, 197, 577
3. J.T. MacGregor. Adv Exp Med Biol 1984, 177, 497
4. B. Stavric. Fed Proc 1984, 43(9), 2454
5. A.M. Pamucku; S. Yalçiner.; J.F. Hatcher; G.T. Bryan. Cancer Res 1980, 40, 3468
6. D. Saito; A. Shirai; T. Matsushima; T. Sugimura; I. Hirono. Teratog Carcinog Mutagen 1980, 1, 213
7. I. Hirono; I. Ueno; S. Hosaka; H. Takanashi; T. Matsushima; T. Sugimura; S. Natori. Cancer Lett 1981, 13, 15
8. K. Morino; N. Matsukura; H. Ohgaki; T. Kawachi; T. Sugimura; I. Hirono. Carcinogenesis 1982, 3, 93
9. R. Kato; T. Nakadate; S. Yamamoto; T. Sugimura. Carcinogenesis 1983, 4, 1301
10. H. Mukhtar; M. Das; W.A. Khan; Z.Y. Wang; D.P. Bik; D.R. Bickers. Cancer Res 1988, 48, 2361
11. A.K. Verma; J.A. Johnson; M.N. Gould; M.A. Tanner. Cancer Res 1988, 48, 5754
12. E.E. Deschner; J. Ruperto; G. Wong; H.L. Newmark. Carcinogenesis 1991, 7, 1193
13. L.W. Wattenberg. Cancer Res 1985, 45, 1
14. W. Bors and M. Saran. Free Rad Res Comms, 1987, 2, 189
15. M. Namiki. Cri Rev Food Sci Nutr 1990, 29, 273
16. K. Hulshof and W.A. Van Staveren. Food Policy 1991, 16, 257
17. M.G.L. Hertog; P.C.H. Hollman; D.P. Venema. J Agric Food Chem, in press.
18. M.G.L. Hertog; P.C.H. Hollman; M.B. Katan. J Agric Food Chem, in press.
19. M.G.L. Hertog; P.C.H. Hollman; M.B. Katan; D. Kromhout (submitted)

THE CONTENT OF THE POTENTIALLY ANTICARCINOGENIC ELLAGIC ACID IN PLANT FOODS

Peter C.H.Hollman, Dini P.Venema
DLO-State Institute for Quality Control of Agricultural Products (RIKILT-DLO), Bornsesteeg 45, NL 6708 PD Wageningen, The Netherlands

1 INTRODUCTION

A number of reports on the antimutagenic and anticarcinogenic properties of ellagic acid in experimental studies have been published[1,2]. The following mechanisms for the inhibition of cancer by ellagic acid have been proposed: inhibition of the metabolic activation of carcinogens, detoxification by stimulation of glutathione s-transferase activity, binding to reactive metabolic forms of the carcinogen, and protection of DNA. Hexahydroxydiphenic acid is very widely distributed in ester form with glucose, called ellagitannins, in flowering plant species. After acid hydrolysis its dilactone ellagic acid is formed[3]. Ellagic acid may also occur in free form[4]. Dietary sources of ellagic acid are fruits of Fragaria and Rubus species, and nuts of Juglans and Caryna species[4,5].

In order to estimate the dietary intake of ellagic acid in the Netherlands, a quantitative HPLC method was developed and applied in the determination of ellagic acid in fruits and nuts.

2 MATERIALS AND METHODS

Sample preparation

All products were purchased at local supermarkets. Fruits were blended in a Waring Blendor within 8 hours and were kept at -18 °C until analysis. Nuts were defatted before analysis with petroleum ether (40-60 °C) by means of Soxhlet extraction

Extraction and hydrolysis

For the combined extraction/hydrolysis, extracts were prepared as follows: To 2 g fruit 25 ml methanol and 10 ml HCl 37% were added (the extraction medium thus contained 3.5 M HCl and 72% methanol). The mixture was refluxed under nitrogen atmosphere for 4 hours at 90 °C. Raspberries were hydrolysed for 6 hours and nuts for 2 hours. After cooling to room temperature samples were made up to 100 ml with methanol, sonicated for 5 minutes and filtered through a 0.45 μm filter.

For the determination of free ellagic acid, extracts were made as follows: 10 g sample and 25 ml methanol were extracted for 30 seconds in a Waring Blendor. After decantation the residue was extracted a second time with 25 ml methanol. Residue and extracts were combined and made up to 100 ml with methanol, sonicated for 5 minutes and filtered through a 0.45 μm filter.

HPLC

10 μl of the extracts or hydrolysates were injected with a autoinjector and were separated at 30 °C on a Novapak C18 column 3.9 x 150 mm, 4 μm, with a Perisorb C18 precolumn, 2 x 75 mm. The mobile phase consisted of methanol/0.025 M KH_2PO_4 pH 2.4 = 40/60, the flow rate was 0.9 ml/min and UV absorption was monitored at 254 nm, 0.1 AUFS For fluorescence detection 0.05 M $Na_2B_4O_7$ was added with a flow of 0.6 ml/min to the mobile phase (post column). Mixing took place in a mixing coil (0.25 x 400 mm), pH in detectorcell was 8.8. Excitation wavelength was 365 nm and the emission wavelength 470 nm, sensitivity 0.5. Integration was performed with a Nelson integrator system. Peak identity and purity was confirmed using a photodiode-array detector.

3 RESULTS

Optimization of the HPLC method

Column choice. Different types of C18 columns and eluents (with modifiers like methanol, acetonitril, tetrahydrofuran and acidifiers like acetic acid, formic acid, KH_2PO_4/H_3PO_4, $NH_4H_2PO_4/H_3PO_4$) were tested but with UV-detection no satisfactory separation of ellagic acid from interfering peaks could be achieved (Fig.1).In addition, excessive peak tailing was observed. The Novapak C18 column proved to be the best compromise. Methanol concentration had to be more than 40 % because otherwise much lower plate counts and severe tailing of the ellagic acid peak occurred, probably due to the poor solubility of ellagic acid in water.

Fluorescence detection. Because attempts to improve the chromatographic separation failed, a different detection principle was chosen. Ellagic acid hardly shows native fluorescence. However, Wolfbeis[7] described the formation of a fluorescent complex of ellagic acid with borax in methanol. This property of ellagic acid was used.

Important is to add sufficient borax to neutralise the low pH of the mobile phase (pH 2.4), because at a low pH no fluorescence is shown. At pH 7.0 and pH 8.8 no differences in fluorescence intensity and no shift in emission maxima of the borax complex were observed. In Fig.1 chromatograms of an identical sample hydrolysate of strawberry obtained with UV-detection and fluorescence detection are shown. Integration of the UV-chromatogram is troublesome and prone to errors.

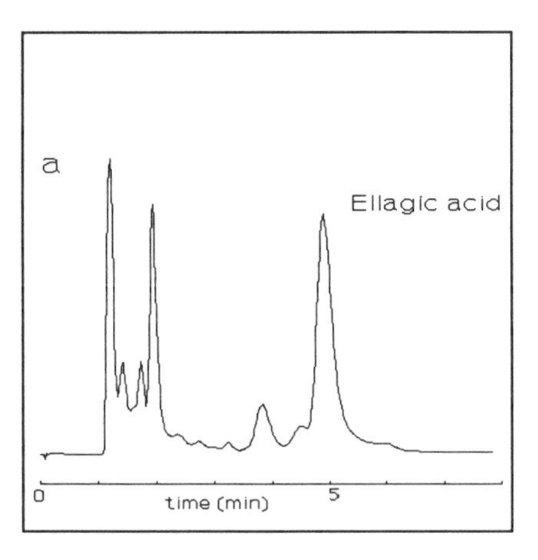

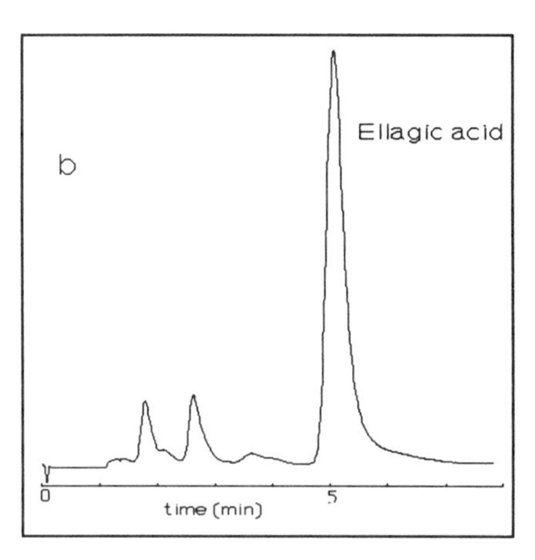

Figure 1 Chromatograms of an identical strawberry hydrolysate; a UV-detection; b fluorescence detection

Extraction and hydrolysis

Extraction of fruits (strawberry, raspberry and blackberry) with methanol showed that free ellagic acid only was present at a low percentage of the total ellagic acid content. After prolonged extraction times, up to 6 hours, this content increased only very slowly.

Hydrolysis was optimized using different HCl and methanol concentrations together with a variation of the hydrolysis period as indicated in Table 1. As is evident from Table 1 the hydrolysis characteristics of the ellagitannins of the walnut differed from those of the fruits.

Daniel[5] applied a separate extraction of ellagitannins followed by hydrolysis of the concentrated extract with trifluoroacetic acid. Results in our laboratory obtained with this method, substituting trifluoroacetic acid with HCl, did not give higher values compared to the single step hydrolysis/extraction method.

Method performance

Standard additions of ellagic acid (25% and 50% of native content) to samples of strawberries, raspberries, blackberries and walnut showed 103-116% (mean 107%) recovery. Standards of ellagic acid passing through the hydrolysis procedure proved to be stable: 93-107% (mean 100%). Coefficient of variation of repeatability was 4%. Limit of detection was 1 mg/kg.

Table 1. Effect of different hydrolysis conditions. Results (duplicates) are expressed as percentage of the highest yield obtained in that food sample

Hydrolysis period in hours	Hydrolysis in 3.5M HCl 72% methanol	Hydrolysis in 5M HCl 57% methanol	Hydrolysis in 3.5M HCl 57% methanol
Strawberries			
0.5	62%	83%	49%
1	71%	88%	61%
2	85%	90%	86%
4	100%	89%	97%
6	90%	90%	99%
Blackberries can			
1	37%	54%	
2	91%	81%	
4	99%	87%	
6	100%	92%	
8	100%	89%	
Raspberries			
2	73%		
4	91%	86%	
6	98%	94%	
8	100%	90%	
Walnut			
0.3	54%	81%	
0.7	67%	96%	
1	91%	100%	
2	99%	95%	
4	91%	98%	
6	99%	97%	

Analyses of foods

Results of the determinations of ellagic acid are summarised in Table 2. Strawberries were sampled from April to July to allow for variation in different varieties available. Two or three major brands of fruit jams were purchased.

4 DISCUSSION

HPLC analysis of ellagic acid in fruits is difficult because of complex chromatograms with many overlapping peaks, forcing the use of gradient elution (Daniel[5]). Complexation of ellagic acid with borax enhances the fluorescence. Using this borax-complex we were able to develop a simple isocratic HPLC method with fluorescence detection after post-column complexation of ellagic acid.

Only strawberries, raspberries, blackberries, walnuts, and pecannuts are relevant dietary sources of ellagic acid.

Table 2. Ellagic acid content in various fruits and nuts

Product	n	Total ellagic acid (mg/kg)		Free ellagic acid (mg/kg)
		Range	Mean (±1SD)	
Strawberry fresh	10	200-510	402 (±85)	20
seeds	1	2440		
pulp without seeds	1	313		
Strawberry jam (35%)*	2	56-118	104	
Strawberry jam (45%)*	3	104-224	160 (±64)	14
Strawberry/cherry juice (45%)*	1	30	30	3
Raspberry fresh	1	1240	1240	
Raspberry jam (45%)*	2	388-686	537	42
Blackberry fresh	2	1930-2090	2010	
Blackberry jam (45%)*	3	246-760	513 (±285)	12
5 fruits jam strawb, raspb, blackb. (50%)*	1	190	190	
4 fruits jam straw- and raspberry (45%)*	1	111	111	
Cake dressing blackb, cherry, blackcurr(55%)*	1	211	211	
Walnut	3	7040-8860	7400 (±1320)	152
skin	1	163000		
nut without skin	1	125		
Pecannuts	1	1980	1980	
Chestnut canned	1	108	108	
In redcurrant, muscadine grapes, blueberry juice, cranberry compote, and rosebud jam <u>no ellagic acid</u> could be detected				

* between brackets the fruit content declared

REFERENCES

1. S. De Flora and C. Ramel, Mutation Res., 1988, 202, 285

2. H. Hayatsu, S. Arimoto and T. Negishi, Mutation Res., 1988, 202, 429
3. E. Haslam, 'Plant polyphenols. Vegetable tannins re-visited', Cambridge University Press, Cambridge, 1989, Chapter 3, p. 127.
4. J.L. Maas, G.J. Galletta and G.D. Stoner, HortScience, 1991, 26(1), 10.
5. E.M. Daniel, A.S. Krupnick, Y-H. Heur, J.A. Blinzler, R.W. Nims and G.Stoner, J. Food Comp. Anal., 1989, 2, 338.
6. J.L. Maas, S.Y. Wang and G.J. Galletta, HortScience, 1991, 26(1), 66.
7. O.S.Wolfbeis, P.Hochmuth, (1986), Monatsheft für Chemie, 117, 369.

INHIBITORY EFFECT OF AN EXTRACT OF LEAVES OF *ROSMARINUS OFFICINALIS* L. ON TUMOR INITIATION AND PROMOTION IN THE SKIN OF CD-1 MICE

M-T. Huang[a], C-T. Ho[b], Z. Y. Wang[a], K. Stauber[a], C. Georgiadis[c], J.D. Laskin[c] and A.H. Conney[a]

[a]Laboratory for Cancer Research, College of Pharmacy, Rutgers University, Piscataway, NJ 08855, [b]Department of Food Science, Cook College, Rutgers University, New Brunswick, NJ 08903, and [c]Department of Environmental and Community Medicine, UMDNJ-RWJMS, Piscataway, NJ 08854, USA

ABSTRACT

The dried leaf of the plant *Rosmarinus officinalis* L. possesses potent flavor and antioxidant activity and is widely used as a spice and food additive. In short term animal studies, topical application of a methanol extract of leaves of *Rosmarinus officinalis* L. (rosemary extract) to the backs of CD-1 mice inhibited the formation of [^{3}H]benzo[*a*]pyrene (BP)-DNA adducts in mouse epidermis and 12-*O*-tetradecanoylphorbol-13-acetate (TPA)-induced increases in inflammation, hyperplasia and ornithine decarboxylase activity in epidermis. In a two-stage skin tumorigenesis model, topical application of rosemary extract to the backs of mice inhibited tumor initiation by BP and tumor promotion by TPA.

INTRODUCTION

The dried leaf of the plant *Rosmarinus officinalis* L. is one of the most widely used spices in food processing because it has a desirable flavor and because it contains high antioxidant activity.[1-3] Rosemary is used in food processing for the preparation of poultry, lamb, veal, shellfish, sausages, and salads as well as soup and breadings.[2,3] Rosemary is also used as a spice in potato chips and french fries. Many antioxidants in rosemary are non-volatile, and the antioxidant activity of rosemary in lard is comparable with that of BHA and BHT.[1,4] Recent studies have indicated that certain compounds with antioxidant properties can inhibit tumor initiation and tumor promotion in mouse skin.[5-10] In this paper, we describe an inhibitory effect of a methanol extract of rosemary leaves on the tumor-initiating activity of BP and the tumor-promoting activity of TPA in mouse skin.

RESULTS AND DISCUSSION

A rosemary extract was prepared according to the previously reported method of Wu *et al.*[1] Fifty g of ground leaves of the plant *Rosmarinus officinalis* L. were extracted twice with 250 ml of methanol at 60° C for 2 hours, and the samples were filtered after each extraction. The combined extract was bleached with 100 g of activated carbon at 60° C and then filtered to yield a light-brown filtrate. The methanol filtrate was concentrated to a final volume of 50 ml with a vacuum rotatory evaporator and then filtered to remove the precipitate. Seventy five ml of water was then added to the filtrate. The precipitate formed after the addition of water was filtered and dried to yield a methanol extract of leaves of *Rosmarinus officinalis* L. (rosemary extract). This preparation of rosemary was used for all experiments.

The formation of [^{3}H]BP-DNA adducts in mouse epidermis is proportional to the dose of [^{3}H]BP and reaches a maximum at 12 to 15 hours after the topical application of 20 nmol [^{3}H]BP.[11] Topical application of 20 nmol [^{3}H]BP to vehicle-treated control mice resulted in the covalent binding of 0.738 pmol [^{3}H]BP metabolites per mg epidermal DNA at 15 hr after the dose. Topical application of 1.2 or 3.6 mg rosemary extract 5 min before the application of 20 nmol [^{3}H]BP resulted in the formation of 0.516 or 0.337 pmol of covalently bound [^{3}H]BP metabolites, respectively, per mg epidermal DNA at 15 hr after the dose (30-54% inhibition).[12]

The effect of rosemary extract on the tumor-initiating activity of BP in mouse skin was evaluated. Female CD-1 mice (30 per group) were treated topically with 200 μl acetone or with rosemary extract in acetone 5 min before each application of 20 nmol BP in 200 μl acetone once weekly for 10 weeks. One week after the last application of BP, the mice were treated with TPA (15 nmol) twice weekly. After 13 or 19 weeks of promotion with TPA, the mice developed 3.4 or 6.9 tumors per mouse, and the tumor incidence was 87 or 100%, respectively (Figure 1). In a parallel group of animals, topical application of 3.6 mg rosemary extract to the backs of mice 5 min prior to the application of BP developed 1.2 or 3.0 tumors per mouse, and the tumor incidence was 48 or 73%, respectively (Figure 1).

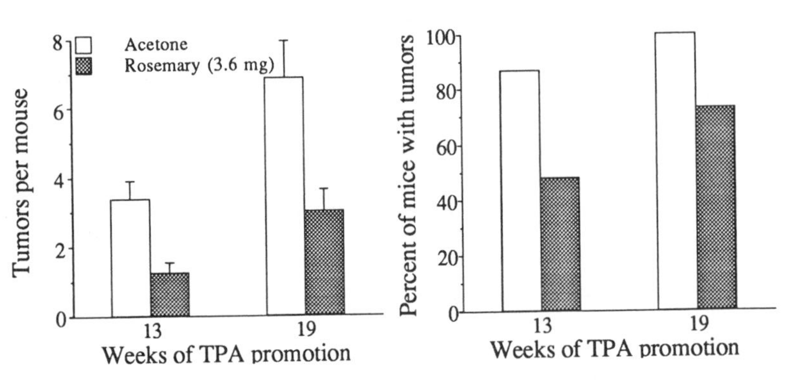

Figure 1. Inhibitory effect of topical application of rosemary extract on the tumor-initiating activity of BP in mouse epidermis. CD-1 female mice (30 per group) were treated topically with 200 μl acetone alone or with rosemary extract (3.6 mg) in acetone 5 min prior to each topical application of 20 nmol BP once weekly for 10 weeks. A week later, the mice were treated topically with 15 nmol TPA twice weekly for 19 weeks. Skin tumors greater than 1 mm in diameter were counted. Tumors per mouse are expressed as the mean ± SE.

Topical application of rosemary extract together with 5 nmol TPA to the backs of mice inhibited TPA-induced increases in epidermal ornithine decarboxylase activity in a dose-dependent manner. Topical application of 0.4 or 3.6 mg rosemary extract together with 5 nmol TPA to the backs of CD-1 mice inhibited TPA-induced increases in epidermal ornithine decarboxylase activity by 66 or 100%, respectively (Figure 2).[13]

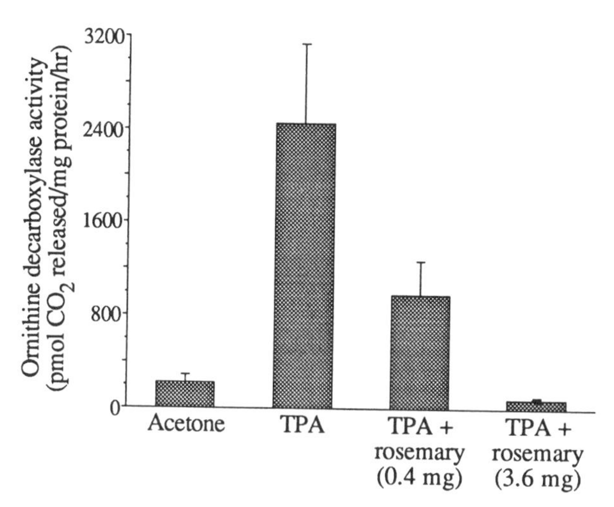

Figure 2. Inhibitory effect of topical application of rosemary extract on TPA-induced increases in epidermal ornithine decarboxylase activity. Mice were treated topically with TPA (5 nmol) alone or TPA together with various amounts of rosemary extract in 200 µl acetone. The animals were sacrificed 5 hr later, and epidermal ornithine decarboxylase activity was determined. Data are expressed as the mean ± S. E. from 3 mice.

Mice that were initiated with 200 nmol 7,12-dimethyl-benz[*a*]anthracene (DMBA) and promoted with 5 nmol TPA twice weekly for 20 weeks developed an average of 17.2 skin tumors per mouse, and 83% of the mice had tumors. Topical application of 0.4 or 3.6 mg rosemary extract together with 5 nmol TPA inhibited TPA-induced tumor formation (tumors per mouse) by 60 or 96%, and the percent of mice with tumors was inhibited by 57 or 92%, respectively (Figure 3).

Topical application of TPA (1 nmol) twice a day for 4 days to the dorsal surface of CD-1 mice resulted in a 4- to 5-fold increase in the number of epidermal cell layers and in the epidermal thickness. Inflammatory cell infiltration in the dermis and intercellular edema in the epidermis were also observed. Topical application of 3.6 mg rosemary extract together with 1 nmol TPA twice a day for 4 days inhibited these effects of TPA.

We isolated carnosol and ursolic acid from rosemary extract, and we studied the biological effects of these compounds. Both carnosol and ursolic acid inhibited TPA-induced ear edema, ornithine decarboxylase activity and tumor promotion in mouse skin. Topical application of 1, 3 or 10 µmol carnosol together with 5 nmol TPA twice weekly for 20 weeks to the backs of CD-1 mice previously initiated with DMBA inhibited the formation of TPA-induced skin tumors per mouse by 38, 63 or 88%, respectively. Topical application of 0.1 or 2 μmol ursolic acid together with 5 nmol TPA twice weekly for 20 weeks inhibited skin tumors per mouse by 52 or 61%, respectively.[12]

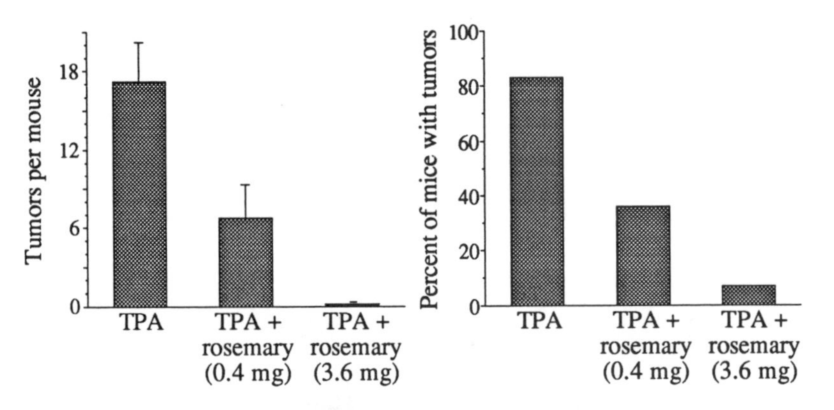

Figure 3. Inhibitory effect of topical application of rosemary extract on TPA-induced tumor promotion in mouse epidermis. Female CD-1 mice (7-8 weeks old; 30 mice per group) were initiated with 200 nmol DMBA. One week later, the mice were promoted with TPA (5 nmol) or TPA (5 nmol) together with 0.4 or 3.6 mg rosemary extract twice weekly for 19 weeks. Skin tumors greater than 1 mm in diameter were recorded. Data are expressed as the mean ± SE.

Recent studies in our laboratory found that rosemary extract (2% of the diet) inhibited BP-induced forestomach and lung tumors in A/J mice as well as azoxymethane-induced colon tumors in CF-1 mice (unpublished results). Dietary rosemary extract also markedly inhibited the toxicity of intraperitoneally administered DMBA in Sencar mice (unpublished results). During the course of our studies, other laboratories have described an inhibitory effect of a rosemary extract or of certain rosemary constituents on tumorigenesis in rodents. Singletary *et al.* reported that administration of 1% crude rosemary extract in the diet to female Sprague-Dawley rats for 3 weeks before a single oral dose of DMBA reduced the mammary gland tumor incidence by 47% at 16 weeks after DMBA treatment.[14] Singletary *et al.* also reported that 0.5% and 1% rosemary extract in the diet inhibited the *in vivo* binding of DMBA to mammary epithelial cell DNA and the formation of two major DNA adducts.[14] Ursolic acid also has been shown to inhibit TPA-induced tumor promotion in mouse skin.[15]

ACKNOWLEDGEMENTS

We thank Thomas Ferraro for his help in the preparation of this manuscript. The research described here was supported by NIH grant CA47956.

REFERENCES

1. J.W. Wu, M-H. Lee, C-T. Ho and S.S. Chang, J. Amer. Oil Chemist's Soc., 1982, 59, 339.
2. C. Fischer, 'Phenolic Compounds in Food and Their Effects on Health I: Analysis, Occurrence, and Chemistry', C-T. Ho, C.Y. Lee and M-T. Huang (eds.), American Chemical Society, Washington D.C., 1992, Chapter 9, (in press).
3. N. Nakatani, 'Phenolic Compounds in Food and Their Effects on Health II: Antioxidants and Cancer Prevention', M-T. Huang, C-T. Ho, and C.Y. Lee (eds.), American Chemical Society, Washington D.C., 1992, Chapter 6, (in press).
4. N. Nakatani and R. Inatani, Agri. Biol. Chem., 1984, 48, 2081.
5. T.J. Slaga and J.D. Scribner, J. Natl. Cancer Inst., 1973, 51, 1723.
6. R. Kato, T. Nakadate, S. Yamamoto and T. Sugimura, Carcinogenesis, 1983, 4, 1301.
7. T.J. Slaga and S.M. Fischer, 'Skin Painting Techniques and *in vivo* Carcinogenesis Bioassays', F. Homburger (ed.), S. Karger, Basel, 1986, 'Progress in Experimental Tumor Research', Vol. 26, p. 85.
8. R.C. Smart, M-T. Huang, Z.T. Han, M.C. Kaplan, A. Focella and A.H. Conney, Cancer Res., 1987, 47, 6633.
9. M-T. Huang, R.C. Smart, C-Q. Wong and A.H. Conney, Cancer Res., 1988, 48, 5941.
10. M-T. Huang, C-T. Ho, Z.Y. Wang, T. Ferraro, T. Finnegan-Olive, Y.-R. Lou, J.M. Michell, J.D. Laskin, H. Newmark, C.S. Yang and A.H. Conney, Carcinogenesis, 1992, 13, 947.
11. R.C. Smart, M-T. Huang, R.L. Chang, J.M. Sayer, D.M. Jerina, A.W. Wood and A.H. Conney, Carcinogenesis, 1986, 7, 1669.
12. M-T. Huang, C-T. Ho, Z.Y. Wang, K. Stauber, C. Georgiadis, J.D. Laskin and A.H. Conney, Proc. Am. Assoc. Cancer Res., 1992, 33, 165.
13. M-T. Huang, C-T. Ho, S.-J. Cheng, J.D. Laskin, K. Stauber, C. Georgiadis and A.H. Conney, Proc. Am. Assoc. Cancer Res., 1989, 30, 189.
14. K.W. Singletary and J.M. Nelshoppen, Cancer Lett., 1991, 60, 169.
15. H. Tokuda, H. Ohigashi, K. Koshimizu and Y. Ito, Cancer Lett., 1986, 33, 279.

VITAMIN A AS A MODULATOR OF *IN VITRO* UNSCHEDULDED DNA SYNTHESIS INDUCED BY 2-AMINO-3-METHYLIMIDAZO[4,5-*f*]QUINOLINE AND 2-AMINO-3,4-DIMETHYLIMIDAZO[4,5-*f*]QUINOLINE IN RAT HEPATOCYTE PRIMARY CULTURES

B. KOCH[1], S. BLOWERS[2], I. ROWLAND[2] and J.F. NARBONNE[3]

[1] Groupe BSN, F-75381 Paris Cedex 08

[2] British Industrial Biological Research Association, Carshalton Surrey, SM5 4DS UK

[3] Laboratoire de Toxicologie Alimentaire, Université Bordeaux I, F-33405 Talence Cedex

INTRODUCTION

The hepatocyte primary culture (HPC)/DNA repair test which measures unscheduled DNA synthesis (UDS) has been shown to be a reliable short-term assay for genotoxic chemical carcinogens as amino acid pyrolysates[1]. Moreover, this test may also be utilized as suitable sreening device for identification of factors possessing anticarcinogenic activity such as vitamin A[2,3]. The inhibitory potential of vitamin A on 2-amino-3-methylimidazo[4,5-*f*]quinoline (IQ) and 2-amino-3,4-dimethylimidazo[4,5 -*f*]quinoline (MeIQ) genotoxicity was investigated in primary rat hepatocyte cultures by autoradiographic measurement of UDS.

II MATERIALS AND METHODS

Experiments were performed either by direct addition of vitamin A (retinol) to hepatocyte cultures from rats provided with a vitamin A adequate diet (20 IU/g diet), or by using cultured hepatocytes from rats fed different vitamin A level diets (0, 20 and 100 IU/g diet, corresponding to deficient, control and supplemented groups, respectively). The HPC/DNA repair test was performed basically in accordance with the method of Butterworth et al[4]. Cytochrome P-450 levels and dependent activities (benzoxyresorufin dealkylase: BROD, aniline hydroxylase: AH and erythromycin demethylase: ERMD) were determined in hepatocytes as indicators of vitamin A-induced changes in xenobiotic biotransformation enzymes.

III RESULTS AND DISCUSSION

Direct addition of retinol to culture medium did not cause any significant increase in UDS compared to solvent control in the range of concentrations tested (1 to 50 μM). DNA repair levels induced by IQ and MeIQ were significantly decreased by in vitro addition of retinol. Maximal inhibitions obtained were 54% and 39% for IQ and MeIQ, respectively with 50 μM retinol. In addition, retinol inhibition was found dose-dependent for both carcinogens (Table 1).

Moreover, rat vitamin A status affected the magnitude of the in vitro IQ- and MeIQ-induced UDS responses. In the DNA repair test using hepatocytes from vitamin A-deficient rats, both IQ and MeIQ elicited a higher response compared with DNA repair levels in control hepatocytes (+52% and +65% for IQ and MeIQ, respectively). In contrast, lower DNA repair levels were measured when hepatocytes from vitamin A-supplemented rats were used (-43% and -27% for IQ and MeIQ, respectively), (Table 2).

Finally, vitamin A-induced changes in IQ and MeIQ genotoxicity levels were closely related to alterations observed in cytochromes P-450 parameters (-35% for AH and cytochrome P-450 level in hepatocytes from deficient rats, and +21% in supplemented rats).

Thus, data reported in our study are consistent with previous findings of a direct effect of vitamin A on amino acid pyrolysate mutagenicity as demonstrated by Ames test[5]. Moreover, our results support a protective effect of vitamin A against IQ and MeIQ genotoxicity in hepatocytes.

Table 1: Effect of in vitro retinol addition on IQ- and MeIQ-induced UDS in rat primary hepatocyte cultures

	UDS net grains/cell£		
Retinol concentration (μM)	Solvent	IQ (5 μM)	MeIQ (2.5 μM)
0	-.523±.368	21.5±6.9	31.5±7.1
10	.799±1.21	19.9±5.1	30.3±6.8
20	.468±.567	18.1±3.9	27.5±5.5
30	.839±1.915	15.9±4.1	22.2±4.8
40	1.21±1.51	11.1±3.1	20.3±3.9
50	.683±1.3	9.8±2.3	19.2±3.6

Table 2: Effect of rat vitamin A status on in vitro IQ- and MeIQ-induced UDS in rat hepatocytes and on some mixed function oxidase activities

		Experimental groups		
Activities		Deficient	Control	Supplemented
UDS net grains	IQ	38.3±5.9*	25.2±5.9	14.3±4.2*
/cell£	MeIQ	55.3±11.8*	33.5±6.7	24.4±3.6*
Cyt. P-450 (pmol/mg prot.)		223±41*	343±49	415±78*
BROD (pmol/min.mg prot.)		5.2±1.4	5.4±1.3	6.1±1.7
AH (pmol/min.mg prot.)		252±33*	388±45	498±47*
ERMD (pmol/min.mg prot.)		382±46*	535±72	592±68

£: Mean±SD of cell-to-cell variation for 3 slides, 50 cells/slide

*: Significantly different from control group

IV REFERENCES

1. A.J. HOWES, J.A. BEAMAND and I.R. ROWLAND, Fd Chem.Toxic., 1986, 24, 383.
2. J.D. BUDROE, J.G. SHADDOCK and D.A. CASCIANO, Environ. Mol. Mutag., 1987, 10, 129.
3. SUSAN A. HALTER, Human Pathology, 1989, 20, 205.
4. E. BUTTERWORTH, J. ASHBY, E. BERMUDEZ, D. CASCIANO, J. MIRSALIS, G. PROBST and G. WILLIAMS, Mutation Res., 1987, 189, 113.
5. C. IOANNIDES, A.D. AYRTON, A. KEELE, D.F.V. LEWIS, P.R.FLATT and R. WALKER, Mutagenesis, 1990, 5, 257.

COMPARISON OF HYDROXYLATED AND NON-HYDROXYLATED NATURAL FLAVONOIDS AS *IN VITRO* MODULATORS OF RAT HEPATIC BENZO(a)PYRENE METABOLISM

A.M. Le Bon, L. Ziegler and M. Suschetet

INRA, Toxicologie Nutritionnelle,
17, rue Sully, 21034 Dijon cedex, France.

1 INTRODUCTION

Flavonoids, a class of polyphenolic compounds, are abundantly found in fruits and vegetables and are ubiquitous components of the food chain. Some flavonoids have been reported to be successful against carcinogenesis induced by chemical carcinogens (polycyclic hydrocarbons, aflatoxin B1).[1,2] Covalent binding of electrophile carcinogenic metabolites to DNA is an essential event in the initiation step of carcinogenesis. Cytosolic and microsomal enzymes generating reactive metabolites are among the factors controlling this critical step. Some previous studies have demonstrated that these events can be modulated by flavonoids. A number of flavonoids have been shown to inhibit *in vitro* the formation of adducts between DNA and microsome activated carcinogens (benzo(a)pyrene (BaP), aflatoxin B1).[3,4] Activities of the cytochrome P-450-dependent monooxygenases can be inhibited or activated by the presence of certain flavonoids in the incubation medium.[5,6] The present report provides additional information on the modulatory effect of a series of hydroxylated and non-hydroxylated flavonoids on the *in vitro* metabolism of BaP by liver microsomes from untreated and 3-methylcholanthrene (MC)-injected rats. A wide range of concentrations was tested on microsomal aryl hydrocarbon hydroxylase (AHH) and epoxide hydrolase (EH) activities and on microsomalcatalysed BaP-DNA adduct formation.

2 EXPERIMENTAL

Twelve seven-week-old male SPF Wistar rats were provided *ad libitum* a purified diet for 4 weeks. Six rats were treated with MC (20 mg/kg body wt, i.p.) dissolved in corn oil for 3 successive days and killed after 14 h fasting. Six control animals received corn oil only. Liver microsomes were prepared by differential centrifugation of homogenized livers as previously described.[7] Protein concentrations were determined by the method of Lowry *et al.*[8]

Flavonoids were purchased from Sigma, France (flavone, 7,8-benzoflavone, quercetin, chrysin) or from Apin, Great Britain (flavanone, tangeretin, pinocembrin).

AHH activity was determined by the radiometric assay of Van Cantford *et al.*[9] using ^{3}H-BaP as substrate. EH activity was measured according to the method of Oesch *et al.*[10] with ^{14}C-styrene oxide as substrate. The reaction mixture for microsome-catalysed DNA binding of 3H-BaP contained 1 mg DNA, 1 mg microsomal proteins, ^{3}H-BaP (80 μM), cofactors (NADPH, $MgCl_2$) and various concentrations of the flavonoids in a total volume of 2 ml 0,1 M potassium phosphate of the buffer (pH 7,4). Reaction time was 20 min. The DNA was then isolated and purified as previously described.[4]

All compounds tested were added in 0.02 ml DMSO. Control received only the solvent.

3 RESULTS AND DISCUSSION

In vitro effects of flavonoids on AHH activity are shown in table 1. Flavonoids inhibit or activate microsomal AHH activity, depending on the treatment of rats and on their structure. Non-hydroxylated flavonoids, flavone and 7,8-benzoflavone, and a polymethoxylated flavonoid, tangeretin, were found to stimulate AHH activity in hepatic control microsomes. This effect was significant at a concentration of 10 μM. However, these same flavonoids were found to inhibit AHH activity in microsomes from rats induced with 3-methylcholanthrene. These differential effects are likely to be due to the different profiles of cytochrome P-450 isozymes present in microsomes. Flavonoids possessing hydroxyl groups (quercetin, pinocembrin, chrysin) were found to be inhibitors of MC-induced or non-induced AHH activity. This effect was dose-dependent.

The effects of these flavonoids on the microsomal EH activity are presented in table 2. Data were quite similar for the two types of microsomes studied. Flavone, flavanone and 7,8-benzoflavone were potent activators of EH activity of 100 μM, as compared with metyrapone, a known activator of EH[11]. Hydroxylated and polymethoxylated flavonoids (quercetin, chrysin, pinocembrin, tangeretin) showed a moderate effect.

Data for the *in vitro* effects of flavonoids on microsome mediated binding of BaP to DNA are shown in figure 1. All flavonoids tested possessed an inhibitory effect. In microsomes from methylcholanthrene-treated rats, flavonoids exhibited a dose-dependent inhibition, ranging from 1 to 100 μM. Quercetin and 7,8-benzoflavone were found to have the greatest effect. In control microsomes, all the flavonoids inhibited the binding of

Table 1 Effects of flavonoids on aryl hydrocarbon hydroxylase activity in hepatic microsomes from untreated and methylcholanthrene-treated rats.

Compounds	Concentration (μM)	Microsomes untreated (% of control[a])	MC
Flavone (FL)	1	ND[b]	109
	10	142	105
	50	175	86
	100	175	74
7,8-Benzoflavone (aBF)	1	ND	109
	10	183	55
	50	133	29
	100	133	29
Flavanone (VA)	1	ND	111
	10	108	105
	50	83	90
	100	58	99
Tangeretin (TG)	1	ND	113
	10	102	104
	50	150	86
	100	142	84
Quercetin (QU)	1	ND	110
	10	75	79
	50	33	39
	100	17	17
Chrysin (CH)	1	ND	109
	10	100	84
	50	75	49
	100	50	31
Pinocembrin (PI)	1	ND	110
	10	92	104
	50	58	92
	100	33	76

a : Control values (without added flavonoid) of AHH activity were 0.12 ± 0.01 and 1.08 ± 0.04 nmol metabolized BaP/mg protein/min in untreated and MC-treated microsomes, respectively (n = 3).
b : ND = Not Determined.

BaP to DNA at the concentration of 1 μM. With higher concentrations, hydroxylated flavonoids were more potent inhibitors than the non-hydroxylated ones. There is a tight relation between the effects of flavonoids on AHH activity and the resulting level of BaP-DNA adducts.

These results suggest that flavonoids may be modulators in the responsiveness of organisms to carcinogens due to their activity at low concentrations. However, little data are available on the amounts of these compounds in tissues when they are orally

Table 2 Effects of flavonoids and metyrapone on epoxide hydrolase activity in hepatic microsomes from untreated and methylcholanthrene-treated rats.

Compounds	Concentration (μM)	Microsomes untreated (% of control[a])	MC
Flavone	1	106	90
	10	167	130
	100	383	294
7,8-Benzoflavone	1	115	92
	10	191	134
	100	314	229
Flavanone	1	103	85
	10	139	108
	100	224	157
Tangeretin	1	106	84
	10	96	111
	100	177	128
Quercetin	1	105	88
	10	139	103
	100	132	109
Chrysin	1	104	94
	10	148	112
	100	234	167
Pinocembrin	1	92	88
	10	139	100
	100	129	111
Metyrapone	1	100	87
	10	131	121
	100	167	147

a : Control values (without added flavonoid) of EH activity were 2.14 ± 0.20 and 3.85 ± 0.55 nmol styrene glycol formed/mg protein/min in untreated and MC-treated microsomes, respectively (n = 3).

administered. Previous studies have demonstrated that, when they are administered to the rat diet, hydroxylated flavonoids do not have any effect on hepatic drug metabolizing enzyme activities,[12] whereas those lacking hydroxyl groups (flavone, flavanone) or with methoxylated groups (tangeretin) have an inducing effect. Furthermore, these latter groups have been shown to protect against liver chemical-induced carcinogenesis in the rat.[2]

The difference between the observed effects of these flavonoids may be explained by the poor absorption of polyhydroxylated molecules, compared to non-hydroxylated flavonoids which are more lipid-soluble, and/or by metabolism of hydroxylated flavonoids by intestinal microflora to give phenolic derivatives which would be inactive as inducers.[13] Additional studies on oral bioavailability and on *in vitro* metabolism of flavonoids are needed to determine why certain flavonoids influence the *in vivo* metabolism of carcinogens and why others do not.

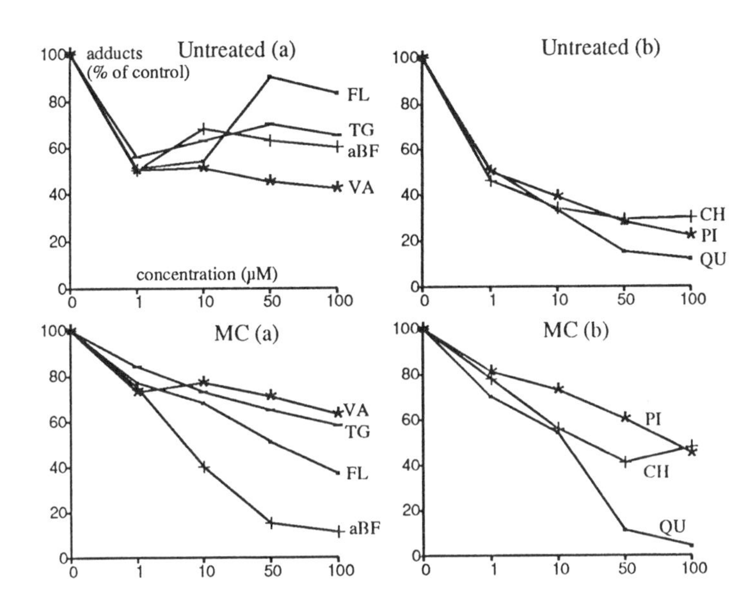

Figure 1 Effects of flavonoids on *in vitro* BaP-DNA adducts formation catalysed by hepatic microsomes from untreated and methylcholanthrene-treated rats. a = non-hydroxylated compounds; b = hydroxylated compounds. Abbreviations : see table 1. Control values (without added flavonoid) of adduct level were 1.27 ± 0.15 and 23.19 ± 0.61 pmol BaP bound/mg protein/min with untreated and MC-treated microsomes, respectively (n = 2).

REFERENCES

1. L.W. Wattenberg and J.L. Leong, Cancer Res., 1970, 30, 1922.
2. M. Suschetet, A.M. Le Bon, C. Frayssinet, B. Rosa-Loridon and M.H. Siess, Proceeding ILSI International Conference Nutrition Cancer, Atlanta, 1991.
3. R.K. Bhattacharya and P.F. Firozi, Cancer Lett., 1988, 39, 85.
4. A.M. Le Bon, M.H. Siess and M. Suschetet, Chem.-Biol. Interact., 1992, 83, 65.
5. F.K. Friedman, D. West, T. Sugimura and H.V. Gelboin, Pharmacology, 1985, 31, 203.
6. M.H. Siess, A. Pennec and E. Gaydou, Eur. J. Drug Metab. Pharmacokinet., 1989, 14, 235.

7. A. Vernet and M.H. Siess, Food Chem. Toxicol., 1986, 24, 857.
8. O.H. Lowry, N.J. Rosebrough, A.L. Farr and R.J. Randall, J. Biol. Chem., 1951, 193, 265.
9. J. Van Cantford, J. De Graeve and J.E. Gielen, Biophys. Res. Comm., 1977, 79, 505.
10. F. Oesch, D.M. Jerina and J. Daly, Biochim. Biophys. Acta, 1971, 227, 685.
11. W.L. Alworth, C.C. Dang, L.M. Ching and T. Viswanathan, Xenobiotica, 1980, 10, 395.
12. M.H. Siess, M. Guillermic, A.M. Le Bon and M. Suschetet, Xenobiotica, 1989, 19, 1379.
13. L.A. Griffiths and G.E. Smith, Biochem. J., 1972, 128, 901.

THE DISTRIBUTION OF QUERCETIN AND QUERCETIN GLYCOSIDES IN VEGETABLE COMPONENTS OF THE HUMAN DIET

Terrance Leighton, Charles Ginther, and Larry Fluss

Department of Biochemistry and Molecular Biology
University of California
Berkeley, CA 94720

1 INTRODUCTION

Flavonols are broadly disseminated in vegetables and fruits found in the human diet.[1] High vegetable content diets can contribute up to 1 g of these compounds daily, primarily in the form of flavonol glycosides.[2] These glycosides are efficiently degraded by glycosidases found in both saliva and the alimentary tract to release free sugars and flavonol agylcones .[3-5] Among dietary flavonols, quercetin (3,3',4',5,7-pentahydroxyflavone) is of particular interest.

Quercetin inhibits the activity of several carcinogens and tumor promoters including bay-region diol epoxides of benzo[a]pyrene, heterocyclic amines, and other carcinogens that require activation by cytochrome oxidases; [6-9] polycyclic aromatic hydrocarbons;[10-12] 12-O-tetradecanoylphorbol-13-acetate (TPA) a phorbol ester;[13-15] and aflatoxin B1.[16]

Quercetin also inhibits enzymatic activities associated with tumor cell metabolism including the calcium and phospholipid-dependent protein kinase (protein kinase C);[17-21] TPA-induced lipoxygenase and ornithine decarboxylase in mouse epidermal tissue;[22] elevated aerobic glycolytic enzyme function;[23] the oncogene pp60 v-src, and other tyrosine kinases;[24] cyclo-oxygenases and 15-lipoxygenase;[25] cyclic GMP phosphodiesterase;[26] and cytochrome P-450/P-448 monooxygenases.[9] Quercetin prevents cigarette smoke inhalation toxicity and ethanol induced gastric damage in rats.[27]

Quercetin enhances the antiproliferative activity of the anticancer drugs cis-diamminedichloroplatinum(II) (cis-DDP), nitrogen mustard, and busulphan in human tumor cell culture systems.[20,28] We have shown that quercetin inhibits the growth of transformed cells containing the activated human oncogene H- *ras*, and prevents malignant transformation of normal cells by H-*ras*.[29] Recently Scambia and coworkers[38-40] have shown that quercetin selectively interferes with the growth of a variety of human tumor cell lines containing type-II estrogen binding sites.

Given the potential impact of quercetin and its glycosides on human cancer risk we have studied quercetin distribution in the *Allium* vegetable family, a group reported to contain high levels of quercetin.[1] We found that quercetin distribution among *Allium* vegetables varied over a fifteen fold range, with some varieties containing no detectable quercetin or its glycosides.[29] These data suggested that a more comprehensive study of vegetables found in the human diet was required to establish which dietary inputs were sources of quercetin.

2 MATERIALS AND METHODS

Flavonoid extraction. 90-300 g of raw vegetable with inedible portions removed were chopped, mixed with butanol containing 0.75% glacial acetic acid (1:1 w/v), blended for 2 min, incubated overnight at 4°C, and filtered through Whatman #1 filter paper. The filtrate was taken to dryness under vacuum at 65°C. The dried material was resuspended in 2.5-10 ml DMSO, and stored in foil covered screw-capped tubes.

XAD-2 column purification of flavonoids for HPLC analysis. 2-5 ml of extract was passed over a XAD-2 column, and then dried with nitrogen gas. The flavonoids were eluted with 10 ml of acetone. The eluted material was dried in a heating block at 67°C under a stream of nitrogen. The dried material was resuspended in 0.2-0.5 ml of DMSO.[30]

Fecalase preparation. We have modified the method of Ames to produce high specific activity human fecal flavonol glycosidase enzyme preparations (fecalase).[29] Briefly, human feces was suspended in buffer (50 mM phosphate buffer, pH 7.4, and 2 mM dithiothreitol) (buffer:feces 2:1 v/v), and sonicated until 95% of the fecal bacteria were disrupted. The suspension was centrifuged (15,000 x g, 20 min), and the supernatant brought to 80% saturation with ammonium sulfate, maintained at pH 7.0. The solution was again centrifuged (18,000 x g for 30 min), and the pellet was resuspended in buffer at 25 mg protein/ml. Following dialysis against buffer, the solution was filtered through a 0.45 micron low protein binding membrane. The sterile fecalase solution was stored at -80°C. The specific activity of the fecalase preparations was assayed by measuring cleavage of the synthetic nitrophenyl-glycoside substrate o-nitrophenyl ß-D-glucoside.[32]

Ames test. Quercetin and several other flavonols are mutagenic in the Ames test. We previously suggested that the mutagenic activity of quercetin in *in vitro* mutagenesis test systems is an artifact resulting from the production of hydroxyl radicals via nonenzymatic Haber-Weiss reactions.[29,31] Only free flavonols, not flavonol glycosides are active in the Ames test. Thus the Ames test provides a convenient screening system to detect free flavonols in untreated vegetable extracts, or total flavonols in fecalase treated extracts.[30]

The Ames test was conducted using strain TA98, which is particularly sensitive to flavonols, as described.[5] When samples were treated with fecalase,

10-25 µl of vegetable extract was mixed with 100 µl of fecalase, 100 µl S9, 300 µl sodium phosphate buffer (0.2 M, pH 7.4). For untreated samples, 10-25 µl of extract was added to 500 µl of phosphate buffer. After addition of bacteria, the mixture was incubated at 37°C for 20 min.

Fecalase treatment of vegetable extracts for HPLC analysis XAD-2 purified vegetable extracts were treated with fecalase by mixing 0.35 ml of each extract with 10 ml of 0.2 M sodium phosphate buffer, pH 7.4; 2.75 ml 7% S9 mix; and 3 ml fecalase. Untreated samples were prepared by adding 0.35 ml of XAD extract to 16 ml of sodium phosphate buffer, pH 7.4. The mixtures were incubated at 35°C for 30 min. The pH was then lowered to 3 by dropwise addition of concentrated HCl, and the extract applied to a XAD column. Flavonols were eluted with acetone, dried, and resuspended in 0.35 ml DMSO.

HPLC analysis of flavonols. Gradient HPLC analysis of flavonols and flavonol glycosides was performed as described.[29] UV-vis spectra were recorded with a diode array detector, and peak areas were quantified. Quercetin identity was established by coelution with purified standards, UV-vis spectra, and by electron ionization mass spectrometery.

3 RESULTS

Ames test screening of vegetable extracts. The mutagenic activities of vegetable extracts with and without fecalase treatment are presented in Table 1. Onion, broccoli, and Italian squash extracts contained mutagenic activity that was increased significantly by treatment with fecalase, suggesting that these three vegetables contained flavonols in the form of flavonol glycosides. The reference flavonol glycoside rutin was included as a positive control.

HPLC analysis of vegetable extracts. Vegetable extracts were also analyzed by gradient HPLC techniques. Because of the chemical complexity of most vegetable samples, identification of flavonols by retention time and diode array spectra was difficult, except in the case of onion extracts where the predominant species were quercetin or its glycosides (Table 2).[29] Careful analysis of HPLC elution profiles suggested that broccoli and Italian squash also contained flavonol glycosides (see Figures 1-2).

Fecalase treatment of vegetable extracts. Treatment of the onion, broccoli and Italian squash extracts with human fecal bacterial glycosides (fecalase) significantly altered the flavonol elution profiles from HPLC columns (Figures 1-2). The treatment resulted in the disappearance of several compounds identified as flavonol glycosides, and resulted in the liberation of new compounds including quercetin.[29] By comparing the quercetin content of the treated and untreated extracts it was possible to estimate the fraction of quercetin compounds present as glycosides (Table 2). A significant fraction of the broccoli glycosides contained quercetin flavonols, while a much smaller proportion of the Italian squash glycosides released quercetin. Fecalase hydrolysis of Italian squash extracts also

Table 1: Mutagenic activity of vegetable extracts with and without fecalase treatment

Extract and treatment	Revertants/plate in Ames test	
	Average	Average-control
Control + 25 µl DMSO	52	0
" + fecalase, S9, DMSO	81	0
Rutin (25 µl, 1 mg/ml)	40	-12
" + fecalase, S9	575	494
Quercetin (25 µl, 1 mg/ml)	620	568
" + fecalase, S9	551	470
Turnips (25 µl)	51	-1
" + fecalase, S9	82	1
Broccoli (25 µl)	66	14
" + fecalase, S9	207	126
Beets (25 µl)	60	8
" + fecalase, S9	87	6
Spinach (25 µl)	54	2
" + fecalase, S9	83	1
Garlic (25 µl)	52	0
" + fecalase, S9	83	2
Italian squash (25 µl)	27	-25
" + fecalase, S9	270	189
Cauliflower (25 µl)	19	-33
" + fecalase, S9	93	12
Red onion (25 µl)	191	139
" + fecalase, S9	TNTC	TNTC
Carrot (25 µl)	51	-1
" + fecalase, S9	89	7
Green beans (25 µl)	66	14
" + fecalase, S9	-	-
Green peppers (25 µl)	71	19
" + fecalase, S9	-	-
Radish (25 µl)	59	7
" + fecalase, S9	86	5
Cabbage (25 µl)	65	13
" + fecalase, S9	-	-

Abbreviations: TNTC = Too numerous to count; - = No significant difference from untreated extracts; Average-Control = mutagenic activity corrected for fecalase and S9 contribution.

Table 2: Relative quantities of quercetin species in selected vegetables

Vegetable	Flavonol glycosides (% total)	Quercetin (% total)
Onion	18920000, 82.0%	2653000, 11.5%
Italian squash	937900, 13.3%	84768, 0.4%
Broccoli	754990, 1.9%	409220, 1.0%

Relative numeric values correspond to integrated peak areas. Relative percentage values correspond to the fraction of the total chromatogram area represented by quercetin or flavonol glycosides.

Figure 1. Gradient HPLC Separation of Broccoli Extract Flavonols and Flavonol Glycosides. Upper Panel - broccoli extract; Lower Panel - broccoli extract treated with fecalase. Abbreviations: a = elution position of quercetin standard; b = elution position of flavonol mono and diglycoside standards.

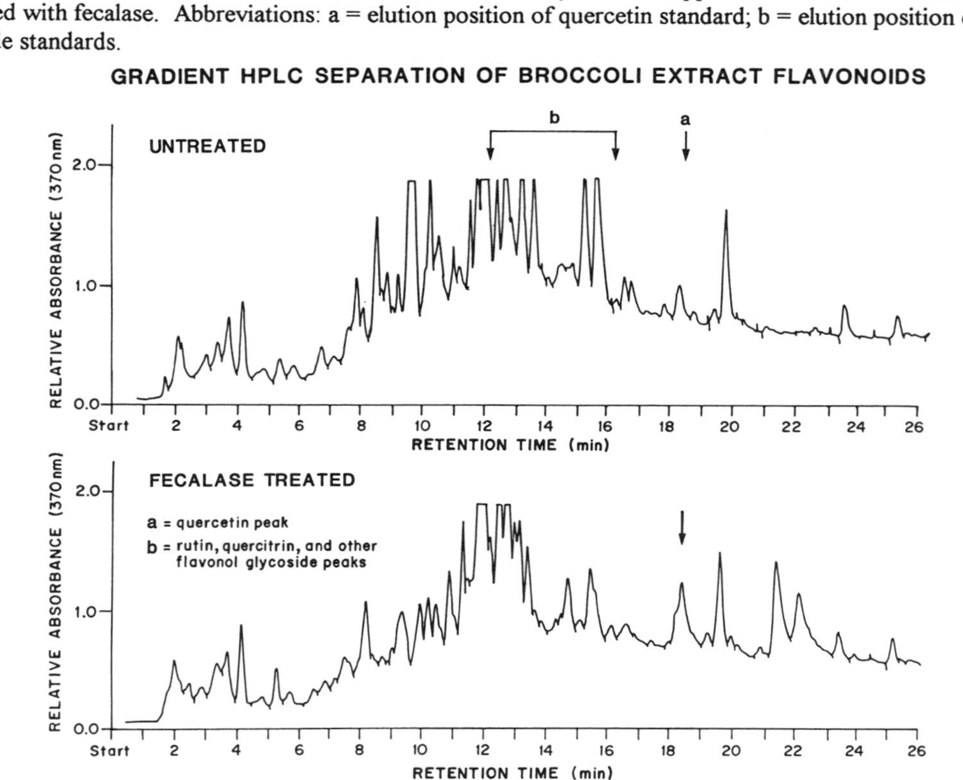

Figure 2. Gradient HPLC Separation of Italian squash Extract Flavonols and Flavonol Glycosides. Upper Panel - Italian squash extract; Lower Panel - Italian squash extract treated with fecalase. Abbreviations: a = elution position of quercetin standard; b = elution position of flavonol mono and diglycoside standards.

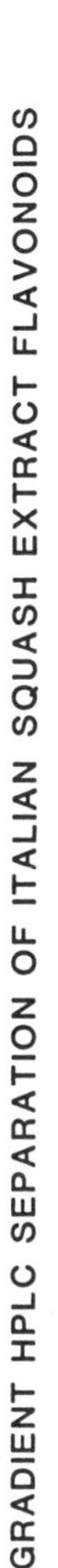

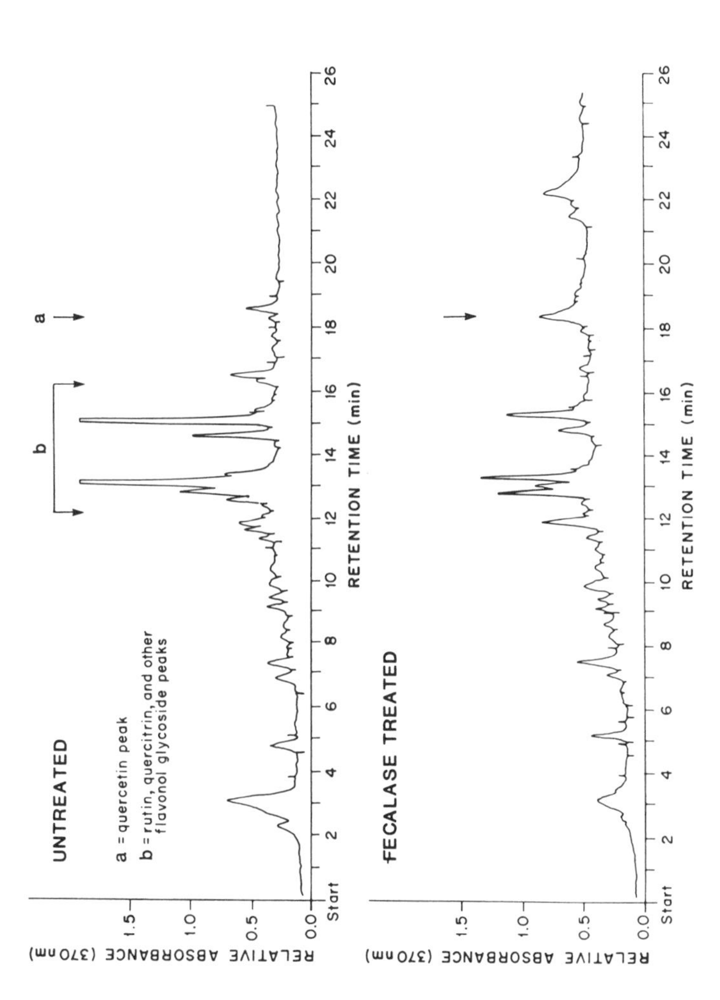

produced the aglycone kaempherol. These results are in good agreement with the Ames test findings which demonstrated that onion, broccoli and Italian squash were the only vegetable extracts to give increased activity following fecalase treatment.

4 DISCUSSION

Epidemiological studies indicate that 35-40% of all cancer mortality may be attributable to dietary factors.[34] Several dietary components may interfere with the initiation or progression phases of carcinogenesis. For example, diets which are high in fruits and green/yellow vegetables, and low in animal fat are low cancer-risk; while diets high in animal fat and low in fruit and green/yellow vegetables are high cancer-risk.[35,36] Because of the apparently beneficial effect of vegetables, several plant derived compounds (vitamin A, vitamin C, carotenes, etc.) have been examined as dietary anticarcinogens.

Our research has focused on the distribution and molecular processing of quercetin, a plant flavonol that has been shown to block the action of a variety of endogenous and exogenous initiators or promoters of cancer cell development. The quercetin content of a variety of vegetables (squash, spinach, cauliflower, broccoli, carrot, green cabbage, green beans, green peppers, beets, turnip, garlic, radish, and onion) were examined using HPLC and diode array spectral analysis. Vegetable flavonols were frequently present as glycoconjugates, which were difficult to resolve by HPLC techniques. Treatment of vegetable extracts with human gut bacterial glycosidases (fecalases) efficiently processed flavonol glycosides to more easily identified free flavonols. These data demonstrate that fecalase treatment of vegetable extracts can be used to deconvolute the phytochemical profile of vegetable flavonols. The quercetin content of vegetables was found to vary from <0.03 to >1 g/kg of vegetable. As shown previously yellow and red onions and shallots contained the highest concentration of total flavonols, up to 1000 mg/kg.[29] Data presented here demonstrates that Italian squash and broccoli also contain significant levels of quercetin. Quercetin could not be detected in leeks, garlic, scallions, cauliflower, green cabbage, green beans, green peppers, beets, spinach, carrot, radish or turnip.[29]

In view of the possible human health benefits which could result from ingestion of quercetin, and epidemiological evidence that *Allium* vegetable consumption reduces the risk of some types of cancer,[37] it is of interest to note (1) the nonuniform distribution of quercetin within major groups of edible vegetables, (2) the particularly high levels of quercetin found in shallots and onions,[29] (3) the significant levels of quercetin compounds in Italian squash and broccoli, and (4) the efficient generation of the anticarcinogen quercetin from dietary flavonol glycosides by human intestinal bacterial enzyme preparations (fecalase).

6 ACKNOWLEDGEMENTS

This research was supported by grants from the National Cancer Institute and the Cancer Coordinating Committee.

7 REFERENCES

1. J. Kuhnau, World Rev. Nutr. Dig., 1976, 24, 117.
2. J.P. Brown, Mutation Res., 1980, 75, 243.
3. I.A. MacDonald, R.G. Bussard, D.M. Hutchinson and L.V. Holdeman, Appl. Environ. Microbiol., 1984, 47, 350.
4. I.A. MacDonald, J.A. Mader and R.G. Bussard, Mutation Res., 1983, 122, 95.
5. G. Tamara, C. Gold, A. Ferro-Luzzi and B.N. Ames, Proc. Natl. Acad. Sci. (U.S.A.), 1980, 77, 4961.
6. M.-T. Huang, A.W. Wood, H.L. Newmark, J.M. Sayer, H. Yagi, D.M. Jerina, and A.M. Conney, Carcinogenesis, 983, 4, 1631.
7. A.J. Alldrick, J. Flynn and I.R. Rowland Mutation Res., 1986, 163, 225.
8. W.A. Khan, Z.Y. Wang, M. Athar, D.R. Bickers, and H. Mukhtar, Cancer Letters, 1988, 42, 7.
9. R.L. Sousa and M.A. Marletta, Arch. Biochem. Biophys., 1985, 240, 345.
10. G.M. Shah and R.K. Bhattacharya, Chem.-Biol. Interactions, 1986, 59, 1.
11. M. Das, W.A. Khan, P. Asokan, D.R. Bickers and H. Mukhtar, Cancer Res., 1987, 47, 767.
12. M. Das, H. Mukhtar, D. Bik and D. Bickers, Cancer Res., 1987, 47, 760.
13. H. Nishino, A. Nishino, A. Iwashima, K. Tanaka and T. Matsuura, Oncology, 1984, 41, 120.
14. K. Tanaka, T. Ono and M. Umeda, Jpn. J. Cancer Res. (Gann), 1987, 78, 819.
15. R. Kato, T. Nakadate, S. Yamamoto and T. Sugimura, Carcinogenesis, 1985, 4, 1301.
16. B.K. Bhattacharya and P.F. Firozi, Cancer Lett., 1988, 39, 85.
17. M. Gschwendt, F. Horn, W. Kittstein, G. Furstenberger, E. Besenfelder and F. Marks, Biochem. Biophys. Res. Commun., 1984, 124, 63.
18. M. Gschwendt, F. Horn, W. Kittstein, and F. Marks, Biochem. Biophys. Res. Commun., 1983, 117, 444.
19. B.K. Mookerjee, H.A. Lipps and E. Middleton, Jr., J. Immunopharmacology, 1981, 8, 371.
20. J. Hofmann, W. Doppler, A. Jakob, K. Maly, L. Posch, F. Uberall and H. Grunicke, Int. J. Cancer, 1988, 42, 382.
21. F. Horn, M. Gschwendt and F. Marks, Europ. J. Biochem., 1985, 148, 533.
22. R. Kato, T. Nakadate, S. Yamamoto and T. Sugimura, Carcinogenesis, 1985, 4, 1301.
23. E.M. Suolina, R.N. Buchsbaum and E. Racker, Cancer Res., 1975, 35, 1825.
24. Y. Graziani, 'Plant Flavonoids in Biology and Medicine: Biochemical Pharmacological and Structural-Activity Relationships', Liss, New York, 1986.

25. W.P. Kingston, Br. J. Pharmacol., 1983, 80, 515.
26. M. Ruckstuhl, A. Beretz, R. Anton and Y. Landry, Biochem. Pharmacol. 1979, 25, 535.
27. T. Harada, K. Maita, Y. Odanaka, and Y. Shirasu, Jpn. J. Vet. Sci., 1984, 46, 527.
28. R. Hoffman, L. Graham and E.S. Newlands, Br. J. Cancer 1989, 59, 347.
29. T. Leighton, C. Ginther, L. Fluss, W.K. Harter, J. Cansado, and V. Notario, "Phenolic Compounds and Human Health", ACS Symposium Series, 1992, in press.
30. T. Nguyen, L. Fluss, C. Ginther, and T. Leighton, J. Wine Res. 1990, 1, 25.
31. W.F. Hodnick, B. Kalyanaraman, C.A. Pristsos, and R.S. Pardini, Basic Life Science, 1988, 49, 149.
32. I.A. Macdonald and J.A. Mader, "Carcinogens and Mutagens in the Environment", Academic Press, New York, 1981, Vol. 2, p. 41.
33. K. Vande Casteele, H. Geiger and C.F. Van Sumere, J. Chromatogr., 1982, 240, 81.
34. R. Doll and R. Peto, J. Natl. Cancer Inst. 1981, 66, 1192.
35. B.N. Ames, "Genetic Toxicity of the Diet", Liss, Inc., New York, NY, 1986, p. 3.
36. T. Hirayama, "Toxicology of the Diet", Liss, Inc., New York, 1986, p. 299.
37. W.-C. You, W.J. Blot, Y.-S. Chang, A. Ershow, Z.T. Yang, Q. An, B.E. Henderson, J.F. Fraumeni, Jr., and T.-G. Wang, J. Natl. Cancer Inst. 1989, 81, 162.
38. L. Telofili, L. Pierelli, M.S. Iovino, G. Leone, G. Scambia, R. De Vincenzo, P. Benedetti-Pancini, G. Menichella, E. Macri, M. Piantelli, *et al.*, Leukemia Research 1992, 16, 497.
39. G. Scambia, F.O. Ranelletti, P. Benedetti-Pancini, M. Piantelli, G. Bonanno, R. De Vincenzo, G. Ferrandina, N. Maggiano, A. Capelli, and S. Mancuso, Gynecologic Oncology, 1992, 45, 13.
40. F.O. Ranelletti, R. Ricci, L.M. Larocca, N. Maggiano, A. Capelli, G. Scambia, P. Benedetti-Panici, S. Mancuso, C. Rumi, and M. Piantelli, Intern. J. Cancer, 1992, 50, 486.

IN VIVO STUDIES ON ANTIGENOTOXIC EFFECTS OF NA-PHYTATE AND *L. CASEI* IN THE GASTROINTESTINAL TRACT OF RATS.

B.L. Pool-Zobel, B. Bertram*, K.D. Jany, U. Schlemmer and W.H. Holzapfel.

Institute for Hygiene und Toxicology, Institute for Nutrition Physiology Federal Research Center for Nutrition Karlsruhe, *Institute for Toxicology and Chemotherapy, German Cancer Research Center, Heidelberg, Germany.

1. INTRODUCTION

A Lactobacillus strain and Na-phytate were studied for antigenotoxic properties in the gastrointestinal (GI) tract of rats. Lactobacilli are a group of rod shaped Gram positive bacteria, present in the intestinal tract of healthy humans and animals, in fermenting vegetables, and they are used for the manufacture of fermented dairy products. They have been associated with beneficial physiological activities, such as maintaining the normal ecological balance in the GI-tract or potential serum cholesterol lowering activities[1,2]. Phytic acid is an ingredient of dormant and germinating seeds, of cereals, and of legumes. It may serve several important physiological functions including storage of phosphorus and cations. It is mainly present in the form of complexes with minerals and proteins and is associated with the soluble fiber components of cereals and vegetables. It has major effects on the balance and availability of several minerals including zinc, iron, calcium[3].

Both phytic acid and lactic acid bacteria have been implied as having potential anticarcinogenic effects, especially in the GI tract[4-8]. Since this effect may be a result of inhibition of initiation or proliferation, it is feasible to study antimutagenic effects when looking for beneficial properties of these food components. In this context, previous studies by Renner and Münzner[9,10] with the Salmonella typhimurium / mutagenicity assay have shown 8 of 10 lactic acid bacterial strains to prevent the growth of his^+ revertants, inducible by nitrosated beef. Also, in cytogenetic assays *in vivo*, one representative strain of lactic acid bacteria, namely *Lactobacillus casei*, inhibited chromosomal damage induced by the strong alkylating agent busulfan in the bone marrow of hamsters and mice. In contrast, Na-phytate has not been shown to be anti-genotoxic. When combined with p.o. application of busulfan, systemic anti-genotoxic properties were not detectable in the bone marrow of hamsters[11].

Following these findings, it was of interest to determine the antigenotoxic effects of *L. casei* in those tissues actually afflicted by tumors and, as is the case for dietary related target organs, it was of foremost interest to study the effects within the gastrointestinal tract. Since effective techniques to achieve this goal were not available, we first further developed several methods to detect genotoxic events in numerous somatic tissues of the rat[12]. This report will present results using one of the most promising systems, the microgelelectrophoresis[13] assay, with cells of the gastrointestinal tract. The investigations were directed at determining the potential of *L. casei* and Na-phytate to act anti-genotoxically in gastric and colon mucosae.

2. MATERIALS AND METHODS:

Somatic cells from gastric or colonic mucosae are explanted via enzyme digestion from animals treated with the genotoxic agent and/or the potential antigenotoxin *per os*, embedded into gels on microscopical slides, lysed, and then subjected to electrophoresis[13,14]. The liberated DNA is subsequently stained with ethidium bromide and analysed microscopically. The tests are evaluated by measuring the migration distance of 101 cells per slide, and 3 slides per organ. The results may either be expressed in terms of the median migration distance of all evaluated cells, or by dividing the cells into different classes according to their degree of DNA damage[12]. Studies were first performed to determine optimal doses and exposure times of the model compound N-methyl-N∩-nitro-nitrosoguanidine (MNNG) in the male Sprague Dawley rat. Combination experiments were then carried out by additionally applying $10x10^9$ *L. casei* per kg b.w. in fresh bacterial broth or 500 mg/kg Na-phytate in NaCl immediately before application of MNNG.

3. RESULTS

It has been found that 5 - 7.5 mg/kg MNNG are effective doses yielding positive responses in the gastric mucosa and in the colon mucosa, without saturating the system. Optimal exposure periods were 1 h for the gastric tissue and 16 h for the colon mucosa, following oral intubation of MNNG. The combination experiments were subsequently performed with *L. casei* and Na-phytate, using the optimal MNNG-exposure times and doses. As shown in Table 1, the simultaneous application of *L. casei* resulted in a clear reduction of induced DNA damage. This reduction was apparent from the increased percentage of intact cells with a migration distance of less than 35 µm. Also, the median migration distance was reduced to control level.

Table 1: Combination effects of MNNG and *L. casei* or Na-phytate *in vivo*. Detection of DNA fragmentation in primary cells of the gastric mucosa, 1h exposure.

Treatment / kg b.w.		N	Viability of cells in (%)	% cells with MD <35μm	median value MD	(C-T)
-	-	7	92±4	95±1	23	./.
Na-phyt. 500 mg	-	4	90±5	96±4	23	0
L. casei $10x10^9$	-	3	95±1	93±1	23	0
-	MNNG 5 mg	12	93±12	43±7	62	39
Na-phyt. 500 mg	MNNG 5 mg	6	88±10	49±8	43	20
L. casei $10x10^9$	MNNG 5 mg	6	92±1	63±5	25	2

C, Value obtained for solvent control; T, Value obtained for differently treated samples; MD, Migration distances; N, Number of animals per group; MD, migration distance, cells < 35μm are considered as still being intact; - untreated control rats, or rats treated only with the respective vehicles (NaCl or fresh bacterial MRS broth).

Na-phytate, however, only caused a partial decrease of the median migration distance and there were no differences in the percentage of intact cells when comparing the MNNG and MNNG + Na-phytate groups.

Table 2 shows similar studies performed with tissues of the colonic mucosa. The cells are not as robust as gastric mucosa cells and this property is reflected by the lower degree of viability and in the somewhat higher basic variation. However, the anti-genotoxic properties of *L. casei* are even more striking in the colon. DNA damage (expressed as percentage of intact cells or as median migration distance) is comparable to the levels of the untreated control. The additional application of Na-phytate does not reveal any differences in comparison to the MNNG-control group.

Even though *L. casei* seems to inhibit the MNNG activity totally (according to the tables), the presentation of the data in the form of bar charts reveals that there is still considerable damage left (Figure 1B).

Table 2: Combination effects of MNNG and *L. casei* or Na-phytate *in vivo*. Detection of DNA fragmentation in primary cells of the colon mucosa, 16 h exposure.

Treatment / kg b.w.		N	Viability of cells in (%)	% cells with MD <35μm	median value MD	(C-T)
-	-	7	78±6	74±10	24	./.
Na-phyt. 500 mg	-	4	87±7	61±10	30	6
L. casei $10x10^9$	-	3	77±7	65±5	25	1
-	MNNG 5 mg	12	83±3	46±9	55	31
Na-phyt. 500 mg	MNNG 5 mg	6	83±7	43±12	54	30
L. casei $10x10^9$	MNNG 5 mg	4	85±3	65±10	24	0

See legend to Table 1

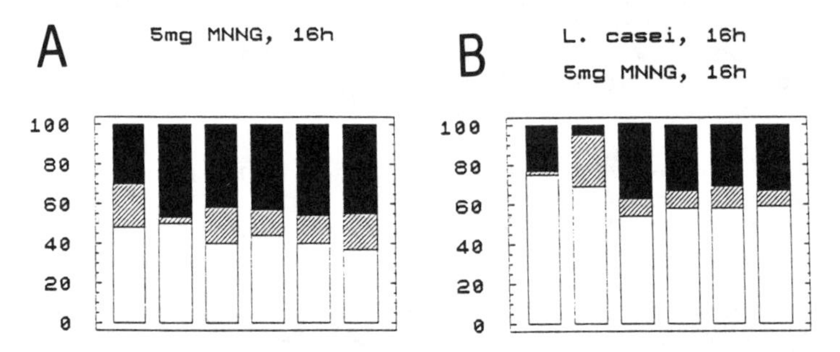

Figure 1: Degree of DNA damage in colon cells 16 h following application of *L. casei*. (See legend Figure 1). Each bar represents results of 1 animal, 3 slides and 101 cells per slide. The bar charts show the % of cells according to their degree of damage (migration distances: 40μm, white; 40-80μm, shaded; >80μm, solid).

Since some types of ingested bacteria may colonize in the colon, we also investigated a sequential treatment schedule. First the bacteria were applied, followed 8 h later by MNNG. After an additional 16 h, the cells were explanted and subjected to electrophoresis. The result was a stronger antigenotoxic effect (Figure 2B), even with higher MNNG doses.

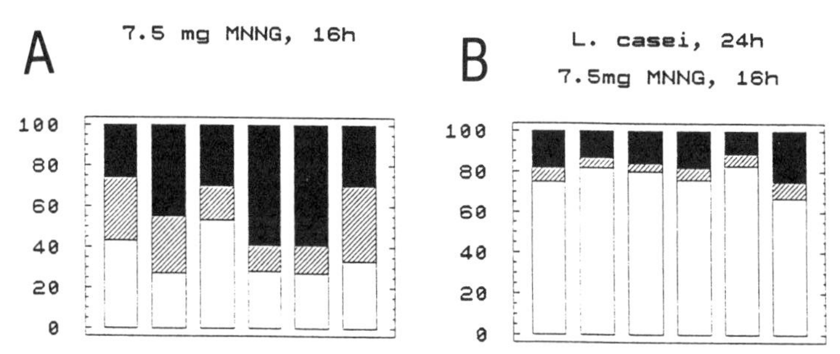

Figure 2: Degree of DNA damage in colon cells 24 h following application of *L. casei* and 16 h after MNNG. (See legend to Figure 1)

These results are interesting not only because of the findings that both agents have protective activities, but also because it will be possible in the future to utilize this new and efficient assay system to study genotoxic and antigenotoxic effects in the GI tract *in vivo*. Accordingly we are presently studying other strains of bacteria, different colon carcinogens and determining dose response relationships. The results of these studies are expected to be of immediate value in determining benefits of lactic acid bacteria also for human health.

REFERENCES

1. V. Botazzi, Biochimie, 1988, 70, 303.
2. W.P. Hammes, N. Weiss, and W.H. Holzapfel, 'The Prokaryotes' Springer, New York, 2nd Ed., 1992, Vol. II, p.1535.
3. M. Torre, A.R. Rogriguez, F. Saura-Calixto, Crit. Revs. Fd. Sc. Nutr., 1991, 1, 1.
4. C.F. Fernandes and K.M. Shahani, J. Fd. Protec., 1990 53, 704.
5. E. Graf and J.W. Eaton, Cancer, 1985, 56, 717.
6. Y. Morishita and K. Shiromizu, Bifidobact. Microfl., 1990, 9, 135.
7. A.M. Shamsuddin and A. Ullah, Carcinogenesis, 1989, 10, 625.
9. P. Van't Veer, J.M. Dekker, J.W.J. Lamers, F.J. Kok, E.G. Schouten, H.A.M. Brants, F. Sturmans, and R.J.J. Hermus, Cancer Res., 1989, 49, 4020.
10. H.W. Renner and R. Münzner, Mutation Res., 1991 262, 239.
11. B. L. Pool-Zobel, et al., unpublished results.
12. B.L. Pool-Zobel, R.G. Klein, U.M. Liegibel, F. Kuchenmeister, S. Weber, and P. Schmezer, Clin. Investig., 1992, 70, 299.
13. N.P. Singh, D.B. Banner, R.R. Tice, L. Brant and E.L. Schneider, Mutation Res., 1990, 237, 122.
14. B. Burlinson, Carcinogenesis, 1989, 10, 1425.

Desmutagenic Effect of Vegetables on Mutagens and Carcinogens and Growth-inhibiting Effect of Spinach Components on Cultured Human Cancer Cells

K. Shinohara[1], M. Kobori[1] and Z-L. Kong[2]

1) Food Functionality Laboratory, Food Nutrition and Physiology Division, National Food Research Institute, The Ministry of Agriculture, Forestry and Fisheries, 2-1-2 Kannondai, Tsukuba, Ibaraki 305 Japan
2) Department of Marine Food Science, National Taiwan Ocean University, 2 Pei-Ning Road, Keelung 20224, Taiwan, R.O.C.

1 INTRODUCTION

Some epidemiological studies revealed that cancer occurrence are closely related to the food habits. Many mutagens and carcinogens have been detected from natural environments. Especially, findings of powerful mutagens and carcinogens in the pyrolyzates of amino acids and proteins, broiled fish and roasted meat have received much attention from the point of view of food-related cancers. On the other hand, it was demonstrated epidemiologically that green- and yellow-colored vegetables reduce the occurrence of cancers. This indicates that such vegetables and fruits contain cancer-preventory constituents. One of the cancer-preventory functions of constituents of vegetables and fruits is an inhibiting function on the formation or activity of mutagenicity of mutagens and carcinogens (desmutagenic and antimutagenic function). Recent studies revealed that a variety of desmutagenic and antimutagenic constituents existed in vegetables and fruits, such as vitamin C, vitamin A, cysteine, polyphenols, peroxidase, fibers, and lignin-like compounds. Most of them have relatively low molecular weight of constituents, except peroxidase and fibers. Desmutagenicity of the high molecular weight of constituents in vegetables and fruits is to be clearly identified yet. Vegetables and fruits comprise a number of constituents, and mutual interactions among those constituents take place during processing, storage and cooking to produce many types of output. It is plausible to expect that unknown desmutagenic substances may exist among these constituents or products.

It is also possible that the constituents in vegetables and fruits may kill or modify the cancer cells directly or activate the immune systems in our body, such as macrophage and lymphocyte cells. These functions are effective for prevention of cancers.

We have now found that new desmutagenic constituents on some mutagens and carcinogens such as 3-amino-1-methyl-5*H*-pyridol[4,3-*b*]indole (Trp-P-2), 3-amino-1,4-dimethyl-5*H*-pyrido[4,3-*b*]indole (Trp-P-1), *N*-methyl-*N*-nitroso-*N*'-nitrosoguanidine (MNNG), benzo-[*a*]pyrene (B[*a*]P), 2-(2-furyl)-3-(5-nitro-2-furyl)acrylamide (AF-2), sterigmatocystin (ST) and aflatoxin B1 (AB1) exist in the non-dialyzable extracts of vegetables and fruits. It was also confirmed that the non-dialyzable extracts of spinach inhibit the growth of human cultured cancer cell lines derived from breast, liver and lung cancers and alter the morphology of a human histiocytic lymphoma cell line, U-937. Activation of biophylactically important macrophage cells and promotion of growth and immunoglobulin production of hybridoma cells by non-dialyzable extracts of spinach were also found.

2 DESMUTAGENICITY OF DIALYZATES OF VEGETABLES AND FRUITS

Non-dialyzable extracts were prepared from various kinds of fresh and freeze-dried vegetables and fruits such as broccoli, burdock, cabbage, carrot, Chinese chive, Chinese cabbage, chingentsuai, cucumber, eggplant, enokitake, green pepper, Japanese radish, kinusayaendo, komatsuna, matsutake, nigauri, onion, potato, pumpkin, spinach, sweet potato, tomato, welsh onion, amanatsu, apple, and natsudaidai, and inhibiting effects of the dialyzate on the mutagenicity of Trp-P-2 toward *Salmonella typhimurium* TA 100 and TA 98 were examined. All of dialyzates of vegetables and fruits inhibited the mutagenicity of Trp-P-2 (1-2). Among the vegetables, the dialyzates of broccoli, burdock, cucumber, eggplant, komatsuna, green pepper and spinach showed a high desmutagenic effect. Some results are shown in Table 1.

The desmutagenic activity of these dialyzates on Trp-P-2 was still retained even after heating them at 100°C for 20 min (Table 1), indicating that heat-stable desmutagens exist in these dialyzates. Heated dialyzates of eggplant, spinach and burdock also inhibited the mutagenicity of MNNG, AF-2, B[a]P, ST, AB1 and Trp-P-1 (Table 2). These dialyzates tended to inhibit greater mutagenicity of the indirect mutagens than the direct ones.

Table 1 Desmutagenic effect of dialyzates of vegetables and fruits on Trp-P-2 (*Salmonella typhimurium* TA 100)

	Inhibition percentage				
Vegetable and fruit	Unheated dialyzate	Heated dialyzate	Vegetable and fruit	Unheated dialyzate	Heated dialyzate
Eggplant	82.5	82.3	Cabbage	35.3	21.7
Broccoli	79.5	74.0	Carrot	24.5	26.3
Komatsuna	77.6	75.7	Potato	25.3	12.3
Spinach	76.7	74.2	Amanatsu	20.0	14.4
Green pepper	73.0	52.0	Apple	58.0	35.4
Cucumber	75.5	58.3	Natsudaidai	50.4	53.2
Burdock	67.8	64.6	Natsudaidai		
Radish	48.3	39.3	pericarp	61.2	61.9
Tomato	46.1	26.8	Natsudaidai		
Onion	35.8	12.1	envelope	41.8	37.2

Table 2 Desmutagenic effect of heated dialyzates of burdock, eggplant and spinach on several mutagens and carcinogens (*Salmonella typhimurium* TA 100)

	Inhibition percentage					
Mutagen	MNNG	AF-2	B[a]P	ST	AB1	Trp-P-1
Burdock	26.9	14.7	40.8	34.5	55.5	75.2
Eggplant	29.5	59.4	76.4	66.4	89.1	86.2
Spinach	21.4	8.0	40.8	24.8	55.5	55.2

In addition to the dialyzate of edible part of eggplant and cucumber, the dialyzates prepared from their leaves also inhibited the mutagenicity of Trp-P-2. Similar high desmutagenic effects on Trp-P-2 were observed in the dialyzates of leaves of sweet potato and Japanese radish and roots of spinach.

Dialyzate of spinach was partially separated by gel-filtrations on Sephadex G-100 and G-25 column. Among four fractions obtained, the SPW2-3 and SPW2-4 fractions which were lately eluted on a Sephadex G-25 gel-filtration were found to have the highest desmutagenicity on Trp-P-2 (3). These fractions also inhibited the mutagenicity of B[a]P and MNNG, suggesting that the fractions of dialyzate of spinach inhibit both direct and indirect mutagens. One of desmutagenic principles of the dialyzate of spinach is suggested to be proteinous, while possible desmutagenic ones of the dialyzates of apple to be polymerized polyphenols (1). Ethanol-soluble portion of dialyzates of vegetables and fruits also exhibited the high desmutagenic activity on Trp-P-2.

3 EFFECT OF DIALYZATE OF SPINACH ON THE GROWTH OF HUMAN NORMAL AND CANCER CELL LINES

To clarify the cancer-preventory effect of vegetables and fruits, the effect of dialyzate of spinach on the growth of human-derived cancer cells at cellular level was examined (4). As shown in Table 3, some fractions of spinach dialyzate, which were separated by a Sephadex G-25 gel filtration, decreased the viability of breast adenocarcinoma cell line (MCF-7)(Table 3). Among the fractions, SPW2-3 and SPW2-4 fractions decreased the viability of MCF-7 cells more significantly. One of active principles of the SPW2-3 fraction is suggested to be a glycoprotein having M.W. of 16 Kda.

Table 3 Effect of the fractions separated by a Sephadex G-25 gel filtration of dialyzate of spinach on the viability of human breast cancer cell line (MCF-7)

Fraction	Viability (%) Dose (μg/ml)			
	0	0.5	1.0	2.0
SPW2-1	100	99.2±0.5	99.3±0.6	98.6±0.6
SPW2-2	100	99.3±0.6	97.8±1.1	93.4±2.6
SPW2-3	100	90.1±2.3	88.2±2.5	68.3±2.7
SPW2-4	100	95.8±1.8	90.4±2.6	79.4±2.2

The effect of SPW2-3 fraction on the viability of various kinds of human-derived normal and cancer cell lines was examined. As shown in Table 4, a tendency that the SPW2-3 fraction lowered the viability of cancer cell lines more significantly than that of normal cell lines was observed. Among the cancer cell lines, the viability of breast adenocarcinoma (MCF-7), differentiated hepatoma (HuH-7), lung carcinomas (PC-8, QG-56 and QG-90) and stomach adenocarcinoma (MKN-28) was markedly decreased by the SPW2-3 fraction of spinach. These findings suggest that the dialyzate of spinach has the ability to kill the cancer cells directly.

Table 4 Effect of SPW2-3 fraction of spinach on the viability of human-derived normal and cancer cells.

Dose (μg/ml)	0	Viability(%) 0.5	1.0	2.0
Normal cells				
Bladder fetus(FHs738Bl)	100	99.4±0.5	97.9±1.6	97.4±1.5
Colon fibroblast(CCD-18Co)	100	99.2±0.6	98.4±1.3	95.3±1.2
Whole embryo(FHs173We)	100	99.3±0.6	94.1±2.2	85.1±2.3
Embryonic lung(WI-38)	100	99.4±0.3	91.6±1.1	81.7±1.9
Cancer cells				
Breast adenocarcinoma(MCF-7)	100	90.3±1.9	88.2±2.2	68.2±2.7
Eidermoid(A431)	100	95.8±1.3	95.1±2.3	80.3±2.4
Differentiated hepatoma(HuH-7)	100	86.3±2.2	75.3±2.6	57.6±3.3
Lung adenocarcinoma(PC-8)	100	93.2±2.2	86.1±2.1	71.4±2.1
Lung squamous carcinoma(QG-56)	100	95.3±1.2	92.3±1.9	76.7±2.3
Lung anaplasticcarcinoma(QG-90)	100	89.6±2.1	84.4±2.4	66.6±2.9
Bladder cancer cell(KU-1)	100	98.2±1.6	97.4±1.6	89.3±2.2
Stomach adenocarcinoma(MKN-28)	100	88.9±2.5	82.7±3.1	77.4±3.5
Melanoma(Bowes)	100	96.7±1.8	91.1±2.2	84.8±2.3

4 MORPHOLOGICAL ALTERING EFFECT OF SPINACH FRACTIONS ON U-937 CELLS

A human histiocytic lymphoma cell line, U-937, is known to be susceptible to morphological alteration in the presence of phorbol esters and vitamin D_3 derivatives and to differentiate into macrophage-like cells which attach to the culture dishes. Such induction of differentiation is used for chemotherapy of leukemia. As shown in Table 5, 1 μg/ml of SPW2-3 fraction of spinach dialyzate was found to cause morphological alteration of U-937 cells and increase in the adhesion on the culture plate (4). The more purified fraction (SPWD5) of SPW2-3 fraction increased the activity.

Table 5 Effect of SPW2-3 fraction of spinach dialyzate on the morphology of U-937 human histiocytic lymphoma cell line

	Viability(%)	Morphologically altered cells(%)
Control(PBS)	98	0
SPW2-3(1 μg/ml)	96	>5
SPWD5(0.5 μg/ml)	95	>20

The active constituents of spinach dialyzate was found to be a glycoprotein having a molecular weight of 16Kda by the following separation procedures with Sephadex G-100 gel column chromatography, 80% ethanol precipitation, 80% ammonium sulfate precipitation, hydroxyapatite column, Butyl-TOYOPEARL 650 hydrophobic column, Glyco-agarose affinity column, Mono-Q FPLC chromatography and SDS-PAGE. The specific activity of the final fraction was 654 folds that of crude extract. The binding of the active glycoprotein to the U-937 cell surface was also confirmed, suggesting that the receptor for the fraction of spinach may exist on the membrane of U-937 cells.

5. ACTIVATING EFFECT OF SPINACH ON MACROPHAGE CELLS

A purified fraction of spinach was found to activate the macrophage-like cell line (U-M) which was established from U-937 cells by TPA treatment (4). As shown in Table 6, the fraction enhanced the nitroblue tetrazolium (NBT) reduction activity and tumor necrosis factor-alpha (TNF-alpha) production of U-M cells, which are markers characteristic of macrophage cells.

Table 6 Effect of purified fraction of spinach on the NBT reducing activity and TNF-alpha production of U-M cells

Dose	NBT reducing activity(%)	TNF-alpha production
PBS	100	-
1 µg/ml	200	+
2 µg/ml	300	+

The fraction were also found to activate the U-M cells to cause a cytotoxic effect on the MCF-7 cells. The secretion of TNF-alpha of U-937 and U-M cell was increased by the treatment with the fraction.

6 OTHER FUNCTIONS OF VEGETABLES AND FRUITS

In addition to these physiological functions of vegetables and fruits, they were also found to have the promoting effect of IgM secretion of hybridoma cells which secrete the antibody to react with the human lung and breast cancer cells specifically (5). It was also observed that some constituents existing in vegetables and fruits, such as flavonoids, inhibited the killing action of UV irradiation on human cells and that spinach extracts reduced the formation of melanin pigments.

7 CONCLUSION

It was thus confirmed that vegetables and fruits have several cancer-preventory functions such as desmutagenicity, cytotoxic effect on human cancer cells, altering effect on morphology of human lymphoma cells, macrophage-activating effect, promoting effect of IgM secretion, UV-trapping effect, and inhibiting effect on melanin pigment formation. These functions of vegetables and fruits may play an important role on the cancer prevention.

REFERENCES

1. K. Shinohara, M. Kurogi, M. Miwa, Z-L. Kong and H. Hosoda, Agric. Biol. Chem., 1988, 52, 1375
2. K. Shinohara, T. Fukuda, K. Iino and Z-L. Kong, J. Jap. Soc. Food Sci. Tech., 1991, 38, 235
3. K. Shinohara, Z-L. Kong, T. Fukuda and K. Iino, J. Jap. Soc. Food Sci. Tech., 1991, 38, 242.
4. Z-L. Kong, H. Murakami and K. Shinohara, Cytotechnology, 1991, 7, 113
5. Z-L. Kong, T. Fukushima, M. Tsutsumi, K. Iino, H. Murakami and K. Shinohara, J. Jap. Soc. Food Sci. Tech., 1992, 39, 79

POTENTIAL ANTI-MUTAGENICITY AND ANTI-CARCINOGENICITY OF SOME PLANT PHENOLS

R. Walker, A.D. Ayrton and C. Ioannides

Division of Toxicology
School of Biological Sciences
University of Surrey
Guildford GU2 5XH UK

Food contains a myriad of structurally diverse chemicals capable of attenuating and even abolishing the tumourigenicity of chemical carcinogens, as repeatedly illustrated in many animal models.[1] Many anticarcinogens are naturally-occurring anutrients, primarily of plant origin, such as flavones and polyhydroxy compounds.

As most chemicals express their carcinogenicity through metabolically formed reactive intermediates that readily interact covalently with DNA, a possible mechanism of action of anticarcinogens is to perturb this process of activation, suppressing the levels of DNA-interacting intermediates. This can be achieved through one or more of the following mechanisms: (a) inhibition of the generation of the reactive intermediates; (b) enhanced detoxication of the reactive intermediates, and (c) direct interaction between the anticarcinogen and the reactive intermediate neutralising its capacity to interact with DNA.

A major group of dietary chemical carcinogens are the heterocyclic primary amines which are formed during the cooking of protein-rich food[2] and to which, therefore, humans are continuously exposed. They are mutagenic in many short term tests and are carcinogenic, at least in rodents.[2] These amines being essentially planar molecules, are activated by hepatic cytochrome P4501 (CYP1)-catalysed N-hydroxylation. The resultant hydroxylamine serves as the proximate carcinogen, and the ultimate carcinogen is believed to be the nitrenium ion which may be generated directly from the hydroxylamine or following the deconjugation of its acetyl and sulphate esters.

It was considered pertinent to investigate the antimutagenic potential of two plant phenols, ellagic acid and anthraflavic acid, using the food carcinogen IQ (2-amino-3-methylimidazo-[4,5-f] quinoline) as the model promutagen. The choice of these plant phenols was dictated by computergraphic studies which revealed that they are both essentially planar structures and thus likely to interact with the CYP1 family leading to inhibition of the IQ activation.[3,4] Moreover, in the case of ellagic acid, it has been claimed to protect against the carcinogenicity of polycyclic aromatic hydrocarbons by inhibiting their activation and by scavenging the diol-epoxides, the ultimate carcinogens, through direct interaction.[5]

Effect of Ellagic and Anthraflavic acids on CYP1 Activity and Bioactivation of IQ

Both ellagic and anthraflavic acids caused a concentration-dependent decrease in the microsome-mediated mutagenicity of IQ in the Ames mutagenicity assay (Table 1). As neither of these compounds interacts with the mutagenic intermediates of IQ,[4,6] presumably the hydroxylamine and nitrenium ion, it was concluded that the likely site of action of both phenols is to inhibit the metabolic activation, and studies were undertaken to evaluate this mode of action. Since IQ is activated specifically by the two proteins of the CYP1 family, namely A1 and A2, the effect of the two phenols on the O-deethylation of ethoxyresorufin, a probe for CYP1A1, and the metabolic activation of Glu-P-1 (2-amino-6-methyldipyrido [1,2-a:3',2'-d] imidazole), a probe for CYP1A2, were investigated. Anthraflavic acid caused a marked and concentration-dependent decrease in the O-deethylation of ethoxyresorufin and Glu-P-1 activation,[3] demonstrating inhibition of CYP1 activity and explaining its suppressive effect on IQ mutagenicity. Ellagic acid, surprisingly as it is also an essentially planar molecule, failed to inhibit either activity, and this was attributed to its hydrophilicity, preventing it from reaching the cytochrome P-450 system which is embedded in lipid.[7] Moreover, ellagic acid did not act through complexation with the magnesium ions present in the activation system.[7] Thus the mechanism by which ellagic acid inhibits the *in vitro* activation of IQ remains elusive. It has been suggested that ellagic acid may interact with DNA in such a way so as to protect binding sites, preventing the interaction of the IQ reactive intermediates with DNA.[8]

Table 1 Effect of anthraflavic and ellagic acids on the mutagenicity of IQ in the Ames test

IQ (100 ng/plate), *Salmonella typhimurium* TA98 and Aroclor 1254-induced hepatic S9 activation system (10% $^{v}/v$) were employed in the test. The spontaneous reversion rate of 25 ± 6 has already been subtracted.

Plant phenol and concentration (M)		Induced mutagenic response (Histidine revertants/plate)
Anthraflavic acid	0	9406 ± 1701
	10^{-7}	8371 ± 356
	10^{-6}	8155 ± 674
	10^{-5}	7536 ± 653
	10^{-4}	1279 ± 417
Ellagic acid	0	10352 ± 860
	10^{-7}	9087 ± 292
	10^{-6}	8520 ± 370
	10^{-5}	7656 ± 495
	10^{-4}	1424 ± 201

Results are presented as Mean ± SD for triplicates.

Effect of treatment with ellagic or anthraflavic acids on rat hepatic CYP1 and glutathione S-transferase activities

Animals were treated with daily intraperitoneal injections of the phenol (100 mg/kg) for five days and were killed 24 hours after the last administration. The objectives were two-fold; (a) to establish whether anthraflavic acid retains its inhibitory effect on CYP1 activity after *in vivo* administration or it behaves like other inhibitors where the inhibitory phase is followed by induction of the same protein(s), and (b) to determine whether the major detoxicating enzyme system, the glutathione S-transferases, is enhanced by treatment with these phenols, thus providing an additional feasible mechanism of the anticarcinogenic effect of ellagic acid.

As presented in Table 2, ellagic acid suppressed the levels of total cytochrome P-450 and inhibited the activity of all the enzymes studied. In contrast, treatment with anthraflavic acid stimulated the O-deethylations of ethoxyresorufin and ethoxycoumarin. These findings indicate that *in vivo* administration of anthraflavic acid increases CYP1 activity and explains the observations that hepatic microsomes from anthraflavic acid-treated rats are more efficient than control microsomes in metabolically converting IQ to mutagens,[7] in marked contrast to the *in vitro* situation. At the dose utilised in the present study, ellagic acid appears to exert a toxic effect on the liver, leading to non-specific destruction of cytochrome P-450 and loss of xenobiotic metabolising capacity. It is worth pointing out that, even during the short duration of treatment employed in the present study, animals exposed to ellagic acid experienced body weight loss (results not shown).

Table 2 Hepatic microsomal and cytosolic xenobiotic metabolism in animals exposed to ellagic and anthraflavic acids

Parameter	Control	Anthraflavic acid	Ellagic acid
Total Cytochrome P-450 (nmol/mg protein)	0.47 ± 0.01	0.52 ± 0.04	0.25 ± 0.01*
Ethoxycoumarin O-deethylase (pmnol/min per mg protein)	42 ± 7	87 ± 13*	20 ± 3*
Ethoxyresorufin O-deethylase (pmol/min per mg protein)	92 ± 1	314 ± 50*	68 ± 10
Glutathione S-transferase (DCNB) (nmol/min per mg protein)	78 ± 5	71 ± 11	54 ± 4*

* $P < 0.05$. Results presented as Mean ± SEM for five animals.

CONCLUSIONS

An approach commonly employed currently to evaluate the antimutagenic/anticarcinogenic potential of chemicals involves incorporating them into the S9-activation system employed in the Ames test, in the presence of various model promutagens and determining mutagenic response. Mechanisms of action are largely ignored and the assumption is made that the *in vitro* findings can be readily extrapolated to the *in vivo* situation. As the studies presented here concerned with anthraflavic acid clearly illustrate, this oversimplistic approach is misleading with possible serious consequences. Anthraflavic acid was a potent inhibitor of the IQ-mediated mutagenicity *in vitro* but, when administered *in vivo*, it enhanced the mutagenic response by virtue of its ability to induce the CYP1 family of proteins responsible for the bioactivation of IQ to the proximate carcinogen. Under such circumstances it would be expected that not only would anthraflavic acid not afford protection, but could actually exacerbate the carcinogenicity of IQ and of other carcinogens that rely on the CYP1 family for their activation.

Ellagic acid is also an effective inhibitor of the *in vitro* IQ-mediated mutagenesis in the Ames test but its mechanism of action is not clear. However, when administered intraperitoneally to rats, at doses previously associated with anticarcinogenicity, ellagic acid displayed a toxic effect which provoked loss of metabolising activity. It is therefore reasonable to infer that the reported protective effect of ellagic acid against chemical carcinogens represents, at least partly, decreased bioactivation as a result of toxicity. As ellagic acid has been shown to be poorly absorbed,[9] ingestion of this phenol in the diet would not be expected to result in serum levels which on the one hand would be anticarcinogenic or on the other, would be hepatotoxic.

ACKNOWLEDGEMENTS

The authors acknowledge with gratitude financial support of part of this work by the Ministry of Agriculture, Fisheries and Food (Grant No.530).

REFERENCES

1. L.W. Wattenberg, Cancer Res., 1992, 52, 2085.
2. E. Overvik and J.-A. Gustafsson, Mutagenesis, 1990, 5, 437.
3. A.D. Ayrton, D.F.V. Lewis, C. Ioannides and R. Walker, Biochim. Biophys. Acta, 1987, 916, 328.
4. A.D. Ayrton, D.F.V. Lewis, R. Walker and C. Ioannides, Fd. Chem. Toxic., 1992, In press.
5. P. Lesca, Carcinogenesis, 1983, 4, 1651.
6. A.D. Ayrton, C. Ioannides and R. Walker, Mutat. Res., 1988, 207, 121.
7. A.D. Ayrton, C. Ioannides and R. Walker, Fd. Chem. Toxic., 1988, 26, 909.
8. R.W. Teel, Cancer Let., 1986, 30, 329.
9. R.C. Smart, M.-T. Huang, R.L. Chang, J.M. Sayer, D.M. Jerina and A.H. Conney, Carcinogenesis, 1986, 7, 1663.

INHIBITION OF NITROSAMINE-INDUCED TUMORIGENESIS BY DIALLYL SULFIDE AND TEA

C. S. Yang, J-Y. Hong, and Z.-Y. Wang

Laboratory for Cancer Research
College of Pharmacy, Rutgers University
Piscataway, NJ 08855, U.S.A.

INTRODUCTION

A large number of food chemicals have been shown or implicated to possess inhibitory activites against tumor formation or growth. Before we can call these compounds anticarcinogens, it is very important for us to understand their mechanisms of action and the possible relevance of this action to human health. In this paper, we shall discuss our work on diallyl sulfide and tea to illustrate some of the mechanisms involved and the issues concerning the relevance of this work.

EFFECTS OF DIALLYL SULFIDE ON CYTOCHROMES P450, CHEMICAL TOXICITY, AND CARCINOGENESIS

Fresh garlic contains a vast number of organosulfur compounds, among which alliin is the major component. Through the action of the enzyme alliinase, cooking, or metabolism, allicin, diallyl disulfide, diallyl sulfide (DAS), methyl allyl sulfide, and other organosulfur compounds are formed [1]. The actions of DAS have been studied extensively and will be discussed herein to illustrate the possible mechanisms of its inhibitory actions against chemically-induced toxicity and tumorigenesis. The specific effects of DAS on different P450 enzymes were demonstrated in the following experiment. After an oral dose of DAS (100 or 200 mg/kg) to the rat, the total P450 content and P450 reductase activity were affected only slightly[2]. However, a clear time-dependent decrease in the P450 2E1-dependent *N*-nitrosodimethylamine (NDMA) demethylase activity in liver microsomes was observed; the activity was lowest (<20% of the control) at 12 h and recovered after 2 days. On the other hand, the pentoxyresorufin dealkylase activity (mainly due to P450 2B1) was greatly enhanced, reaching a plateau of 100-fold increase between 24 to 48 h. When diallyl sulfone ($DASO_2$) was given to the rat, the NDMA demethylase activity decreased very rapidly [2]. Subsequent studies demonstrated that DAS was metabolized to diallyl sulfoxide and then to $DASO_2$ which was a suicide inhibitor of P450 2E1 [3]. In addition, DAS, $DASO_2$, and diallyl sulfoxide were all competitive inhibitors of P450 2E1. The structures and the metabolism of these compounds are shown in Fig. 1. A weaker activity in inactivation of P450 2E1 was observed with methyl allyl sulfide, but diallyl disulfide or dipropyl sulfide did not inactivate P450 2E1.

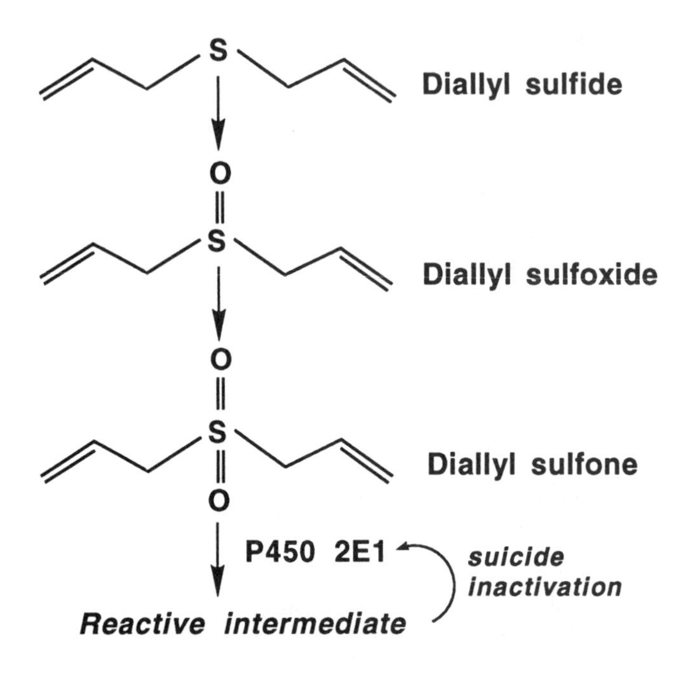

Figure 1. Structure and Metabolism of Diallyl Sulfide

Since P450 2E1 is vital in catalyzing the activation of NDMA, 1,2-dimethylhydrazine (DMH), benzene, alkanes, halogenated hydrocarbons, and many other low molecular weight environmental chemicals [4,5], inhibition of this enzyme is expected to block the toxicity and carcinogenicity of these compounds. The inhibition of NDMA- and CCl_4-induced hepatotoxicity by DAS has been demonstrated [2]. The inhibition of P450 2E1-dependent activation of carcinogens is the most likely molecular mechanism for the reported inhibitory action of DAS against DMH-induced hepatotoxicity and colon carcinogenesis in rats [6,7] as well as DMH-induced colon nuclear aberrations in mice [8].

In theory, inhibition of the metabolic activation of a toxicant or a carcinogen in the liver, could reduce hepatotoxicity and hepatocarcinogenesis. However, it may increase the exposure of nonhepatic tissues to this toxic compound and thus enhance carcinogenesis in the nonhepatic organs [9]. In the following example, however, a net benefit without increased risk is possible. Acetaminophen (APAP), a widely-used analgesic, is mostly metabolized by the formation of glucuronide and sulfate conjugates and is subsequently excreted. A small percent of APAP can be oxidized by P450 2E1 and other enzymes to a toxic intermediate, *N*-acetyl-*p*-benzoquinone imine. If not promptly removed by reacting with glutathione, this intermediate could react with key cellular components and lead to hepatotoxicity, as in the case of overdose. In alcoholics, toxicity may be produced even with therapeutic doses of APAP. Because of the inhibitory actions of DAS and $DASO_2$ against P450 2E1-catalyzed reactions, we predicted that these compounds would prevent APAP induced hepatotoxicity. This prediction has been confirmed recently in both rats and mice [10]. At a dose of 15 or 50 mg/kg, a protective effect of $DASO_2$ was observed when given prior, concomitantly with, or within 3 h after a toxic dose of APAP in the rat. In mice, the protective effect could also be observed if $DASO_2$ was given within 20 min of the APAP dose. $DASO_2$ is water soluble, devoid of the garlic smell, and with low toxicity; it has a potential for practical application.

INHIBITION OF 4-(METHYLNITROSAMINO)-1-(3-PYRIDYL)-1-BUTANONE-INDUCED LUNG TUMORIGENESIS BY DAS AND $DASO_2$

4-(Methylnitrosamino)-1-(3-pyridyl)-1-butanone (NNK) is a potent tobacco carcinogen which may be important in human cancer etiology. It was observed that oral adminstration of DAS markedly decreased the rate of NNK bioactivation in rat lung and nasal mucosa microsomes [11, 12]. This decrease in metabolic activation activity appears not to be related to P450 2E1 inactivation, and the mechanisms remain to be elucidated. However, this result suggested that DAS would inhibit NNK-induced lung tumorigenesis. This activity was demonstrated experimentally. When a single dose of NNK (2 mg/mouse, i.p.) was given to female A/J mice, almost all the animals developed lung adenomas after 16 weeks with an average of 9 tumors per mouse. When DAS was given to the mice orally at a daily dose of 200 mg/kg for 3 days before the NNK dosing, the tumor incidence was reduced by 60% and tumor multiplicity was decreased by 90% [13]. A similar inhibitory action was also produced with $DASO_2$ at a dose of 100 mg/kg; at a dose of 20 mg/kg the inhibitory action was weaker.

INHIBITION OF NNK-INDUCED LUNG TUMORIGENESIS BY TEA

Using the same animal model, we studied the effects of tea on tumorigenesis [14]. When decaffeinated green or black tea extracts (0.6%) were given to female A/J mice as the sole source of drinking water from 2 weeks prior to and until 1 week after the NNK treatment, tumor multiplicity was reduced by 65%. When the tea extract was given one week after the NNK-treatment until the end of the experiment, 0.6% green tea extract decreased the tumor incidence and tumor multiplicity by 30 and 85%, respectively. In this protocol, 0.6% black tea extract reduced tumor multiplicity by 63% but did not significantly affect the tumor incidence [14]. In a similar experiment, oral administration of 0.6% green or black tea extracts during the NNK-treatment period was found to inhibit the NNK-caused DNA methylation in the lung by about 30% [15]. When added to microsomal incubation mixtures, green or black tea polyphenol fractions or (-) epigallocatechin-3-gallate inhibited the bioactivation of NNK [15].

INHIBITION OF *N*-NITROSOMETHYLBENZYLAMINE (NMBzA)-INDUCED ESOPHAGEAL TUMORIGENESIS BY TEA

In this study, male S.D. rats were given NMBzA (2.5 mg/kg, s.c.) twice weekly for 5 weeks. At 39 weeks after starting the NMBzA treatment, 65% of the rats developed esophageal tumors with an average of 1.4 tumors per rat. When given to rats as the sole source of drink water during the carcinogen-treatment period, decaffeinated green or black tea extracts (0.6%) were equally effective, decreasing tumor incidence and tumor multiplicity by 74% and 71%, respectively[16]. When given after the NMBzA-treatment period until the end of the experiment, tumor incidence and multiplicity were decreased, but the result was not statistically significant. The tumor size, however, was drastically decreased due to tea adminstration, especially with black tea in the latter protocol[16].

MECHANISTIC CONSIDERATIONS AND RELEVANCE TO HUMAN HEALTH

The preventive activity of DAS against NNK, DMH, and NMBzA-induced tumorigenesis is most likely to be due to inhibition of the bioactivation of these carcinogens. DAS is the most active compound from garlic tested so far. However, other mechanisms may also be involved. Wattenberg *et al.* [17] suggested that some of the organosulfur compounds may serve as scavengers for electrophilic intermediates of carcinogens. The anticarcinogenic components in tea still remain to be identified. In green tea, (-)epigallocatechin-3-gallate, (-)epicatechin, (-)epigallocatechin, and (-)epicatechin-3-gallate are the major polyphenols. In the manufacture of black tea, theaflavins and thearubigins are formed through polyphenol oxidase-catalyzed oxidation and polymerization. The structures of these polyphenols are shown in Fig. 2. These compounds are strong antioxidants. The antioxidative activity and perhaps antiproliferative activity may be important for the antitumorigenic effects of tea. The inhibition of 8-hydroxydeoxyguanosine formation by green tea administration has been reported recently [18]. In addition, the inhibition of NNK bioactivation by green and black tea has also been demonstrated *in vivo* and *in vitro* [15].

The present work demonstrates interesting biological activities of chemicals in garlic and tea in the inhibition of chemically-induced tumorigenesis in animals. Caution must be applied when relating these results to the possible prevention of human cancer. Although epidemiological studies have shown an inverse correlation between the consumption of garlic (and other allium vegetables) and the incidence of gastric cancer in certain areas [19, 20], broad-based strong protective effects against other cancers have not been reported. Even if garlic can be demonstrated to have clear-cut effects against carcinogenesis, the role of DAS in such a protection function still remains to be determined because it does not occur in large quantities in our diet. The possible application of $DASO_2$ or related compounds as prophylactics against chemical toxicity and carcinogenesis remains to be explored. On the other hand, tea is taken in rather large quantities by many individuals in certain areas. The estimated levels of human consumption are still lower than the levels used in the present studies, but they may be in the same order of magnitude. Nevertheless, there is no clear-cut human data to indicate a protective function of tea against lung or esophageal cancer. It is reasonable to suggest that the possible protective function of tea against certain types of cancer is related to the specific causative factors involved. Thus, conclusions obtained on one cancer from one population may be different from those on other cancers or on other populations. Concerns also exist on whether the consumption of tea increases the incidence of certain cancers. A recent review of the literature indicates that there is inadequate evidence for the carcinogenicity of tea drinking in humans and experimental animals [21]. It would be a challenge for researchers to systematically and repeatedly study certain populations to delineate the etiology and to assess the possible protective effect of tea against specific cancers.

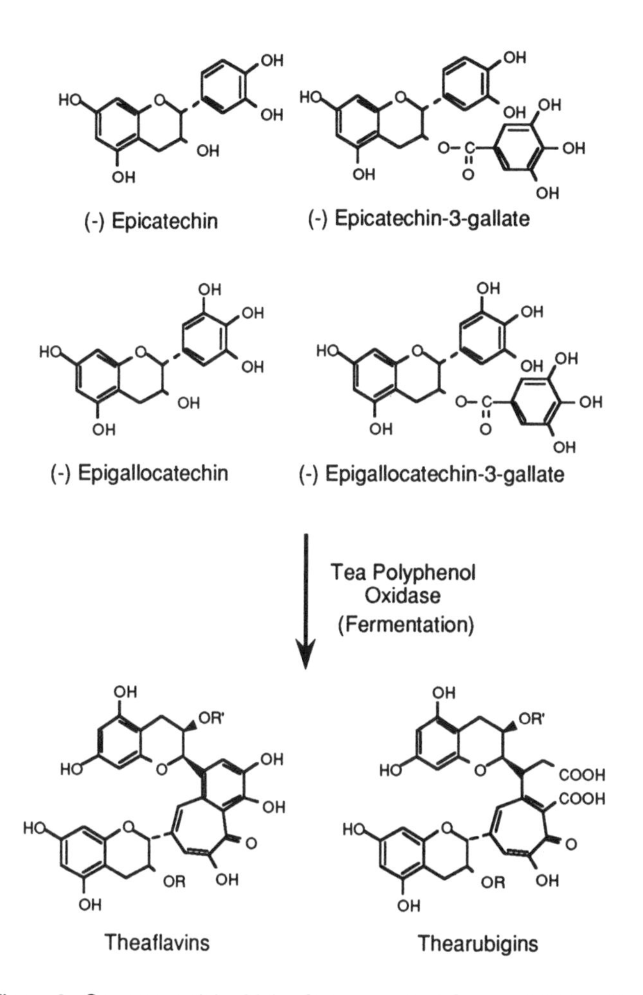

Figure 2. Structures of the Major Components of Green and Black Tea

REFERENCES

1. E. Block *Scient. Am.* 1985, *252*, 114-119.
2. J. F. Brady; M.-H. Wang; J.-Y. Hong; F. Xiao; Y. Li; J.-S. H. Yoo; S. M. Ning; J. M. Fukuto; J. M. Gapac and C. S. Yang *Toxicol. Appl. Pharmacol.* 1991, *108*, 342-354.
3. J. F. Brady; H. Ishizaki; J. M. Fukuto; M. C. Lin; A. Fadel; J. M. Gapac and C. S. Yang *Chem. Res. Toxicol.* 1991, *4*, 642-647.
4. C. S. Yang; J.-S. H. Yoo; H. Ishizaki and J.-Y. Hong *Drug Metab. Rev.* 1990, *22*, 147-160.
5. C. S. Yang; J. F. Brady and J.-Y. Hong *FASEB J.* 1992, *6*, 737-744.
6. M. A. Hayes; T. H. Rushmore and M. T. Goldberg *Carcinogenesis (Lond.)* 1987, *8*, 1155-1157.
7. M. J. Wargovich *Carcinogenesis (Lond.)* 1987, *8*, 487-489.
8. M. J. Wargovich and M. T. Goldberg *Mutat. Res.* 1985, *143*, 127-129.
9. L. M. Anderson *Carcinogenesis (Lond.)* 1988, *9*, 1717-1719.
10. M. C. Lin; E.-J. Wang; C. Patten; M.-J. Lee; F. Xiao; K. Reuhl and C. S. Yang *Toxicol. Appl. Pharmacol.* 1992, (submitted for publication).
11. J.-Y. Hong; T. Smith; J. F. Brady; M. Lee; B. Ma; W. Li; S. M. Ning and C. S. Yang *Proc. Am. Assoc. Cancer Res.* 1990, *31*, 120.
12. J.-Y. Hong; T. Smith; M.-J. Lee; W. Li; B.-L. Ma; S.-M. Ning; J. F. Brady; P. E. Thomas and C. S. Yang *Cancer Res.* 1991, *51*, 1509-1514.
13. J.-Y. Hong; Z.-Y. Wang; T. Smith; S. Zhou; S. Shi and C. S. Yang *Carcinogenesis (Lond.)* 1992, *13*, 901-904.
14. Z. Y. Wang; J.-Y. Hong; M.-T. Huang; K. Reuhl; A. H. Conney and C. S. Yang *Cancer Res.* 1992, *52*, 1943-1947.
15. S. T. Shi; Z. Y. Wang and C. S. Yang 1992, (manuscript in preparation).
16. Z. Y. Wang; L. D. Wang; W. F. Cheng; M. T. Huang; A. H. Conney and C. S. Yang 1992, (manuscript in preparation).
17. L. W. Wattenberg; V. L. Sparnins and G. Barany *Cancer Res.* 1989, *49*, 2689-2692.
18. Y. Xu; C.-T. Ho; S. G. Amin; C. Han and F.-L. Chung *Cancer Res.* 1992, *52*, 3875-3879.
19. W.-C. You; W. J. Blot; Y.-S. Chang; A. G. Ershow; Z.-Y. Yang; Q. An; B. Henderson; G.-W. Xu; J. F. J. Fraumeni and T.-G. Wang *Cancer Res.* 1988, *48*, 3518-3523.
20. E. Buiatti; D. Palli; A. Decarli; D. Amadori; C. Avellini; S. Bianchi; R. Biserni; F. Cipriani; P. Cocco; A. Giacosa; E. Marubini; R. Puntoni; C. Vindigni; J. J. Fraumeni and W. Blot *Int. J. Cancer* 1989, *44*, 611-616.
21. International Agency for Research on Cancer "Coffee methylxenthines, and methylglyoxal." *IARC Monographs* 1991, *51*, 207-271.

PART 5 SUPPRESSING TUMOUR DEVELOPMENT: THE ROLE OF DIET IN THE MODULATION OF CELL PROLIFERATION

ROLE OF DIETARY FACTORS IN THE MODULATION OF CANCER INDUCTION

M. B. ROBERFROID

UNIVERSITE CATHOLIQUE DE LOUVAIN, SCHOOL OF PHARMACY,
UNIT OF BIOCHEMICAL TOXICOLOGY AND CANCEROLOGY,
UCL 7369, B-1200 BRUSSELS BELGIUM

1 INTRODUCTION

Differences in cancer rates between countries and changes in rate among migrants are classical indirect evidences in favor of the implication of diet as potentially important. (1) In addition to epidemiology, experimental research has also given support to the hypothesis of a role of diets in the etiology of cancer mainly breast and colon cancers.

Both approaches have identified specific dietary factors as primary targets for preventive recommendations. Content and/or nature of fats , fibre and micronutrients (vitamins and oligoelements e.g., Se) as well as calorie intake are the most frequently quoted candidates. (2-5)

By quoting these data from epidemiologic and animal studies, health authorities both in Europe and in North America are advocating recommendations for reduction in dietary fat intake and increase in dietary fiber content as major clues for cancer prevention. However the scientific basis for such recommendations have been repeatedly questioned and controversial arguments have been developed. (5-10)

To study experimentally the influence of diets containing low vs high fat, saturated vs unsaturated lipids, low vs high fibre, fermented vs non-fermented polysaccharides, low vs high calorie, chemical carcinogenesis is most frequently used as a model process. By reference to the two (multi) step theory of carcinogenesis, such dietary factors are classified as promoter, antipromoter, co-carcinogen, anticarcinogen ... according to some characteristics of their effects as proposed by Wattenberg. (11) To review the experimental evidences pro-and con an etiological role of these dietary factors in breast and colon carcinogenesis can thus not be made without reference to this theory. The objectives of the present communication are : (a) to discuss, in some details, the two stage theory of chemical carcinogenesis with the aim, (b) to introduce the concept of modulation as a new tool, (12-16) (c) to review these experimental evidences with the hope it might help resolving the argument.

2. PATTERNS OF EXPERIMENTAL NEOPLASTIC DEVELOPMENT, THE MULTISTAGE HYPOTHESIS

Nearly all proposed definitions of cancer emphasize the characteristically progressive, disproportionate and seemingly purposeless overgrowth of a tissue that continues indefinitely after all known or suspected inciting stimuli have ceased to operate. (17)

Chemical carcinogenesis, a reference model to study neoplastic development

During many years (up to the early fifties), experimental study of cancer has most exclusively been limited to either "spontaneous" tumor development (mostly mammary tumors) or, tumor induction (mostly in skin) by repeated administration of a chemical or a mixture of chemicals (e.g. tar). Since the fifties, after the pioneering works of Rous and Kidd, (18) Berenblum, (19, 20) Berenblum and Shubik, (21, 22) chemically induced carcinogenesis has become a reference model to study neoplastic development. These studies have all confirmed the long lasting and progressive nature of neoplastic development as well as, in many cases, the existence of qualitatively different stages that preceed the appearance of malignancy. They are at the origin of two (multi) stage theory of carcinogenesis.

The concept of initiation (I)

In that framework, initiation (I) is the necessary event without which neoplasia would never occur. It can even be the sufficientevent since a single dose of some carcinogens induces a full neoplastic development without any subsequent treatment. (23-27) "I" is the treatment that induces latent neoplastic potentialities in cells which then advance, at varied, often extremely slow rates, towards the neoplastic state(s).

The concept of promotion (P)

Promotion (P) which, as opposed to "I", might not obligatorily be a step in neoplastic development, means selection and clonal proliferation of initiated cells induced by a chemical compound or an other factor applied repeatedly or acting chronically. As a consequence, less trivial-transient lesions may be formed whereas more frequent clonal foci of phenotypically altered cells emerge some of which being more prone to malignancy, so that the risk as well as the kineticsof their progression to malignancy may increase. According to the classical theory, such a definition applies only to treatment occurring after "I". (28)

The two stage theory of carcinogenesis : a critical attitude

Based on such observations, a simplified view of neoplastic development describes it as a two (multi) step process resulting from two fundamentally different mechanisms : initiation and promotion. But this view ignores : (a) that "spontaneous" carcinogenesis exists; (b) that a single dose of a carcinogen is, in some cases, (23-27) sufficient to induce a full neoplastic development; (c) that most reports on so-called promotion of carcinogenesis rely on the counting of phenotypically altered lesions (papilloma on skin, foci and nodules in liver...) without any evaluation of incidence and/or yield of subsequent malignant tumors which are the only true end point of neoplastic development; (d) that treatments do exist which, even though they reduce the incidence of phenotypically altered lesions, still shorten the latency period for malignant tumor development and increase its kinetics; (29) (e)that surgical and dietary manipulations performed before (e.g. partial hepatectomy), during and/or after (e.g. porto caval shunt) "I" enhance neoplastic development as evaluated by incidence and yield of malignant tumors. (30-32) All these treatments, which are not obligatory to, but can qualitatively and/or quantitatively modify the outcome of neoplastic development in experimental animals, are not strictly equivalent to promotion. They are more general because their effect(s) is (are) on the neoplastic development as a whole. Futhermore they can be applied before, during and/or after "I" and finally (and most importantly), their effects are on incidence and/or yield of malignant tumors not on neoplastic lesions. Moreover "promotion" is only seen as a treatment which enhances neoplastic development not considering the possibility that it might hinder it by slowing down its progression or by reducing the incidence and/or the yield of tumors. Expressions like "inhibition of carcinogenesis, anticarcinogenesis, antitumor promotion, chemoprevention of cancer,..." are used to cover these aspects. (11, 33, 34)

3. MODULATION OF NEOPLASTIC DEVELOPMENT

With all that in mind we have recently proposed the term <u>modulation</u> to account for these modifications/ changes in the pattern(s) of neoplastic development as evaluated by counting histologically identified malignant tumors as end point. (12-15, 35) <u>Modulation</u> is then defined as the effect of any treatment which given before, during and/or after "I" modifies the pattern of neoplastic development as evaluated by the kinetics of appearance, the incidence, the yield (quantitative effects) and/or the nature (qualitative effects) of malignant tumors emerging at one particular site. In our terminology, <u>modulation</u> is said to be either positive or negative if its effect(s) is (are) respectively as described in table 1. Based on our present understanding of this concept we hypothesize that any treatment or feeding protocol which creates a metabolic or proliferative unbalance (a rupture in homeostasis) will have the potential to positively modulatle carcinogenesis. On the contrary, any treatment or feeding protocol which restores or helps restoring metabolic or proliferative balance (homeostasis) will have the potential to negatively modulate it.

Table 1 Summary of the effect of positive and negative modulation on neoplastic development.

Criteria to evaluate modulation of neoplastic development	Nature of the modulator	
	Positive	Negative
Malignant tumor		
Kinetics of formation	speading up	slowing down
Incidence	higher	lower
Yield	higher	lower
Degree of malignancy	= or +	= or -
Invasiveness	= or +	= or -

One effect is sufficient to conclude to modulation.

4. DIETARY MODULATION OF NEOPLASTIC DEVELOPMENT

Diet is an essential element of health. Nutritionists have advocated the concept of "balanced diet" that, if eaten regularly, provides what is required for a healthy life. This concept implies that any dietary unbalance due either to nutrition deficiencies or to changes in the intake of selected macronutrients may cause physiological disturbances and disequilibria that are potentially pathogenic. For cancer more than for any other diseases the role of these factors, in particular fat, calorie or fiber intake, has been questioned repeatedly.

Dietary fat and modulation of neoplastic development

Both the nature (saturated vs unsaturated/animal vs vegetal) and the amount of fat in diet have been modified experimentally with the aim to study the influence of fat on neoplastic development. Skin, mammary glands, the pancreas and the colon were the most frequent targets of spontaneous or chemically induced cancers in these studies (for review on Fat and Tumorigenesis see 2, 36, 37). Due to differences in strain of animals, in protocol of carcinogenesis (in particular the nature and the dose of the carcinogen but also the timing of sacrifices), in the composition of food, in source and nature of fat, in protocol for anatomo-pathological analysis... the results of most of these studies are difficult to compare. Moreover the results are somehow contradictory and they are regarded by many authors as highly questionable so that the relationship between fat intake and the occurrence of tumors in experimental animals remains controversial. (5, 9, 38)

The results of carefully protocoled investigations with correctly designed diets that provide equivalent nutrient over calorie ratio and that are supplemented with some vitamins consistently show no significant differences in tumor incidence or yield between animals fed low-or high fat diets. (5, 39-41) Working in our laboratory for her Ph D thesis, Masereel M.(personal communication, manuscripts in preparation) has similarly demonstrated that isocaloric diets containing 5, 10, 15 and 20% of a mixture of vegetable fats (1/3rd saturated, 1/3rd monounsaturated, 1/3rd polyunsaturated) given to rats that had previously been treated with 15 weekly s.c. injections of 13.6 mg/kg b.w. 1,2 dimethylhydrazine do not differently modulate neoplastic development. Indeed, the kineticsof development, the incidence and the yield of malignant tumors, at any sacrifice, were not significantly different in the 4 groups of rats.

It seems thus reasonable to conclude that dietary fat per se does not act simply as a modulator of neoplastic development. That does not mean however that high fat diet does not either. Indeed, modifications of food composition that : (a) do not take into account the difference in calorie density of fats as compared to carbohydrates and proteins; (b) that lead to dilution of micronutrients due to increase in fat content; or (c) that create deficiencies in essential nutrient such for example as essential fatty acid due to the use of animal fat as sole source of lipids, (43) all create dietary unbalances that, due to physiological disturbances, may indirectly modulate tumorigenesis at various sites including skin, breast, pancreas, colon,... In particular, the conclusion that the enhancing effects of high fat diet on chemically induced skin and breast carcinogenesis could mainly be due to higher calorie rather than to higher fat intake was already known in the early forties. (43-45) It has been confirmed more recently by Kritchevsky et al. (46, 47) and Pariza. (48)

Calorie intake and modulation of neoplastic development

Already in the late forties, Boutwell et al. proposed that the net energy value of a high fat diet could account for its enhancing effect on carcinogenesis. (49) As a tentative explanation, it has been argued (50) that : (a) an animal fed a high fat diet spends less energy for heat but retains more energy in the carcass than an animal fed a low fat diet; (b) the body uses calories from fat more efficiently than calories from carbohydrates or proteins; (c) fat can also increase intestinal transit time, which may favor increased nutrient absorption; (d) high levels of dietary fat depress blood flow through and heat production by brown adipose tissue; (e) all these effects would increase the efficiency of energy utilization. The concept has thus emerged that calorie restriction could be an effective way to prevent cancer.

Recent reports have successfully adressed this question and they have provided convincing arguments including hypotheses for mechanism of action (for reviews see 51, 52). By comparing the effects of calories and fat (low fat vs high fat calorie diets) in virgin female Sprague-Dawley rats treated with a single oral dose of 7,12 dimethylbenz(a)anthracene (DMBA), Kritchevsky et al. have shown that feeding a low fat-high calorie diet prior to DMBA feeding led to the greatest number of tumors per tumor bearing rat. (46, 47) When rats were maintained, after DMBA feeding, on a calorie restricted (by 40%) regimen that provided the same amount of vitamins, minerals and fiber but 2.15 times as much fat as the controls, the incidences of mammary tumors was 0% in the restricted group as compared to 58% in the control group.

Boissonneault et al. have reported that rats can consume a high fat diet and yet develop fewer tumors than rats fed a low-fat diet if net energy, as distinct from percent of fat or calories per se, is restricted. (50) They concluded that tumor appearance depends upon a complex interaction involving energy intake, energy retention and ultimate body size.

By multivariate regression analyses of the data from 82 published experiments involving several tumor sites in mice, Albanes showed that, regardless of the level of dietary fat, tumor incidence increased with increasing calorie intake and body weight over a wide range of intakes. (4) This author concluded that calorie intake is an important determinant of tumorigenesis in mice. He further hypothesized that body weight may be a more sensitive indicator for this effect than is calorie intake alone.

Similar results have been obtained with protocols in which spontaneous pulmonary tumors (in A mice), (53) leukemia (in AK mice), (54) and lymphomas (in mice), (55) (leukemia induced by whole body X-ray irradiation of rats (56) and azoxymethane-induced colon tumors in male F344 rats (57) were used as end-points of neoplastic development. Underfeeding consistently lowered the incidence of cancers. But, since it is not always clearly demonstrated that these were malignant tumors, we cannot always definitely conclude on a negative modulation.

The mechanisms by which the decreased intake of nutritional energy affects the cancer incidence and/or mortality rate are probably complex and, as yet, not fully understood.(52) One of the hypothesis is that dietary restriction may lead to a changed hormonal balance that may contribute to the inhibition of tumorigenesis.(58) It has also been suggested that animals on restricted food intake have lower metabolic rates, an enhanced immuno-competence, a reduced rate of cell proliferation, a higher level of enzymatic defense mechanisms against free radicals and that they absorb a significantly higher amount of Vitamin A through the small intestine (for a review see 52).

All these data as well as the hypothetical mechanisms are consistent with our proposal that calorie restriction negatively modulates neoplastic development in experimental animals. It is most effective if it is applied very early in life and if it is maintained for most of the lifespan. Its effect through hormonal balance, metabolic regulation, control of cell proliferation and increased immunocompetence, if confirmed, would agree with our hypothesis of negative modulation via a reinforced stability of the physiological behavior of cells or tissues in a more resistant environment.

Dietary fibers and modulation of neoplastic development

It is generally accepted that dietary fiber may have the property of negatively modulating neoplastic development in the large bowel. However, dietary fiber being a generic term that includes a number of substances, one has to be very cautious when making such claim because the effect of one particular substance might not be that of an other. Such a remark is even reinforced by the results of experimental studies (most exclusively in the rats in which intestinal tumors were chemically induced) which have examined the possible role of various types of dietary fiber. Indeed, these results are conflicting. As pointed out by Reddy (37) this discrepancy might have been, in part, due : to the nature, the dose and the number of doses of the carcinogen used, to differences in the susceptibility of rat strain to carcinogen treatment, to variation in the composition of diets, to qualitative and quantitative differences in administered intact fibers and their components, to relative differences in food intake and/or in rate of body weight growth, to differences in experimental design and duration of the experiment, to absence of clearly defined criteria for histological identification of the tumors.

Among the various dietary fibers which are available, wheat bran has received much of the attention. The majority (9 out of 13) of the studies designed to test its effect have concluded on a reduced risk of chemically induced colon cancer provided the wheat bran-rich diet was given before, during and after or, at the least after, the exposure to the carcinogen. Other products like corn, rice, soybean or oat brans have also been tested at least once but, in general, they are not very active in inhibiting neoplastic development. For the pectins, 5 out of 8 studies show no inhibition or even (in 3 out of 8 studies) an enhancement of chemically induced colon carcinogenesis. With cellulose, the results are contradictory if the fiber rich diet is given only during the period that follows the exposure to the carcinogen. But this product is protective in most of the studies (5 out of 7) in which it has been given before, during and after the exposure to the carcinogen. With miscellaneous products like Guar gum, carrageenan or alfalfa the results are disappointing and contradictory. Either they have no effect (3 studies out of 7), an enhancing effect (3 studies out of 7) or an inhibitory effect (1 study out of 7).

By computing the results of all available studies one obtains the following figures : ± 50% show inhibiton, ± 30% show no effect and ± 20% show an enhancement of chemically induced neoplastic development on the rat colon. It must be underlined however that in most of the positive studies (±80%) the inhibitory effect appears only when the fiber rich diet contains at least 15% of the product (bran, cellulose, ...). Only a few studies (±20%) have shown an effect at concentration of 10% or less. (59)

The mechanisms by which fiber rich diet could act as negative modulator of neoplastic development in the colon are still a question of much debate. It is generally accepted that consumption of high fiber diet is associated with increased stool bulk and faster intestinal transit. It has thus been hypothesized that these effects would lead to a dilution of any carcinogens or promoters present within the intestinal lumen while decreasing the time available for their interaction with the intestinal epithelium. (60) Among the potential promoters of colonic carcinogenesis that may be diluted by fiber rich diet are the secondary biliary acids that furthermore could bind to certain dietary fibers. (61) Other hypotheses tend to relate the effects of fiber with : (a) modulation of pancreatic enzyme activity; (b) change in large bowel mucosal growth cell proliferation and crypt cell migration; (c) alterations in epithelial cell nutrient transport and absorption or epithelial cell metabolic processes; (d) deficiencies of certain nutrients, in particular minerals such as zinc, iron and possibly calcium known to affect cell proliferation and differentiation.

Such effects are however not always clearly related to inhibition of carcinogenesis (for a review and a discussion see 62). More recently (for further discussion see 5) however, it has become recognized that a high content of fiber can alter the availability of other nutrients in the diet and, in general, may influence the availability of calories. (63) Furthermore, the feeding of excessively high levels of fiber can compromise food intake and body growth (64) because of a decreased availability of nutrients for digestion and assimilation from the intestine, because of increased fecal loss of fat and nitrogen and therefore because of a reduced availability of calories. (65) Finally and most importantly,dietary fibers undergo fermentation in the large bowel resulting in the production of short chain fatty acids principally acetate, propinate, butyrate and lactate.(66) These fiber-derived energy substrates could modulate the development of both normal colonic mucosa and neoplastic colonic cells, a dual effect that could explain both the inhibition and the enhancement of neoplastic development by fiber rich diet.

The results of the experiments designed to demonstrate an inhibition of colonic neoplastic development by fiber rich diet can, as a whole, be taken as convincing. But much work remains to be done to fully characterize these effects and to identify the active ingredients. By reference to our terminology, it is worth considering these products as potentially active negative modulator of neoplastic development. Most likely this effect could be due to a change in availability of nutrients and calories as well as a modulation of growth, proliferation and differentiation of colonic mucosa. With regard to the effect on availability of nutrients and calories, it is proposed that high fiber diet could be, at least partly, equivalent to caloric restriction (see above). Further work is needed to test this hypothesis.

5. CONCLUSIONS

That diet may influence neoplastic development is a well established and valid hypothesis. Neoplastic development is a long lasting process during which incipient neoplasia progresses slowly up to the emergence of malignant tumors. Such a process can be modulated either positively or negatively if conditions are created that either disturb or reinforce the stability of the physiological behavior (homeostasis) of cells and/or tissues respectively. From the results of experimental studies, it can be concluded that chemically induced carcinogenesis can be modulated by calorie restriction and high fiber diet. Both effects are consistent with the definition of negative modulation, they might even have in common a (reduced or) decreased availability of nutrients and/or calories with as a consequence a retarded body weight increase and lower rate of cell proliferation at certain sites. Fat per se has most probably no direct effect on carcinogenesis, but increasing fat content in food might create indirect dietary unbalances that might effect neoplastic development at various sites. Such effects could be due to increased nutritional efficiences and available calories.

If this turns out to be the case, both negative and positive modulation of neoplastic development by dietary manipulations could have the same common basis: dietary balance. Improving it would protect against cancer whilst disturbing it would increase the risk. By broadening the view on neoplastic development, the concept of modulation may thus clarify the debate by focusing the question marks.

REFERENCES

1. B. Amstrong and R. Doll, Int. J. Cancer, 1975, 15, 617.
2. D.B. Clayson, Cancer Res., 1975, 35, 3292.
3. B.S. Reddy, L.A. Cohen, G.D. Mc Coy, P. Hill, J.H. Weisburger and E.L. Wynder, Adv. Cancer Res., 1980, 32, 237.
4. D. Albanes, Cancer Res., 1987, 47, 1987.
5. K.M. Nauss, L.R. Jacobs and P.M. Neuwberne, Am. J. Clin. Nutr., 1987, 45, 243.
6. M.G. Enig, R.J. Munn and M. Keeney, Fed. Proc., 1978, 37, 2215.
7. M.E. Shils, Med. Clin., 1979, 63, 1027.
8. J.E. Enstrom, Cancer Res., 1981, 41, 3722.
9. M. Mogadam, Am. J. Gastroenterol., 1988, 88, 1346.
10. L.K. Heilbrun, A. Nomura, J.H. Hanking and G. Stemmermann, Int. J. Cancer, 1989, 44, 1.
11. L. Wattenberg, Cancer Res., 1985, 45, 1.
12. M.B. Roberfroid, "Concept and theories in Carcinogenesis", A. Maskens, Amsterdam, 1987, p157.
13. M. Roberfroid, "Experimental Carcinogenesis", M. Roberfroid and V. Préat, New York, 1988, p29.

14. M. Roberfroid and V. Préat, "Theories of Carcinogenesis, O.H. Iversen, Washington, 1988, p319.
15. M. Roberfroid and V. Préat, Bull. Cancer, 1990, 77, 467.
16. M. Roberfroid, N. Delzenne and V. Préat, Annu. Rev. Pharmacol. Toxicol;, 1991, 31, 163.
17. L. Foulds, "Neoplastic development", Academic Press, London & New York, 1969, Vol.1, 225pp.
18 P. Rous and J.G. Kidd, J. Exp. Med., 1941, 73, 365.
19. I. Berenblum, Arch. Pathol., 1944, 38, 233.
20. I. Berenblum, J. Natl. Cancer Inst., 1949, 10, 167.
21. I. Berenblum and P. Shubik, Br. J. Cancer, 1947, 1, 383.
22. I. Berenblum and P. Shubik, Br. J. Cancer, 1947, 1, 383.
23. B. Terracini, P. Shubik and G. Della Porta, Cancer Res., 1960, 20, 1538.
24. P. Shubik, Cancer, 1977, 40, 1821.
25. A. Maskens, Cancer Res., 1981, 41, 1240.
26. N. Shivapurkar, K.L. Hoover and L.A. Poirier, Carcinogenesis, 1986, 7, 547.
27. H.P. Glauert and J.A. Weeks, Toxicol. Lett., 1989, 48, 283.
28. P. Schulte-Hermann, Arch. Toxicol., 1985, 57, 147.
29. V. Préat, J. de Gerlache, M. Lans, H.S. Taper and M. Roberfroid, Carcinogenesis, 1986, 7, 1025.
30. V. Préat, J.C. Pector, H.S. Taper, M. Lans, J. de Gerlache and M. Roberfroid, Carcinogenesis, 1984, 5, 1151.
31. J. de Gerlache, H.S. Taper, M. Lans, V. Préat and M. Roberfroid, Carcinogenesis, 1987, 8, 337.
32. H. Bartsch, V. Préat, A. Aitio and M. Roberfroid, Carcinogenesis, 1988, 9, 2315.
33. T.J. Slaga, A.J.P. Klein-Szanto, S.M. Fisher, C.E. Weeks, K. Nelson and S. Major, Proc. Natl. Acad. Sci. USA, 1980, 77, 2251.
34. S. De Flora, Mutation Res., 1988, 202, 279.
35. V. Préat and N. Delzenne, "Experimental hepatocarcinogenesis", M. Roberfroid and V. Préat, New York, 1988, 41.
36. K.K. Caroll and H.T. Khor, Prog. Biochem. Pharmacol., 1975, 10, 308.
37. B.S. Reddy, Prog. Food Nutr. Sci., 1985, 9, 257.
38. W. Willet, Nature, 1989, 338, 389.

39. K.M. Nauss, M. Locniskar and P.M. Newberne, Cancer Res., 1983, 43, 4083.
40. K.M. Nauss, M. Locniskar, D. Sondergaard and P.M. Newberne, Carcinogenesis, 1984, 5, 255.
41. M. Locniskar, K.M. Nauss, P. Kaufmann and P.M. Newberne, Carcinogenesis, 1985, 6, 349.
42. G.J. Hopkins and K.K. Caroll, J. Natl. Cancer Inst., 1979, 62, 1009.
43. A. Tannenbaum, Cancer Res., 1942, 2, 468.
44. A. Tannenbaum, Cancer Res., 1945, 5, 616.
45. P.S. Lavik and C.A. Baumann, Cancer Res;, 1943, 3, 749.
46. D. Kritchevsky, M.M. Weber and D.M. Klurfeld, Cancer Res., 1984, 44, 3174.
47. D. Kritchevsky, M.M. Weber, C.L. Buck and D.M. Klurfeld, Lipids, 1986, 21, 272.
48. M.W. Pariza, Am. J. Clin. Nutr., 1987, 45, 261.
49. R.K. Boutwell, M.K. Brush and H.P. Rusch, Cancer Res., 1949, 9, 41.
50. G.A. Boissonneault, C.E. Elson and M.W. Pariza, J. Natl. Cancer Inst., 1986, 76, 335.
51. D. Kritchevsky and D.M. Klurfeld, Am. J. Clin. Nutr., 1987, 45, 236.
52. G. Hocman, Comp. Biochem. Physiol., 1988, 91A, 209.
53. C.D. Larsen and W.E. Heston, J. Natl. Cancer Inst.,, 1945, 31.
54. C.H. Barrows and G.L. Kokkonen, Age, 1978, 1, 131.
55. R. Weindruch, R.L. Walford, S. Fligiel and D. Guthrie, J. Nutr., 1986, 116, 641.
56. L. Gross and Y. Dreyfus, Proc. Natl. Acad. Sci. USA, 1984, 1, 7596.
57. B.S. Reddy, C.X. Wang and H. Maruyama, Cancer Res., 1987, 47, 1226.
58. M.W. Pariza and R.K. Boutwell, Am. J. Clin. Nutr., 1987, 45, 151.
59. M.B. Roberfroid, CRC Critical Rev. in Food Sci. Nutr., 1992, in press.
60. D. Burkitt, Am. J. Clin. Nutr., 1978, 31, S58.
61. J.H. Weisburger, B.S. Reddy, L.A. Cohen, P. Hill and E.L. Wynder, Carcinogen. Compr. Surve., 1982, 7, 175.
62. L.R. Jacobs, Adv. Exp. Med. Biol., 1986, 206, 105.
63. A.P. Kaur, C.M. Bhat and R.B. Grewal, Nutr. Rep. Int., 1985, 32, 383.
64. K. Watanabe, B.S. Reddy, J.H. Weisburger and D. Kritchevsky, J. Natl. Cancer Inst., 1979, 63, 141.

65. J.H. Cummings, M.J. Hill, D.J. Jenkins, J.R. Pearson and H.S. Wiggins, Am. J. Clin. Nutr., 1976, 29, 1468
66. J.H. Cummings, Lancet, 1983, 1206.

DIET AND BREAST CANCER

H Leon Bradlow, Nitin T Telang, Jon J Michnovicz* and Michael P Osborne

Strang Cornell Cancer Research Laboratory
Institute for Hormone Research
New York, NY 10021 USA

1. INTRODUCTION

A causative role for estrogens in breast cancer has been evident since the pioneering studies of Beatson in 1890 showing remission after ovariectomy.[1] The low incidence of breast cancer following early hysterectomy is additional confirmation for the role of ovarian hormones in breast cancer. More recent observations, particularly international comparisons of fat consumption and breast cancer incidence, have also confirmed a role for diet both in the induction and promotion of breast cancer and in its possible prevention.

Any effect of diet in the response to estrogen must act in one of two ways; it can act on the synthesis of estradiol or it can act on the metabolism of estradiol leading to more or less active metabolites which differ in their effect on the initiation and promotion of tumors. Examination of the disposition of estrogens suggests a way in which diet might act to alter estrogenic actions on tumors. Estradiol metabolism is predominantly oxidative in nature going sequentially from $E_2 \rightarrow E_1 \rightarrow 16\alpha\text{-OHE}_1$ or 2-OHE_1. The latter steps are mediated by P-450 isozymes. The key points are that the C-2 pathway leads to a biologically inactive product with a touch of antiestrogenic activity,[2] while the C-16 pathway leads to biologically active fully potent estrogens[3] and also possesses genotoxic activity.[4]

In addition to its estrogenic activity which is significantly prolonged relative to estradiol, $16\alpha\text{-OHE}_1$ also has genotoxic properties[4] which are related to its unique ability to form covalent bonds to amino groups on receptors of DNA.[5] The C-17 keto function initially forms a Schiff base with a free amino group on peptides or DNA followed by spontaneous rearrangement to form 17-amino, 16-keto products, resulting in a covalent link to cellular elements until their ultimate degradation.

2. *IN VIVO* STUDIES

The first significant evidence for an alteration in estradiol metabolism was reported by Schneider *et al.*[6] in 1980 who reported an increase in 16α-hydroxylation in postmenopausal women with breast cancer relative to matched control subjects. Since the possibility exists that this increase may be related to the presence of a tumor we carried out additional studies in women at high risk for breast cancer but who were free of detectable disease. These women show a statistically significant increase in 16α-hydroxylation relative to women at low risk for this disease.[7] *In vivo* studies were also carried out in murine strains with widely varying rates of mammary tumor formation.[8] These studies showed a highly significant correlation between tumor incidence and the extent of 16α-hydroxylation with the rate greatest in the R111 and C3H lines with very high tumor rates and lowest in the C-57 lines with a low tumor rate. The rate of reaction was not sex-linked. Studies on stabilized F-11 sublines derived from a cross between high risk C3H mice and low risk C-57 mice showed that the rate of 16α-hydroxylation was inherited autosomally. Prior studies showed that the mouse mammary tumor virus (MMTV) which is transmitted by nursing plays a key role in tumor risk with the incidence decreased in virus free mice. There is a tightly linked interaction between the virus and estrogens since ovariectomized mice carrying the virus showed a low tumor incidence. Finally foster nurturing studies showed that the presence of the virus resulted in a higher level of 16α-hydroxylation while a lower level was found in virus free mice of the same strain.

3. *IN VITRO* STUDIES

In vitro studies have also been carried out in terminal end buds from mice and in terminal duct lobular units obtained after mammoplasy (TDLU-LR) and after mastectomy but distal to the tumor site (TDLU-HR). These organelles can be maintained in organ culture for up to 42 days and biochemical studies can be carried out.[9] These studies showed that 16α-hydroxylation occurs directly in breast tissue and that it is correlated with Ras P21 expression. Comparison of TDLU-HR and TDLU-LR showed that the TDLU-HR have a higher basal rate of reaction at C-16 as well as of Ras P21 expression than the rate in low risk TDLU.[10] In addition the TDLU-HR showed a greater responsiveness than TDLU-LR to various stimuli such as BP, DMBA and linoleic acid for both parameters while ω-3 fatty acids inhibited this increase in reaction at C-16.[11]

Transfection of normal mouse mammary epithelial cells with either ras or myc oncogenes, resulted in increased reaction at C-16 and an increase in tumorigenicity. This increase at C-16 is paralleled by a decrease in reaction at C-2.[12] Treatment of normal murine mammary cells with 16α-OHE_1 established that this compound is uniquely genotoxic and capable of causing increased unscheduled DNA repair and anchorage independent growth.[4]

4. DIETARY STUDIES

In light of these findings it would clearly be desirable to decrease the extent of 16α-hydroxylation as a tumor preventive measure. Attempts to reduce the extent of 16α-hydroxylation by biochemical intervention directly, failed completely despite a massive effort. On the other hand an alternative approach by inducing a increase in 2-hydroxylation served to reduce the level of 16α-hydroxylated metabolites very effectively. This succeeds because with a finite pool of estrogens available for metabolic transformations an increase in one pathway effectively serves to decrease the extent of transformation by the alternative pathway;[13] i.e. increased 2-hydroxylation results in a decrease in 16α-hydroxyestrone and estriol. This has been found experimentally.[14] Practically this approach is attractive because it has proven to be relatively easy to induce an increase in 2-hydroxylation by a variety of methods. Thus increasing the protein content of the diet results in a marked increase in C-2 hydroxylation with no change in reaction at C-16,[15] while taking cimetidine, which causes a decrease in C-2 hydroxylation results in an increase in C-16 metabolites.[16] Marked increases in body fat in fat intake both result in a decrease in C-2 hydroxylation,[17] and at sufficiently high levels of fat intake an increase in reaction at C-16.[18]

Smoking also proved to be a potent inducer of reaction at C-2[19] which correlates with the reported protective effect of smoking against endometrial cancer.[20] Dioxin exposure also results in an increase in C-2

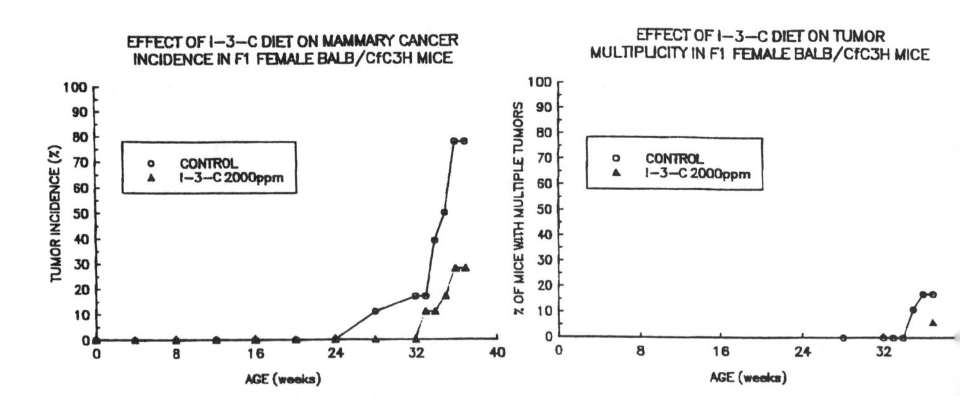

Fig. 1. Suppression of tumors in female Balb/CfC3H mice. Groups of mice[20] were fed AIN76A containing 0, or 2000 ppm of I3C. A = increase in % tumors with time in weeks; B = % of mice bearing multiple tumors at different time interva

hydroxylation[21] which correlates with the report by Bertazzi[22] that following the Sevaso incident in which women were exposed to dioxins the breast cancer rate was reduced by 50%. Proceeding on this approach we sought other substances which would increase estradiol 2-hydroxylation without the negative effects of smoking or dioxin exposure. The most satisfactory choice proved to be indole-3-carbinol (I3C), a substance presence as a complex in cruciferous vegetables. Dietary studies in cell cultures, mice, rats and humans (23-25) established that administration of this compound results in a marked increase in 2-hydroxylation and a decrease in the excretion of 16-hydroxylated metabolites. Finally administration of I3C to mice with high rates of spontaneous mammary tumors results in a marked decrease in the incidence of these tumors.[24]

REFERENCES

1. G. Beatson, Lancet, 1898, 2, 104.
2. J. Schneider, M.M. Huh, H.L. Bradlow and J. Fishman, J. Biol. Chem., 1984, 259, 4840.
3. J. Fishman and C. Martucci, J. Clin. Endocrinol. Metab., 1980, 51, 611.
4. N.T. Telang, A. Suto, G.Y. Wong, M.P. Osborne and H.L. Bradlow, J. Natl. Cancer Inst., 1992, 84, 634.
5. G.E. Swaneck and J. Fishman, Proc. Natl. Acad. Sci., 1988, 85, 7831.
6. J. Schneider, D. Kinne, A. Fracchia, V. Pierce, K.E. Anderson, H.L. Bradlow and J. Fishman, Proc. Natl. Acad. Sci. USA, 1982, 79, 3047.
7. M.P. Osborne, R.A. Karmali, R.J. Hershcopf, H.L. Bradlow, I.A. Kourides, W.R. Williams, P.P. Rosen and J. Fishman, Cancer Invest., 1988, 629.
8. H.L. Bradlow, R.J. Hershcopf, C.P. Martucci and J. Fishman, Proc. Natl. Acad. Sci. USA, 1985, 82, 6295.
9. N.T. Telang, H. Leon Bradlow, Hiroaki Kurihara, and Michael P. Osborne, Breast Cancer Res. and Treatment, 1989, 13, 173.
10. M.P. Osborne, N.T. Telang, H. Kurihara and H.L. Bradlow, Proc. AACR, 1988, 29, 236.
11. N.T. Telang, A. Basu, M.J. Modak, H.L. Bradlow and M.P. Osborne, S. Nigam and T. Walden, Eicosanoids, eds. Kluwer Academic Publishers, Boston 1991.
12. N.T. Telang, R. Narayanan, H.L. Bradlow and M.P. Osborne, Breast Cancer Research and Treatment, 1991, 18, 155.
13. R. Lustig, R.J. Hershcopf and H.L. Bradlow, In Adipose Tissue and Reproduction, ed. R. Frisch, Karger Press, Zurich, 1989, pp.119-132.
14. B.R. Goldin, S.L. Gorbach, Am. J. Clin. Nutr., 1988, 48, 787.
15. K.E. Anderson, A. Kappas, A.H. Conney, H.L. Bradlow and J. Fishman, J. Clin. Endocrinol. Metab., 1984, 59, 103.
16. R. Galbraith and J. Michnovicz, New Eng. J. Med., 1989, 321, 269.

17. J. Schneider, H.L. Bradlow, G. Strain, J. Levin, K. Anderson and J. Fishman, J. Clin. Endocrinol. Metab., 1983, 56, 792.
19. J.J. Michnovicz, R.J. Hershcopf, H. Naganuma, H.L. Bradlow and J. Fishman, N. Engl. J. Med., 1986, 315, 1305.
20. S.M. Lesko, L. Rosenburg and H. Morgenstern, N. Engl. J. Med., 1985, 313, 593.
21. J. Gierthy, D. Lincoln, J. Kampcik, H. Dickerman, H. Bradlow, T. Niwa and G. Swaneck, Biochem. Biophys. Res. Commun., 1988, 157, 515.
22. P.A. Bertazzi, C. Zocchetti, A.C. Pesatori, S. Guercilena, M. Sanarico and L. Radice, Am. J. Epidemiol., 1989, 129, 1187.
23. Jon J. Michnovicz and H. Leon Bradlow, J. Natl. Cancer Institute, 1990, 82, 947.
24. H.L. Bradlow, J.J. Michnovicz, N.T. Teland and M.P. Osborne, Carcinogenesis, 1991, 12, 1571.
25. J.J. Michnovicz and H.L. Bradlow, Nutrition and Cancer, 1991, 16, 59.

PROLIFERATIVE ACTIVITY IN THE COLON OF HEALTHY SUBJECTS IN TWO ITALIAN CITIES WITH DIFFERENT DIETARY HABITS.

Giovanna Caderni, Franca Bianchini, M.Teresa Spagnesi

Department of Pharmacology,
University of Florence
50134 Florence, Italy.

1 INTRODUCTION

Colon cancer risk has been associated with dietary habits in both epidemiological and experimental studies[1,2] . In particular, consumption of diets rich in fat and meats and poor in vegetables and fibers has been repeatedly associated with an increased risk of colon cancer[1-4].

To explain how diet may affect colon cancer risk, it has been suggested, mainly on the basis of experimental studies, that some diets may act as promoters in colon cancerogenesis increasing the proliferative activity of the colonic mucosa[5,6]. It has been demonstrated in fact that high proliferation in the colon is associated with increased risk of colon cancer [6]; in addition, some studies suggest that a shift of the proliferative activity from the lower to the upper part of the colon crypts is also associated with a high risk of colon cancer[6].

In Italy traditional dietary habits differ from Region to Region, starchy foods and fruits being consumed more frequently in the Southern and Central part of the Country as compared to the North [7]. In Italy, moreover colon cancer mortality varies with geographical zones, being higher in the North-Center when compared to the South [8].

It seemed interesting therefore, to study whether healthy subjects from two italian cities from the North and the Center (Trieste and Florence, respectively) have different proliferative activity in the colorectal mucosa and whether these subjects also differ in dietary habits.

2 MATERIALS AND METHODS

The subjects were recruited in the Gastroenterology Units of Public Clinical Centers in the two cities, among subjects aged 40-70, referred by their general practitioner to the Clinics for endoscopic control of reported disorders of intestinal function. Subjects with colon cancer, multiple polyps, acute or chronic inflammatory diseases or undergoing drug therapy, were excluded from the study. We studied 44 subjects: 18 in Trieste (10 males and 8 females) and 26 in Florence (17 males, and 9 females).

All the subjects included in the study were found negative for colon pathology (polyps or cancer) by colonoscopy. During the endoscopic examination three mucosal biopsies were taken in all subjects at about 15 cm from the anal verge.

The proliferative activity was determined by ^{3}H-thymidine incorporation and autoradiography as previously described [9]. Full longitudinal crypts were examined microscopically and scored for the number of mitoses, the number and the position of the labelled cells in the crypt, and the total number of cells/crypt section. Proliferative activity was expressed as mitotic index (number of mitoses/ number of cells counted in that crypt section x 100). To analyze the distribution of the proliferative activity along the crypts, we ideally divided each crypt in three equal compartments: low, middle and upper, and in each compartment we determined the percentage of labelled cells over total labelled cells in that crypt.

To assess dietary habits, the subjects under study were interviewed by dietitians using a quali-quantitative questionnaire relative to the dietary habits of the month preceding the endoscopic examination[10].

3 RESULTS AND DISCUSSION

The results of the determination of the mitotic activity in the colorectal mucosa in the group of subjects from Trieste and Florence indicated that subjects in Trieste had significantly higher mitotic activity when compared with subjects in Florence (Table 1).

We also analyzed the distribution of the proliferative activity along the crypt; the results of this analysis indicated that in the different compartments of the crypt the percentage of labelled cells over the total labelled cells, was similar in the two groups (Table 2).

In Table 3 we report the intake of nutrients in the subjects in Trieste and Florence; these results show that the intake of proteins, starches and fibers in the group of Trieste was significantly lower when compared to the group of Florence.

We also calculated the percentage of the energy

provided by proteins, starches, simplex carbohydrates (CHO) and lipids in the two groups of subjects. The results (Table 4) indicate that the subjects living in Trieste, given their overall lower caloric intake, derive more energy in % from lipids and less from starches than the subjects in Florence.

Table 1. Mitotic activity in the colorectal mucosa in the groups of Trieste and Florence.

	Trieste	Florence
mitotic index	0.17 ± 0.04	0.089 ± 0.02 *

Data are means ± S.E. * significantly different from the values in Trieste using the non-parametric Wilcoxon 2-sample test Z = 0.0227. n=18 in Trieste and n=21 in Florence.

Table 2. Distribution of the proliferative activity along the crypt in the two groups of subjects living in Trieste and Florence.

	Trieste	Florence
low compartment	57.3 ± 4.8	64.2 ± 2.1
middle compartment	35.3 ± 3.2	32.1 ± 1.9
upper compartment	7.4 ± 3.1	3.7 ± 0.7

Data are means ± S.E. n = 17 in Trieste and n = 26 in Florence.

Table 3. Daily nutrient intake in the two groups of subjects living in Trieste and Florence.

	Trieste	Florence
proteins (g)	69 ± 4.4 *	83 ± 3.7
lipids (g)	90 ± 5.1	94 ± 3.9
carbohydrates(g)	254 ± 19.5	293 ± 15
starches (g)	157 ± 15.4 *	199 ± 12.1
fibers (g)	28 ± 2.6 *	40 ± 2.8
Kcalories	2188 ± 127	2476 ± 93.8

* = $P<0.05$ as compared to values in the group of Florence by Wilcoxon-two samples test. n=18 in Trieste and n=21 in Florence.

Table 4. Percentage of the total Energy intake derived from the different nutrients in the two groups of subjects living in Trieste and Florence.

% Energy from	Trieste	Florence
proteins	12.78 ± 0.45	13.43 ± 0.36
lipids	37.72 ± 1.67 *	33.56 ± 1.29
starches	29.39 ± 1.86 *	35.10 ± 1.86
simplex CHO	20.37 ± 1.52	18.09 ± 1.54

* $P<0.05$ compared to the groups of Florence by analysis of variance. Data are means ± SE. n= 18 in Trieste and n=23 in Florence.

Several studies with rodents and some epidemiological studies have shown that dietary components affect the proliferative activity in the colon [5,11,12]. However, in the present study, correlating individual mitotic activity with nutrient intake in the different subjects we did not find any significant correlation (data not shown).

A higher proliferative activity in the colorectal mucosa has been associated with higher risk of developing colon cancer [6]. Studies with humans have shown that populations at very high risk (patients with familial adenomatous polyposis, ulcerative colitis, or people with colorectal carcinoma) have a higher and disarranged proliferative activity in the colon when compared with normal healthy subjects or with very low risk populations such as Seventh Day Adventist vegetarians [6,12].

Although the incidence of colon cancer in Trieste and Florence is different for males, 37/100,000 and 19/100,000, respectively, is similar for females, 16.4 /100,000 and 17.1 /100,000 in Trieste and Florence, respectively [13]. Since the subjects studied were of both sexes and a small number, it would be difficult and arbitrary to correlate these few observations on colonic proliferation with the incidence of colon cancer in the two cities.

In conclusion, we have found that a group of healthy subjects living in Trieste have higher mitotic activity when compared to a similar group of subjects living in Florence. We also found that the subjects in Trieste have a lower intake of starches, fibers, and proteins, and that they derive more energy from lipids and less from starches as compared to the group of Florence. However, no statistical correlation existed between the individual consumption of these nutrients and intestinal proliferation.

ACKNOWLEDGMENTS

This work has been supported by a Grant from "Regione Toscana Italy".

REFERENCES

1. W. Willet, Nature, 1989, 338, 389.
2. W.R. Bruce, Cancer Res., 1987, 47, 4237.
3. W.C. Willet, M.J. Stampfer, G.A. Colditz, B.A. Rosner, and F.E. Speizer, N. Engl. J. Med., 1990, 323, 1664.
4. S.A. Bingham, Proceedings of the Nutrition Society, 1990, 49, 153.
5. H.L. Newmark, M. Lipkin, N. Maheshwari, J. Natl. Cancer Inst., 1990, 82, 491.
6. M. Lipkin, Cancer Res., 1988, 48, 235.
7. F. Fidanza, J. Amer. Dietetic Assoc., 1980, 77, 133.
8. C. Cislaghi, A. Decarli , C. La Vecchia , and M. A. Vigotti Cancer, 1988, 61, 1262.
9. F. Tonelli, F. Bianchini, M. Lodovici, R. Valanzano, G. Caderni, and P. Dolara, Diseases colorectum, 1991, 34, 385.
10. E. Buiatti, D. Palli, A. Decarli, D.Amadori, C. Avellini, S. Bianchi, R. Biserni, F. Cipriani, P. Cocco, A. Giacosa, A. Marubini, R. Puntoni,C. Vindigni, J. Fraumeni, and W. Blot, Int. J. Cancer, 1990, 45, 896.
11. G. Caderni, F. Bianchini, P. Dolara , and D. Kriebel, Cancer Res.,1989, 49, 1655.
12. M. Lipkin, K. Vehara, S. Winaver, A. Sanchez, C. Bauer, R. Phillips, H.T. Lynch, W.A. Blattner, and J. Fraumeni, Cancer Letters, 1985, 26, 134.
13. E. Buiatti, M. Geddes, A. Amorosi, D. Balzi, A. Berchielli, A. Biggeri, S. Carli, R. Cecconi, R. Gaspari, B. Sorso, G. Vannucchi,Quaderni di Oncologia 1992, 4, Lega Italiana per la Lotta contro i Tumori, Firenze, Italy.

EFFECTS OF SHORT CHAIN FATTY ACID INFUSION ON THE GASTROINTESTINAL EPITHELIUM OF INTRAVENOUSLY FED RATS.

RA Goodlad, R Chinery, CY Lee, MA Ghatei*, SR Bloom* & NA Wright.

Imperial Cancer Research Fund,
Histopathology Unit,
35-43 Lincoln's Inn Fields,
London WC2A 3PN.

* Endocrinology Department,
Royal Postgraduate Medical School,
DuCane Road,
London W12 ONN.

INTRODUCTION

Dietary fibre can have a multitude of effects on the gastrointestinal physiology, which include several trophic actions. While viscous fibres may stimulate the small bowel [1], we have found that the most pronounced effects of fibre feeding occur in the colon[2]. Recently a direct effect on the stomach has also been observed (see chapter in this book). Nevertheless, the most dramatic effects are seen in the colon, and these colonic effects have been shown not to be due to the bulking actions of fibre alone[3]. The proliferative effects of fibre on the mucosa of the colon are completely abolished in germ-free rats [4] in both an acute starvation-refeeding model and in a chronic steady state model (see chapter in this book). The logical conclusion of these studies and those of Sakata [5] is that it is the products of fibre breakdown in the hind gut, namely the short chain fatty acids (SCFA's) that are the trophic agents. A similar proliferative role for the SCFA's has also been indicated in the foregut of ruminants[6], where SCFA production can contribute 70% of energy needs[7]. In man the contribution is more modest, even so estimates of 10% of the energy supply are not unreasonable [8]. In this chapter we describe the results of two studies, in which SCFA mixtures were continuously infused into the hind gut of rats maintained by total parenteral nutrition (TPN). The TPN rat is a very useful model as intestinal function is reduced to basal levels, thus proliferative effects should be more prominent and the several potentially confounding consequences of dietary manipulation, such as altered food intake or feeding patterns, abolished.

Methods

A two-channel continuous perfusion system was used to infuse intravenously fed, unrestrained rats continuously for one week. The rats were anaesthetised and silastic cannulae inserted into the jugular vein and into the caecum [9](see fig 1)

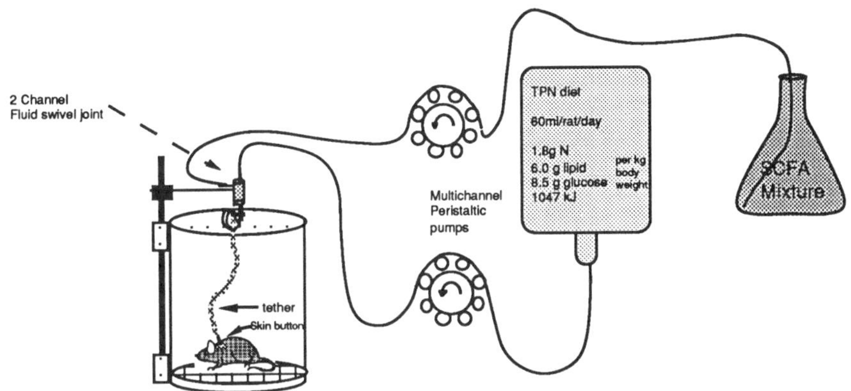

Fig 1 Diagram of 2-channel infusion system. Up to 32 rats are housed individually in wire-bottomed cages and the TPN diet infused into the jugular vein. A second cannulae is inserted into the gut. Both cannulae are taken subcutaneously and exit via a stainless steel tether to a fluid swivel joint, allowing the rat considerable freedom of movement. The TPN diet and the infusion solution are kept in a fridge.

<u>The SCFA mixture</u> In the first investigation rats were either infused intravenously with the TPN diet or infused into the colon for 7 days. In the second experiment SCFA's were infused into the caecum for 5 days. The colonic/caecal infusions gave 4.5% of the daily calorific intake, whilst the intravenous gave 2%. The molar ratios of actetate/propionate/butyrate were 75:35:20 and if given luminally, were administered in a salt solution designed to mimic hind gut contents[10].

Rats were injected with 1mg/kg of vincristine at the end of the investigations (to arrest cells as they entered metaphase) and killed 2 hours later. The gastrointestinal tract was removed, rinsed, blotted and weighed. Samples from all the regions of the gut were fixed in Carnoy's fluid and stored in 70% alcohol. The tissue was stained with the Feulgen reaction and intestinal and colonic crypts were displayed by microdissection and gently squashed with a coverslip. The number of arrested metaphases in 20 crypts was then counted[11].

Results are presented as the mean ± standard error of the mean.

* = $p < 0.05$, ** = $p < 0.01$, *** = $p < 0.001$.

Results

A significant increase in colonic and small intestinal tissue weight was observed in the luminal infused group, there was also an indication of an effect in the venously infused group, See fig 2.

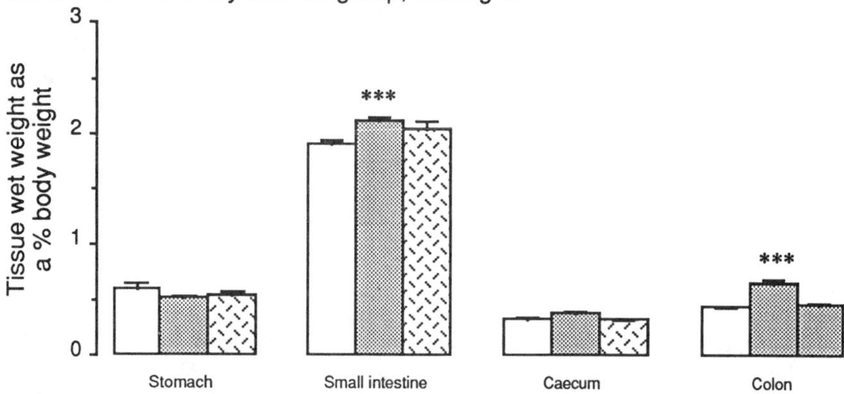

Fig 2 The effects of 7 days SCFA infusion (either into the colon or into jugular vein) on intestinal wet weight. Plain bars were the controls, shaded bars colonic infused, and hatched bars were intravenously infused.

A modest, but significant effect on cell proliferation, in the small bowel and in the colon, was seen in the intraluminally infused group, and again there was an indication, although not a significant one, of an effect in the intravenously infused. See fig 3.

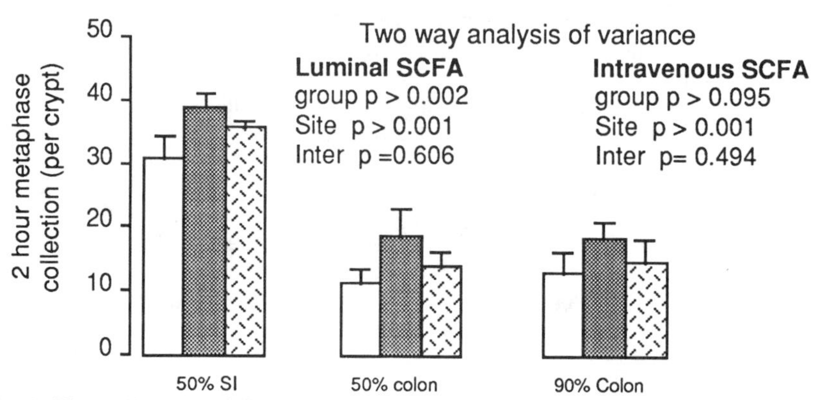

Fig 3 The effect of SCFA infusion (into colon or into jugular vein) on intestinal proliferation. Shaded bars were intraluminally infused, hatched bars were intravenously infused.

No effect on plasma gastrin or insulin were observed, but enteroglucagon and PYY appeared to be decreased by SCFA infusion.

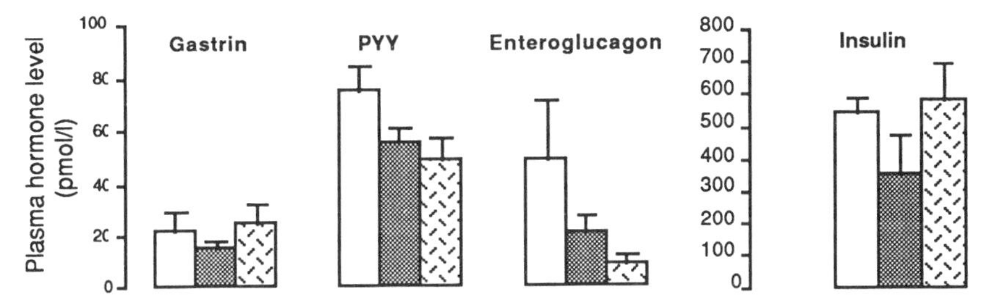

Fig 4 Plasma hormone levels after SCFA infusion. Shaded bars were intraluminally infused, hatched bars were intravenously infused

The second study, in which the SCFA's were pumped into the colon, showed a modest proliferative response in the small intestine, no effect was seen in the colon, nevertheless, a different proliferative response was seen, in which crypt branching, rather than metaphase accumulation occurred (see fig 5). This group also demonstrated increased expression of gastrin and TGFα, as determined by the RNase protection assay technique, in the distal ileum and throughout the colon

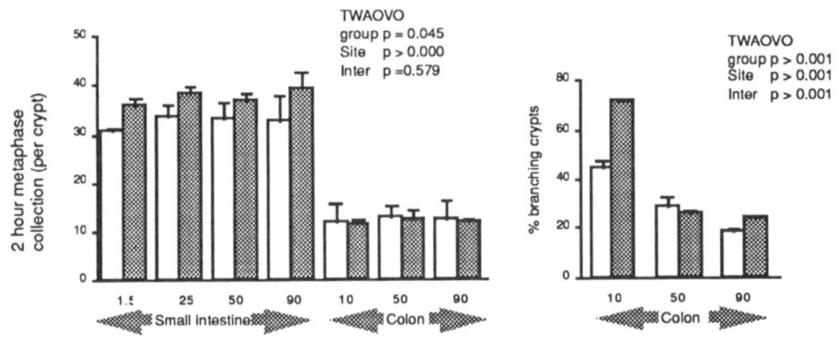

Fig 5. The result of the second infusion study. Control infusion are the plain bars, shaded bars were the SCFA infusion.

Discussion

While the results of the present study confirm that SCFA's can significantly stimulate intestinal epithelial cell proliferation[12-14] the magnitude of the response was not as great as our previous work, and the published literature had led us to expect. Although the advantages of TPN feeding have been alluded to, it is possible that the lack of luminal contents in the hind gut in these investigations may have altered the uptake and hence exposure of the epithelium to the SCFA's. The choice of an experimental model is always a difficult one, especially when it would appear that Cleave's concept of fibre 'what God had put together let no man put asunder' [15] is gaining importance, nevertheless, there are still many advantages in our extreme reductionist approach[16]. Some of the differences may also be attributed to the difference between bolus and continuous administration.

The different nature of the results obtained in the first and second experiments may reflect the different times of administration or the different sites of administration. Propionate and butyrate are metabolised by the colonocytes or by the liver[17], thus only actetate is likely to have a systemic role. It is of interest that no effect on metaphase accumulation was observed in the second investigation, nevertheless there was a dramatic increase in the number of branching crypts. Increased crypt branching has been shown to precede an increase in mitotic activity in a human study[18]. The potential importance of crypt branching as a method of increasing cell mass is only recently being appreciated[19], however, the number of branched crypts in the colon suggests that they are a permanent feature, especially in the proximal colon, where the crypt base is also a functional compartment.

In conclusion the results of our study, while demonstrating that SCFA can indeed stimulate cell renewal rates in the gastrointestinal tract, both at the site of administration and abscopally, also indicate that there is a urgent need for further research.

REFERENCES

1. Johnson IT, Gee JM, Brown JC. Am J Clin Nutr 1988, 47, 1004.
2. Goodlad RA, Lenton W, Ghatei MA, Adrian TE, Bloom SR, Wright NA. Gut 1987, 28, 171.
3. Goodlad RA, Wright NA. British Journal of Nutrition 1983, 50, 91.
4. Goodlad RA, Ratcliffe B, Fordham JP, Wright NA. Gut 1989, 30, 820.
5. Sakata T, Yajima T. Q J exp Physiol 1984, 69, 639.
6. Goodlad RA. Quart J Exp Physiol 1981, 66, 487.
7. Stevens CE, Argenzio RA, Clemens ET. Microbial digestion: rumen versus large intestine. In: Ruckebusch Y, Thivend P, ed. *In Digestive physiology and metabolism of ruminants.* Lancaster: MTP Press, 1980: 685.
8. McNeil NI. Am J Clin Nutr 1984, 39, 338.
9. Goodlad RA, Wilson TG, Lenton W, Wright NA, Gregory H, McCullagh KG. Gut 1987, 28, 573.
10. Sakata T, Englehardt WV. Comp Biochem Physiol 1983, 74A.
11. Goodlad RA, Wright NA. Quantitative studies on epithelial replacement in the gut. In: Titchen TA, ed. *Techniques in life sciences. Digestive physiology.* Ireland: Elsevier Biomedical Press., 1982: p212.
12. Koruda MJ, Rolandelli RH, Settle RG, Zimmaro DM, Romneau JL. Gastroenterology 1988, 95, 715.
13. Kripke SA, Fox AD, Berman JA, Settle RG, Rombeau JL. J Parenteral and enteral nutrition 1989, 13, 109.
14. Sakata T. Br J Nutr 1987, 58, 95.
15. Heaton KW. Concepts of dietary fibre. In: Southgate DAT, Waldron K, Johnson IT, Fenwick GR, ed. *Dietary fibre: Chemical and biological aspects.* Cambridge: Royal Society of Chemistry, 1990: 3.
16. Goodlad RA, Wright NA. Bailliere's Clinical Gastroenterology 1990, 4, 97.
17. Frankel WL, Rombeau JL. Prob Gen Surg 1991, 8, 118.
18. Sullivan PB, Brueton MJ, Tabara Z, Goodlad RA, Lee CY, Wright NA. Lancet 1991, **338**, 53.
19. Cheng H, McCulloch C, Bjerknes M. Anat Record 1986, 215, 35.

IN VITRO STUDIES INTO THE SELECTIVE TOXICITY OF ALLYL ISOTHIOCYANATE TOWARDS TRANSFORMED HUMAN TUMOUR CELLS

S. R. R. Musk and I. T. Johnson

AFRC Institute of Food Research
Norwich Laboratory
Norwich Research Park
Colney
Norwich NR4 7UA

1 INTRODUCTION

Cruciferous vegetables such as cabbage, broccoli and Brussels sprouts contain significant quantities of a group of compounds known as glucosinolates (1) which, upon disruption of the tissue are broken down by the endogenous enzyme myrosinase (thioglucosidase) to yield isothiocyanates (ITCs). Experimental evidence shows that ITCs and glucosinolates can protect laboratory animals from the tumourigenic effects of model carcinogens (2) and it has been suggested that these compounds may play a role in the anticarcinogenic effect of cruciferous vegetables revealed in epidemiological studies.

The mechanism(s) by which ITCs may exert an anticarcinogenic effect remains unclear. However it has been demonstrated that the presence of cabbage in the diet can inhibit the development of mammary tumours in MNU-treated rats at a stage subsequent to initiation (3) and reduce the yield of pulmonary metastases in mice injected intravenously with BALB/c mammary tumour cells (4). This suggests that consumption of cruciferous vegetables may exert an anticarcinogenic effect in humans by modifying the growth of cells in a pretumourous state, and preventing them from becoming established as a fully-fledged tumour. In this study we attempted to obtain evidence that ITCs can exert an antitumourigenic activity by examining the cytotoxic and cytostatic activities of allyl ITC upon the human colon carcinoma HT29 cell line *in vitro*. This cell line can be induced to differentiate and detransform in culture by treatment with agents such as sodium butyrate (BUT) and dimethylformamide (DMF).

2 MATERIALS AND METHODS

AITC was purchased from Aldrich Chemical Co. Ltd. (Gillingham), BUT and DMF from Sigma Chemical Co. Ltd.

(Poole). AITC was dissolved in ethanol at a concentration of 1mg/ml immediately prior to use, further dilutions being made in complete medium before addition to the cultures. The final concentration of ethanol in the cultures was less than 1% and had no effect on the survival of the cells. Stock solutions of BUT and DMF were prepared in complete medium at concentrations of 50mM and 8% respectively and stored at 4°C.

Cell culture

HT29 cells were a gift from Dr. I. Gibson (University of East Anglia). The cells were grown in Eagle's Minimum Essential Medium (ICN Flow) supplemented with 2mM glutamine and 10% foetal calf serum (Imperial). Cultures were incubated in 5% CO_2 at 37°C in a humidified incubator and split 1:3 (using a mixture of 0.05% trypsin + 0.02% EDTA) every 8 days, conditions under which the cell cycle is about 30 hours. The medium was changed in stock cultures every 2 days.

Detransformation of HT29 *In Vitro*. Cultures of HT29 were detransformed by exposure to 0.8% DMF or to 2mM BUT. The medium was changed daily in cultures exposed to detransforming agents for longer than 24 hours and in their corresponding controls; populations exposed to DMF and BUT for longer than 24 hours underwent a certain amount of cell death and subsequent morphological transformation (data not shown) following which the growth rate was reduced.

Determination of clonal survival. Cells were harvested from log-phase cultures and plated out at the required low densities 4 hours before exposure to AITC, which was presented concurrently with detransforming agent where appropriate. The exposure time was 24 hours following which the cells were given fresh medium (without BUT or DMF) and incubated for 10-12 days until colonies were visible with the naked eye. At this point the cultures were fixed, stained with Crystal violet and scored for colonies of over 50 cells. Each experiment was carried out in triplicate.

Determination of mass growth rate. Cells were harvested from log-phase cultures and plated out at 2.5×10^5 per 10mm dish. At 24 hour intervals for 7 days the cells were exposed to AITC in fresh medium, detransforming agents being added 3 hours before the first application of AITC and at each subsequent application. The numbers of cells in certain dishes were counted at daily intervals (using a haemocytometer) and growth curves constructed. Each count was made from duplicate dishes.

3 RESULTS AND DISCUSSION

Table 1 presents the parameters of the survival curves

of HT29 exposed to AITC and the effects of a 3 hour preexposure to BUT or DMF thereupon. Detransformation rendered the cells more resistant to the cytotoxic effects of AITC, more than doubling the D_q from 0.32 μg/ml to 0.74 μg/ml (a ratio of 2.31) and increasing the D_0 from 0.74 μg/ml to 0.84 and 0.96μg/ml for DMF and BUT respectively (ratios of 1.14 and 1.30). The survival of the transformed cells at the D^q concentration for the detransformed populations was 56%. Increasing the length of pre-exposure from 3 to 72 hours had no further effect upon the survival curves (data not shown).

Figure 1 presents the results of a typical experiment in which the growth of mass populations of transformed and detransformed HT29 cells was measured and the effects of exposure to AITC assayed. Clearly, cells detransformed with either BUT or DMF grew more slowly and were contact inhibited at much lower densities than the transformed controls. However, what growth there was in the detransformed populations was more resistant to the cytostatic effects of AITC. Table 2 shows the results combined from 3 such experiments, expressing the final number of cells for a given concentration of AITC as a percentage of the number in the corresponding population that had been grown for a week in the absence of any AITC. Whilst only 19% inhibition of the growth of cells detransformed with DMF was observed at 1.6 μg/ml (the highest dose used) and BUT-treated cells were only slightly more sensitive to AITC, the transformed cells were severely retarded in growth at 1.2 μg/ml AITC and at 1.6 μg/ml inhibition was as high as 62%.

The results demonstrate that detransformation of HT29 protects the cells against the cytotoxic and cytostatic activities of AITC. Both BUT and DMF were effective in protecting the cells although they induced quite different morphological changes in the cultures. The protective effect was fully operational after 3 hours of exposure. Given that a slowing of growth rate is also not observed until at least 24 hours after exposure to BUT or DMF it would appear that protection is not induced simply by an increase in cell cycle length allowing the cells more time to repair AITC-induced damage before crucial points in the cycle.

4 CONCLUSION

Clearly it would not be valid to extrapolate directly from the *in vitro* experiments described here to the human gastrointestinal tract. However, the results allow us to tentatively advance the hypothesis that the slower rate of progression of colonic neoplasms in patients consuming high levels of cruciferous vegetables (5) might be partly due to the presence of

Table 1 Parameters of Survival Curves of HT29 Treated with AITC

TREATMENT	D_q	D_o	D_{37}
	(all in µg/ml)		
CONTROL	0.32±0.04	0.74±0.07	1.06±0.08
SODIUM BUTYRATE	0.74±0.06	0.96±0.09	1.70±0.10
DIMETHYLFORMAMIDE	0.74±0.05	0.84±0.11	1.58±0.13

Table 2 Inhibition of Growth of HT29 Cells by AITC

TREATMENT	CELL NUMBER AS % OF THAT IN UNTREATED CULTURE AFTER EXPOSURE TO GIVEN CONCENTRATIONS OF AITC		
	0.8	1.2	1.6
	(µg/ml)		
CONTROL	0.88±0.02	0.60±0.07	0.38±0.07
SODIUM BUTYRATE	0.94±0.04	0.79±0.05	0.77±0.07
DIMETHYLFORMAMIDE	1.12±0.10	1.03±0.04	0.81±0.03

Figure 1 Growth Curves of HT29 Cells Treated with AITC

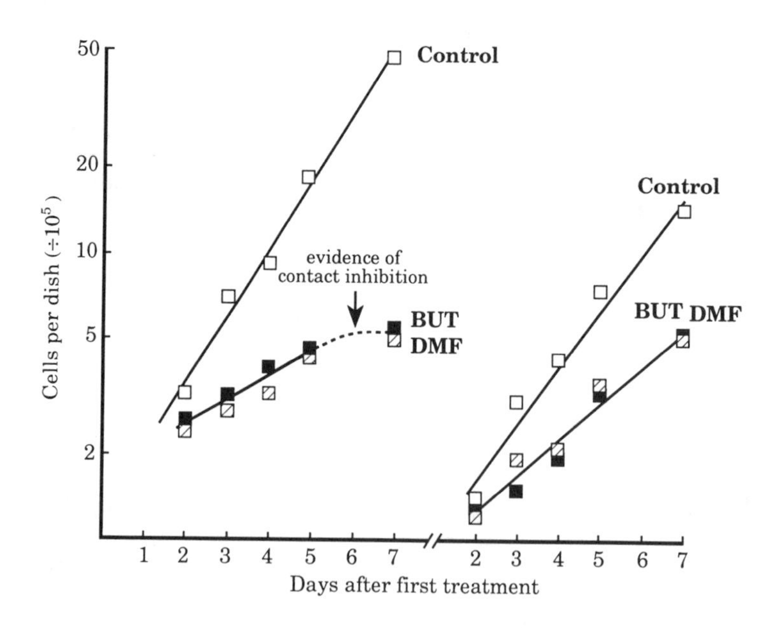

dietary AITC inhibiting the growth of transformed cell clones within the colorectum whilst having little or no effect on the "normal" epithelial population.

REFERENCES

1. G.R. Fenwick and R.K. Heaney, Food Chem., 1983, 11, 249.
2. G.D. Stoner, D.T. Morrissey, Y.-H. Heur, E.M. Daniel, A.J. Galati and S.A. Wagner, Cancer Res., 1991, 51, 2063.
3. E. Bresnick, D.F. Birt, K. Wolterman, M. Wheeler and R.S. Markin, Carcinogenesis, 1990, 11, 1159.
4. E.M. Scholar, K. Wolterman, D.F. Birt and E. Brensick, Nutr. Cancer, 1989, 12, 121.
5. G. Hoff, I.E. Moen, K. Trygg, W. Frolich, J. Sauar, M. Vatn, E. Gjone and S. Larsen, Scand. J. Gastroenterol, 1986, 21, 199.

CANCER PREVENTIVE AGENTS IN PROCESSED GARLIC

Hoyoku Nishino

Department of Biochemistry
Kyoto Prefectural University of Medicine
Kawaramachi-Hirokoji, Kamigyoku, Kyoto 602, Japan

1 INTRODUCTION

Preventive effect of garlic on human cancer has been reported; for example, in Shandong Province (China), Gangshan County, where residents consume a lot of garlic (an average of 20 g of garlic daily), had the lowest gastric cancer death rate (3.45/100,000) and by contrast, Quixia County, where little garlic is eaten, had the highest (40/100,000).[1] Furthermore, it has been proved in animal experiments that garlic constituents showed anti-tumorigenic activity.[2,3] Therefore, garlic seems to provide promising agents with the potential to protect against cancer, and thus extensive studies in this field of food science must be warranted for public health.

In the present study, we confirmed that the extract prepared from aged garlic suppressed the promoting stage of carcinogenesis, and identified some of the effective principles in garlic extract.

2 MATERIALS AND METHODS

Chemicals

Allixin (isolated and purified as described previously[4]) and eruboside-B were provided by Wakunaga Pharmaceutical Co. 7,12-Dimethylbenz[a]anthracene (DMBA) was purchased from Wako Pure Chemical Industries. 12-O-Tetradecanoylphorbol-13-acetate (TPA) was obtained from Pharmacia PL Biochemicals, Inc. Radioactive inorganic phosphate (^{32}Pi, carrier-free) was purchased from Japan Radioisotope Associations.

^{32}Pi Incorporation into Phospholipids of Cultured Cells

Incorporation of ^{32}Pi into phospholipids of cultured HeLa cells was assayed by a method described previously.[5]

In Vivo Carcinogenesis Experiments

Initiation of skin carcinogenesis was carried out by

a single application of 100 μg DMBA on the shaved back of 8-week-old female ICR mice (purchased from Shizuoka Laboratory Animal Center). For promotion, TPA (0.5 μg or 1.0 μg per painting) was applied twice weekly for 18 weeks. Garlic extract (5 mg per painting), allixin (1 mg per painting), or vehicle as control, was applied just before the TPA treatment. The number and incidence of tumors were determined each week.

3 RESULTS

Inhibitory Effect of Garlic Extract on ^{32}Pi Incorporation into Phospholipids of Cultured Cells

It has been reported that the exposure of mammalian cells to tumor promoters caused a rapid enhancement of phospholipid metabolism.[6] Interestingly, it was found that various kinds of chemicals which showed the inhibitory effect on this earliest phenomenon induced by tumor promoters, suppressed also in vivo carcinogenesis at the stage of promotion. Thus, we examined the effect of extract prepared from aged garlic (extracted with 20% ethanol and subsequently with ethyl acetate) on tumor promoter-enhanced phospholipid metabolism of cultured cells as the screening test to evaluate the potency of anti-tumor promoter activity. As shown in Table 1, garlic extract inhibited TPA-stimulated ^{32}Pi incorporation into phospholipids of HeLa cells in a dose-dependent manner. The potency of inhibitory effect of garlic extract was comparable to those of naturally occurring or synthetic anti-tumor-promoting agents, such as glycyrrhetinic acid[7] and eperisone.[8]

Inhibition of Tumor Promotion by Garlic Extract

We further investigated the effect of garlic extract on two-stage mouse skin carcinogenesis. It was proved

Table 1 Inhibitory effect of garlic extract and various kinds of anti-tumor-promoting agents on TPA-enhanced ^{32}Pi incorporation into phospholipids of cultured HeLa cells

Samples	Concentration μg ml^{-1}	Inhibition %
Garlic extract	25	9.7
	50	20.1
	100	42.3
Glycyrrhetinic acid	50	36.8
Eperisone-HCl	50	39.1

that the treatment with garlic extract (5 mg per painting) during the promoting stage resulted in complete suppression of tumorigenesis; at week 18 of the tumor promotion, the control group, in which TPA alone without garlic extract was applied, induced 10.9 tumors per mouse, while the group treated with garlic extract just before each TPA painting produced no tumor at all.

Anti-Tumor-Promoting Principles in Aged Garlic

These results of in vitro and in vivo experiments prompted us to survey anti-tumor-promoting principles in the extract of aged garlic. As the result, we found that allixin is one of the effective principles. Allixin is produced as a stress compound in garlic processed by physical- and/or chemical-treatment.[3] As shown in Figure 1, allixin showed significant inhibitory effect on TPA-enhanced ^{32}Pi incorporation into phospholipids of HeLa cells; its potency was about 4 times higher than that of garlic extract.

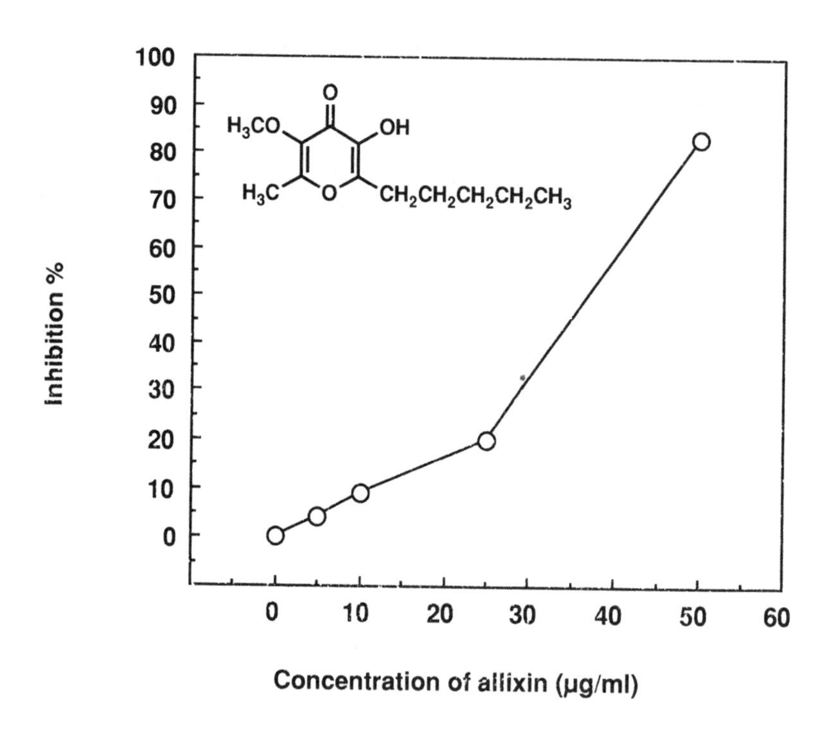

Figure 1 Effect of allixin on TPA-enhanced ^{32}Pi incorporation into phospholipids of cultured HeLa cells

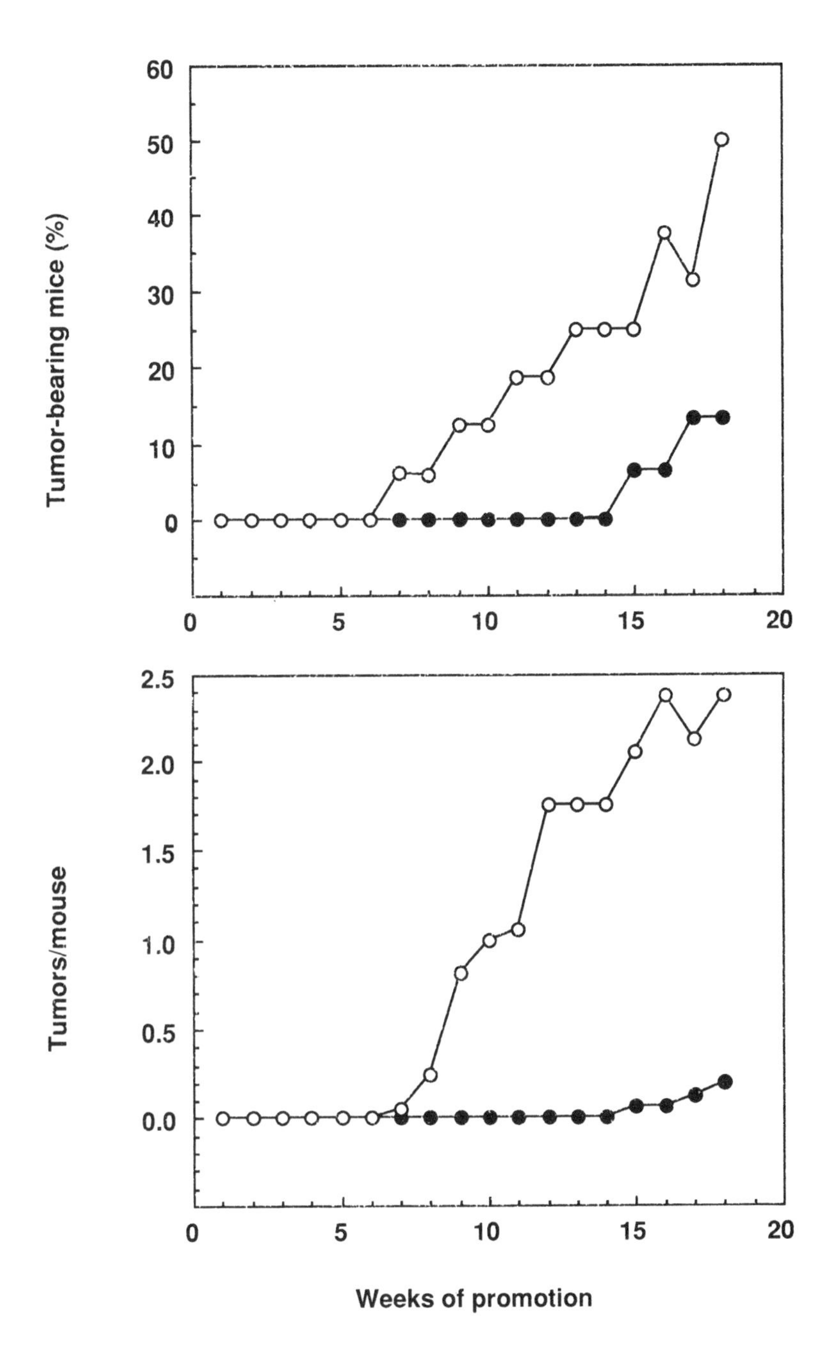

Figure 2 Effect of allixin on the promotion of skin tumor formation by TPA in DMBA-initiated mice.
o, Group treated with DMBA plus TPA;
●, group treated with DMBA plus TPA and allixin.

In the mouse skin two-stage carcinogenesis experiment, allixin showed significant inhibitory effect on tumor promotion (Figure 2). Anti-tumor-promoting activity of allixin was also demonstrated in two-stage lung carcinogenesis experiment (Data not shown).

Besides allixin, processed garlic contains other effective factors; for example, a steroidal glycoside eruboside-B.[9] We found that eruboside-B, which is one of the constituents of aged garlic, showed relatively high activity in the in vitro screening test. Eruboside-B was proved to have about 2 times higher potency than that of allixin; at the concentration of 25 µg/ml, eruboside-B inhibited TPA-enhanced ^{32}Pi incorporation into phospholipids of HeLa cells by 39.4%.

4 DISCUSSION

In the present study, allixin and eruboside-B were demonstrated to be active anti-tumor promoters in garlic. Besides allixin and eruboside-B, processed garlic seems to contain several other cancer-preventive agents. Thus, further investigation to survey anti-carcinogenic principles in processed garlic is now in progress. In any case, the sum of inhibitory actions of these preventive factors seems to result in a potent suppression of carcinogenesis.

ACKNOWLEGEMENTS

I would like to thank Prof. A. Iwashima, Department of Biochemistry, Kyoto Prefectural University of Medicine, Kyoto, for his kind encouragement during the course of this study. This work was accomplished by the collaboration with Wakunaga Pharmaceutical Co. Research Center, Hiroshima.

REFERENCES

1. N. Horwitz, Medical Tribune, August 12, 1981.
2. S. Belman, Carcinogenesis, 1983, 4, 1063.
3. M. J. Wargovich, Carcinogenesis, 1987, 8, 487.
4. Y. Kodera, H. Matsuura, S. Yoshida, T. Sumida, Y. Itakura, T. Fuwa and H. Nishino, Chem. Pharm. Bull., 1989, 37, 1656.
5. H. Nishino, H. Fujiki, M. Terada and S. Sato, Carcinogenesis, 1983, 4, 107.
6. L. R. Rohrschneider and R. K. Boutwell, Cancer Res., 1973, 33, 1945.
7. H. Nishino, K. Yoshioka, A. Iwashima, H. Takizawa, S. Konishi, H. Okamoto, H. Okabe, S. Shibata, H. Fujiki and T. Sugimura, Jap. J. Cancer Res., 1986, 77, 33.
8. J. Takayasu, Y. Yamaoka, Y. Nakagawa, H. Nishino and A. Iwashima, Oncology, 1989, 46, 58.
9. H. Matsuura, T. Ushiroguchi, Y. Itakura, N. Hayashi and T. Fuwa, Chem. Pharm. Bull., 1988, 36, 3659.

OMEGA 3 FATTY ACIDS SUPPRESS MUCOSAL CRYPT CELL PRODUCTION IN RATS

J.D. Pell, J.C. Brown and I.T. Johnson

AFRC Institute of Food Research, Norwich Research Park, Colney Lane, NORWICH, NR4 7UA, UK

1 INTRODUCTION

Intake of dietary fat has a positive correlation with colon cancer, in both epidemiological and animal studies (1). In experimental tumour systems linoleic acid has tumour promoting effects which seem in part to be mediated by the production of eicosanoids (2). However recent reports indicate that marine (n-3) polyunsaturated fatty acids inhibit the development and growth of tumours induced in mice by azoxymethane (3). The consumption of fish oils leads to the incorporation of the n-3 fatty acids eicosapentaenoic and docosahexaenoic acids, into plasma membranes of rapidly proliferating tissues including platelets (4), erythrocytes (5) and intestinal mucosal cells (6). Such changes modify prostaglandin metabolism and may thereby influence carcinogenesis.

Evidence suggests that increasing crypt cell production rates (CCPR) enhances the fixation and promotion of genetic lesions occurring in the colonic mucosa and therefore constitute a risk-factor for the development of neoplasia (7). Patients with adenomatous polyps, or with existing colorectal cancer, show evidence of hyperproliferation throughout the entire colorectal mucosa (8). Moreover groups at low risk of developing these diseases tend to have relatively low rates of colonic mucosal cell proliferation (9). In this study we have examined CCPR throughout the gastrointestinal tract of rats fed fibre-free diets containing three types of fat, namely corn oil (n-6 polyunsaturated fatty acids), lard (saturated fatty acids) and fish oil (n-3 fatty acids). Circulating levels of the putative gastrointestinal growth hormone enteroglucagon, together with selected morphological parameters, were also measured.

2. MATERIALS AND METHODS

Thirty male Wistar strain rats (150-180g) were obtained

Table 1. (g/Kg)

	Corn Oil	Lard	Fish Oil
Corn starch	360	360	360
Sucrose	300	300	300
Casein	200	200	200
Mineral Mix*	40	40	40
Vitamin Mix*	20	20	20
Corn Oil	80	-	-
Lard	-	80	-
Fish Oil	-	-	80
Total Energy (kJ/g)	18.1	18.1	18.1

* Formulated to provide all micronutrients essential for growth in the rat.

from a commercial supplier and housed singly, in wire-bottomed cages, in an animal house with controlled temperature, humidity and light-cycle (12h light/12h dark). The animals were randomly assigned to 3 groups of 10, and fed semi-synthetic diets containing 8g/100g of corn oil, fish oil or lard. The detailed composition of the diets is given in Table 1. Food intake in all groups was restricted to that of the rats fed fish-oil in order to ensure equal consumption of total dietary energy.

After 28d food was withdrawn at 09.00 h on the day of the experiment. Each animal received an intra-peritoneal injection of the anti-mitotic drug vincristine sulphate (1mg/kg). Individual animals were deeply anaesthetized at approximately 12 min intervals for 2h. The abdomen was opened with a ventral incision and a sample of blood was obtained from the vena cava. The intestinal organs were removed and measured, and samples (1 cm) were removed at 10% and 90% of the total small intestinal length, and from the caecum and proximal and distal colon. The epididymal fat pads were also removed and weighed. Samples of plasma were prepared, and both total glucagon-like immunoreactivity and pancreatic glucagon were assayed using a commercial assay kit containing specifically active antisera (Novo Laboratories, Basingstoke, UK).

The samples of intestinal tissue were fixed with acetic acid:ethanol (25:75) and subsequently stained in bulk with Feulgen's reagent. Crypt cell production rate (CCPR) was calculated from the slope of the regression line obtained by plotting the average number of blocked mitoses in 10 microdissected crypts from each animal against the time elapsed after treatment with vincristine (10). Results were expressed as cell divisions per crypt/h, and the significance of differences between slopes was determined by a t-test utilising a pooled estimate of the standard deviation.

The significance of other differences was assessed by one-way analysis of variance and calculation of the least significant difference at a probability level of 0.05.

3. RESULTS

All animals gained weight over the feeding period and there were no significant differences in the final body-weights of the groups. However the epididymal fat pads of the rats fed fish oil (6.62g +/- 0.30g) were significantly lighter than those of the rats corn oil (7.67g +/- 0.28g) or lard (8.30g +/- 0.38g). The small intestinal length in the fish oil group (120.7 cm +/- 0.93) was significantly greater than that of the corn oil group (116.8 cm +/- 1.1cm) and the lard group (114.2 cm +/- 1.37cm). Plasma enteroglucagon levels, integrated over the 2h period following removal of food, were lowest in rats fed fish oil and highest in those fed lard (Fig 1).

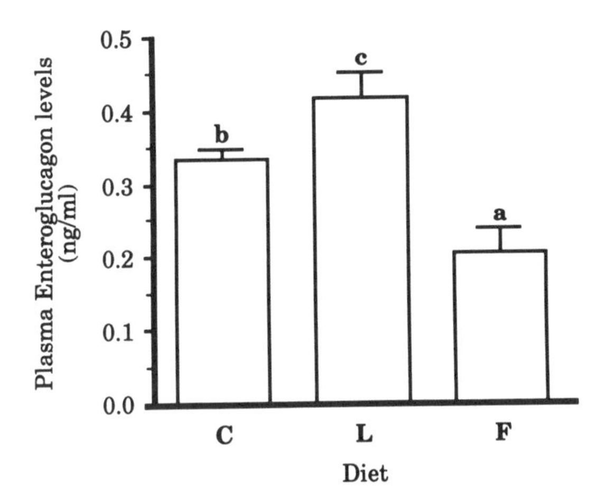

Figure 1 Plasma enteroglucagon in rats fed corn oil (C), lard (L) or fish oil (F). Values are means and SEM for 10 rats. Columns with similar hatching but different index letters differ significantly ($p<0.05$).

The rates of crypt cell production at two sites in the small intestine and in the caecum, proximal and distal colon are shown in Fig 2. Animals fed corn oil or lard had similar CCPR in the jejunum and ileum, but the rate was lower at both sites in the rats fed fish oil. In all three groups, the CCPR was substantially lower in the large intestine compared to the small intestine. In the proximal and distal colon, the rats fed fish oil had the lowest rates of proliferation. However the pattern was different in the caecum, where animals fed corn oil had the lowest rates.

4. DISCUSSION

This study has demonstrated a significant effect of varying dietary fatty acid sources on mucosal cell proliferation and morphology in the alimentary tract of

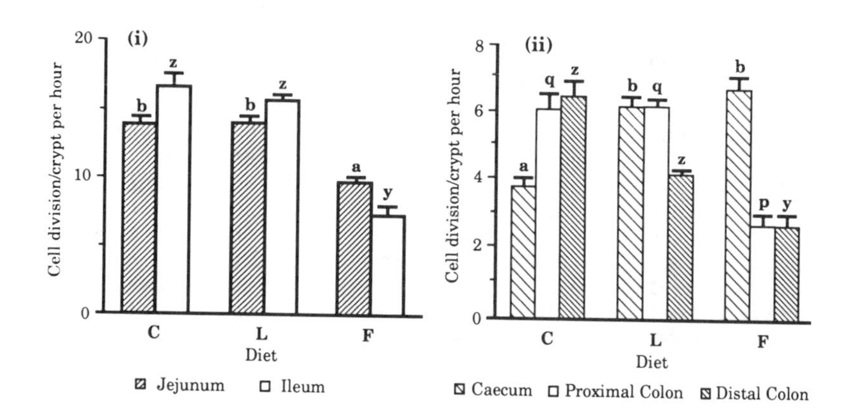

<u>Figure 2</u> CCPR in small (a) and large (b) intestine in rats fed corn oil (C), lard (L) or fish oil (F). Columns with similar hatching but different index letters differ significanctly ($p<0.05$).

growing rats, in the absence of fermentable dietary fibre. The lowest rates of mucosal cell replication at most sites were observed in rats fed diets containing fish oil. The reasons for this are unclear however because the mechanisms controlling mucosal crypt cell proliferation are complex and incompletely understood. EPA and DHA inhibit the cyclo-oxygenase pathway for prostaglandin synthesis, and this mechanism has been proposed as a means by which dietary fish oil may inhibit carcinogenesis (3). Prostaglandins may also contribute to the control of normal cell proliferation. Alternatively the various fatty acids may differ in their ability to stimulate the release of endocrine factors controlling the growth of the intestinal mucosa. The intestinal peptide enteroglucagon is widely recognised as a probable mucosal growth hormone. In previous studies we have shown that both the CCPR and the release of this peptide depends upon the fat content of the diet (11). In the present study the lowest levels of enteroglucagon were seen in the fish-oil fed rats. Further studies on the release and action of enteroglucagon would be needed to verify this hypothesis.

Apart from the effects of fish oil on mucosal cell replication, this study suggests important differences in the post-absorptive metabolism of the different fatty acids. Body weight-gain did not differ amongst the groups, but the deposition of epididymal fat pads, was relatively low in rats fed fish oil. This may indicate a difference in the rate of absorption and subsequent metabolism of fish oil. Triglycerides from marine sources have been shown to resist hydrolysis by pancreatic lipase (12). The relatively long small intestines seen in the fish oil group may indicate an adaptive response to lipid malabsorption. Further studies are needed to explore the effects of fish oil on human gastrointestinal growth and susceptibility to carcinogenesis.

REFERENCES

1. W. Willett, Nature 1989, 338, 389.
2. R.A. Karmali, J. Intern. Med. Suppl. 1989, 225, 197.
3. B.S. Reddy, Cancer Res. 1991, 51, 487.
4. G.J. Nelson, P.C. Schmidt and L. Corash, Lipids, 1991, 26, 87.
5. C. Popp-Snijders, J.A. Schouten, W.J. van Blitterswizk and E.A. van der Veen, Biochim. Biophys. Acta. 1986, 854, 31.
6. T.A. Brasitus, P.K. Dudeja, R. Dahiya and A. Halline, Biochem. J. 1987, 248, 455.
7. S. Preston-Martin, M.C. Pike, R.K. Ross, P.A. Jones and B.E. Henderson, Cancer Res. 1990, 50, 7415.
8. M. Ponz de Leon, L. Roncucci, P. Di Donata, L. Tassi, O. Smerieri, M.G. Amorico, G. Malagoli, D. DeMaria, A. Antonioli, N.J. Chahin, M. Perini, G. Rigo, G. Barberini, A. Manenti, G. Biasco and L. Barbara, Cancer Res. 1988, 48, 4121.
9. M. Lipkin, K. Uehara, S. Winawer, A. Sanchez, C. Bauer, R. Phillips, H.T. Lynch, W.A. Blattner, J.F. Fraumeni Jr., Cancer Lett. 1985, 26, 139.
10. N. Wright and M. Alison, In: The Biology of Epithelial Cell Populations Vol.1, pp. 97-202, Clarendon Press 1984, Oxford, UK.
11. J.D. Pell, J.M. Gee, G.M. Wortley and I.T. Johnson, J. Nutr. 1992, (in press)
12. N.R. Bottino, G.A. Vandenburg and R. Reiser, Lipids, 1967, 2, 489.

WORKSHOP REPORT: INCREASED CELL PROLIFERATION AS A CAUSE OF HUMAN CANCER

R. Goodlad

Imperial Cancer Research Fund
Histopathology Unit
35-43
Lincoln's Inn Fields
London
WC2A 3PN

The discussion of the Workshop veered from rodent to human studies and back. The justification for this being that estimates in cell proliferation in most human studies left much to be desired: although it was agreed that microdissection-based techniques could now provide valid, robust measures of proliferation in animals and in man.

Proliferation is a prerequisite for carcinogenesis, as non-dividing cells have little clonogenic potential, and continually renewing cells are at a statistical disadvantage, nevertheless, the dearth of tumours in the small bowel, the most proliferative part of the gastrointestinal tract, shows that proliferation is not the only factor.

There is a considerable body of evidence from animal studies demonstrating increased tumour yield in hyperproliferative studies, however, many of the models are extreme. Increased proliferation and also increased carcinogenesis are seen near sites of damage and near gut associated lymphoid tissue. It has also been demonstrated that greater nutrient load causes proliferative activity which is associated with enhanced intestinal carcinogenesis.

Proliferation is increased in many human diseases in which there is an increased risk of cancer: ulcerative colitis, gastric cancer, gastritis (with or without Helicobacter pylori) and colon cancer were discussed in some depth. General agreement was reached that in most systems proliferation would promote, or positively modulate, previous initiation (mutation) events, supporting the two step or multistage theories of carcinogenesis. Cell division could fix mutations before repair or genetic housekeeping could occur, and increased proliferation would thus increase accumulation of genetic errors and hence eventually might lead to neoplastic transformation. Although some cancers may arise by spontaneous mutation, especially in childhood, it was agreed that most would involve the action of an exogenous mutagen. The implications of the recent work of Bruce Ames on the ubiquity of natural mutagens in our diet was mentioned and while it was agreed to be controversial, it was generally accepted.

Little conclusion was reached on the role of putative stem cells in carcinogenesis, or on the implications of alteration in the distribution of dividing cells within the proliferative compartments (the growth fraction).

Consensus was reached that the original title (increased cell proliferation as a cause of human cancer) overstated the case. Nevertheless no-one suggested that increased cell proliferation was not related to carcinogenesis and in fact it was agreed to be closely associated with cancer in humans. However, the involvement of other modulators was not discounted.

A suggestion was made that prospective studies could be performed providing that "normal" humans could be found to volunteer for chronic biopsy, perhaps as part of a sponsored screening programme.

WORKSHOP REPORT: DIETARY PROTECTIVE FACTORS - NEW CANDIDATES

L. Wattenburg

University of Minnesota
Department of Laboratory
Medicine & Pathology
6-133 Jackson Hall
321 Church Street E., Minneapolis
Minnesota

The report on the identification of new candidate compounds has two components. The first deals with suggestions as to strategies for identifying new protective factors and the second some candidate groups or specific agents. The Workshop began with a discussion of suppressing agents. One group of compounds that offers promise are those that may prevent hormone driven neoplasia in women at increased risk of cancer of the breast. For this purpose a general strategy of using agents that inhibit 16α-hydroxylation of estradiol and induce increased 2-hydroxylation appears attractive. These hydroxylations are carried out by cytochrome P_{450} enzymes. Precise information pertaining to which P_{450} isozymes have the capacity to carry out these reactions is important to obtain. With this information it should be possible to evaluate foods for the presence of constituents inducing increased 2-hydroxylation and reducing 16α-hydroxylation. An additional process of obtaining protection for women at increased risk of breast cancer entails the consumption of foods containing phytosteroids with antiestrogen activity. A systematic identification of foods with this property is desirable.

A second group of suppressing agents that were discussed are compounds that can reduce proliferation of mucosal cells of the large bowel in individuals at increased risk of cancer of this site. Inhibitors of the arachidonic acid cascade, in particular polyphenolic compounds, fall into this category. The studies of combinations of antioxidant nutrients merit further investigation.

The Workshop subsequently began consideration of blocking agents. The major focus was on Phase 2 enzymes. Numerous studies have demonstrated that evaluation of electrophile-processing Phase 2 enzymes can protect rodents and cultured cells from the toxic, mutagenic, and neoplastic effects of carcinogens. Since virtually all Phase 2 enzyme inducers are protective under the appropriate experimental circumstances, the use of Phase 2 enzyme induction as a surrogate marker for anticarcinogenic activity may be a rapid method for identifying novel synthetic and naturally occurring anticarcinogens. Although the chemical signals that endow xenobiotics with the ability to induce Phase 2 enzymes is now understood (see Talalay *et al.*, this volume) undoubtedly many unrecognised Phase 2 enzyme inducers exist. Moreover, vegetables that induce Phase 2 enzymes are known to reduce cancer risk in man. Thus, it is of considerable interest to develop an economical, rapid, and systematic approach for the identification of dietary sources rich in Phase 2 enzyme inducer activity.

The technology of rapid screening for inducers of NAD(P)H: (quinone-acceptor) oxidoreductase (EC 1.6.99.2) as a marker for Phase 2 enzyme induction has been developed in a recent series of superb investigation[1]. It is now feasible to screen foods for their content of Phase 2 enzyme inducer activity as well as to assess the fate of inducer activity after cooking, storage, and other processing techniques. Moreover, the constituents responsible for enzyme induction can be isolated and studied. After a capital investment of $50,000 for specialized equipment (tissue culture facilities, microtiter spectrophotometer, and computer), 1000 food samples could be screened in less than a year at a cost of approximately $50,000. This screening would not only provide information of great interest for epidemiology and possibly intervention, but it would also be a prototype for further investigations for screening foods for putative inhibitors of carcinogenesis.

A miscellaneous group of compounds was put forth as meriting investigation. These include phytate, and some of its less phosphorylated derivatives, in particular those formed during fermentation. Other compounds are α-carotene, cell wall polysaccharides, tyrosine kinase inhibitors such as genistein and naturally occurring inhibitors of angiogenesis. In addition, protective effects of various strains of *Lactobacillus* would be of interest to evaluate.

I would like to thank the participants of the Workshop. They worked hard, interacted vigorously as one always hopes will occur. I believe some excellent suggestions were made and it was all done with a sense of scientific camaraderie and good humour.

REFERENCES

1. Y.S. Zhang, P. Talalay, C.G. Cho and G.H. Posner, *Proc. Natl. Acad. Sci.*, 1992, 2399.

PART 6 IMMUNE MECHANISM: THE ROLE OF FOOD COMPONENTS AS IMMUNOREGULATORS

BIOACTIVE CELL WALL AND RELATED COMPONENTS FROM HERBAL PRODUCTS AND EDIBLE PLANT ORGANS AS PROTECTIVE FACTORS

K. W. Waldron and R. R. Selvendran

AFRC Institute of Food Research
Food Molecular Biochemistry Department
Norwich Research Park
Colney
Norwich NR4 7UA
UK

1 INTRODUCTION

In the treatment of disease, the approach taken by Sino-Japanese and Chinese traditional medicine takes into account various factors such as the age and constitution of the patient. However, little attempt is made to identify the specific cause of the disease[1]. The success of this strategy has largely relied on the use of extracts from herbal sources which, after oral administration, are thought to bring about a general improvement in the health of the individual, and a subsequent cure.

Over the past 30 years, there has been considerable scientific interest in the active components of herbal drugs and there is increasing evidence that many polysaccharides of plant origin are responsible for their bioactive properties[2,3]. These are normally of high molecular weight, usually between 10^3 and 10^6 daltons[1,4-6] and may be associated with small amounts of protein. A range of bioactivities has been identified including anti-tumour activity, anti-viral activity, anti-bacterial activity, anti-complementary activity, anti-inflammatory activity, hypoglycemic activity, anti-coagulatory activity and phagocytotic activity[1].

2. ANTI-TUMOUR POLYSACCHARIDES

Identification of anti-tumour polysaccharides in herbal extracts has been facilitated by the development of *in vivo* bioassays. These usually involve solid or ascites allogeneic and syngeneic murine tumours that have been implanted subcutaneously or injected into mice, and sometimes autochthonous tumours. The bioactive extract, or a subfraction, is administered orally, intraperitoneally, (i.p.), intravascularly or subcutaneously and the growth of the tumour and longevity of the host assessed. Such assays have facilitated the fractionation and purification of anti-tumour polysaccharides from plant materials such as fungi[6,7] algae[8,9] and gymnosperms[10] traditionally used in oriental medicine. In addition, screening programmes have assisted in the identification of anti-tumour polysaccharides from a wide range of alternative sources including fungi, yeasts, lichens, algae and higher plants[2]. The composition and structural features of these polysaccharides are comparable to those found in mucilages, gums and plant cell walls, the structures of which are fairly well documented[11,12]. Selected examples of anti-tumour polysaccharides are shown in Table 1 along with the effective doses. It is clear that anti-tumour polysaccharides can vary considerably in composition, glycosidic linkage type and molecular weight.

Mode of action of anti-tumour polysaccharides

There are few examples of anti-tumour polysaccharides that are directly cytotoxic towards tumour cells[21]. In the vast majority of cases, the mode of action of anti-tumour polysaccharides is host mediated, i.e. their activity is dependent on the reaction of the host[2,6,9,22-24]. Preliminary theories to explain such activity included the lowering of blood pressure in arteries supplying the tumour, thus resulting in a reduction in blood supply and associated tumour necrosis[25-27] and increased permeability to water of the tumour cell plasma membrane and endoplasmic reticulum, resulting in massive vacuolisation and associated damage[2,28]. Subsequently, evidence has emerged suggesting that anti-tumour polysaccharides might act by altering the immune response of treated animals. For example, pre-treatment of mice with specific polysaccharides such as gum arabic and O-methyl cellulose prevented them from accepting tumour grafts[29,30]; furthermore, administration of some anti-tumour polysaccharides was associated with increased phagocytotic activity within the tumour[32]. Additional examples have been documented by Whistler et al[2]. The potential for such bioactive polysaccharides to modulate the immune response was seized upon by researchers since it could offer explanations not only to the workings of Sino-Japanese medicine, particularly the way in which it focuses on the health of the individual, but also why the polysaccharides could exhibit other beneficial properties listed above.

In the recent past research in this area has concentrated on the immunomodulatory activities of anti-tumour polysaccharides, particularly in murine model systems. There is evidence that anti-tumour polysaccharides can influence aspects of both innate (natural) and adaptive immunity.

(i) Innate Immunity. Innate immunity includes numerous nonspecific elements and is present from birth. It is the first line of defence against invasive organisms and tumour cells and includes physical barriers such as skin and mucous membranes, soluble factors including enzymes (e.g. of the alternative complement pathway), acute phase proteins and α and β interferons, and cells such as macrophages, polymorphonuclear neutrophils (PMN)

Table 1. Antitumour activity of polysaccharides against subcutaneously implanted Sarcoma 180 in mice.

Glycan	Source*	Sugar Composition and/or linkage	Effective dose (mg/kg x No.)	Route of administration	Complete regression	Inhibition Ratio (%)**
Lentinan[13]	F: *Lentinus edodes*	β-D-Glucose, mainly (1-3)-linkage	1x10 5x10	i.p i.p	7/10 6/10	97.5 95.1
Lichenan[14]	L: *Cetraria islandica*	β-D-Glucose, mainly (1-3) and (1-4)-linked	15x10	i.p	8/8	100
Mannan[15]	Y: *Saccharomyces cerevisiae*	Mannose	100x10	i.p	7/8	100
Glucomannan[16]	Y: *Candida utilis*	Mannose (90%) and glucose (10%)	100x10	i.p	8/10	99
Arabinoglucoxylan[17]	AN: Wheat (Straw)	Xylose, arabinose and glucose	25x10	i.p	8/10	95
Arabinoxylan[18]	AN: Bamboo (leaf)	Xylan Arabinose, glucose and galactose	200x10	i.p	3/9	93.2
Rhamno-galacturonan[19] (fraction AR-4-E)	AN: *Angelica acutiloba* (roots)	Rha: Ara: Gal: GalA 11: 61: 15: 12	3.1x10	i.p	-	>99%†
Rhamno-galacturonan[5] (fraction S1A)	AN: *Cassia angustifolia* (leaves)	Rha:Ara:Gal:Glc:GalA 19:32:28:4:15	5x10	i.p	4/10	52%
Acidic (pectic) polysaccharide[20] (fraction VII)	G: *Pinus parviflora* (cones)	Ara:Man:Gal:Glc:UA 7:7:26:11:60	10x5 20x3	i.p i.p	- 5/10	170%† 77%†

Key
* F: fungus; L: lichen; Y: yeast; AN: angiosperm; G: gymnosperm.
** Inhibition ratio is calculated on the basis of tumour weights as reported by the authors, and as calculated by Whistler et al.[2]
† Increase in life expectancy (ILS) over that of the control (%)

and natural killer (NK) cells. The way in which these cells may be affected by anti-tumour polysaccharides are discussed below.

Macrophages are derived from blood monocytes. Their functions in tumour immunity include their activity both as antigen-presenting cells (see below) and as effector cells to mediate tumour lysis[33]. The mechanisms by which macrophages can recognise tumour cells and mediate lysis are not fully understood. However, since they only become cytolytic if activated by macrophage activating factors (MAF), which are commonly produced by T cells following antigen-specific stimulation, their participation as effector cells may be T cell-regulated. A range of anti-tumour polysaccharides has been shown to stimulate the activity of murine macrophages both *in vitro* and *in vivo*. *In vitro*, cytotoxicity of mouse macrophages towards allogeneic and syngeneic tumours has been enhanced by Viva Naturel, an anti-tumour polysaccharide extracted from seaweed[34] and DMG, a degraded glucomannan[35]. This increase may be due to the increased production of biocidal superoxide (O2-) as demonstrated for murine peritoneal macrophages after i.p. administration of cellulose and pectic polysaccharides[36]. In addition, the ß-(1-3)-linked fungal glucan lentinan has been shown to activate the pinocytotic function of murine macrophages, apparently via specific ß-glucan receptors. Furthermore, it has been reported that certain anti-tumour polysaccharides can stimulate the secretion of physiologically active molecules from mouse intraperitoneal macrophages. For example, DMG enhances the production of interleukin 1 (IL 1), a peptide messenger important in stimulating the T cell mediated immune response, and the production of differentiation-inducing-factor (DIF) has been promoted by PSK, a protein-containing polysaccharide preparation isolated from the basidiomycete *Coriolus versicolor*[37], and also by acidic polysaccharide from cones of pine (*Pinus parviflora*)[10]. *In vivo*, the stimulation of murine peritoneal macrophage cytotoxicity by Lentinan has been shown to be dependent on the prior stimulation of T cells[6], i.p. administration of a polysaccharide NMF-5N has been reported to increase the cytotoxicity of peritoneal macrophages to syngeneic tumour cells[38]. Also, PSK has been found to stimulate the recovery of macrophage cytotoxicity lost after inoculation with either allogeneic or syngeneic tumours (see references in reference 7).

Polymorphonuclear neutrophil (PMN) cells are a subtype of the granulocytic leukocytes. They have been shown to act as effector cells in tumour cell cytotoxicity and tumour rejection[39-41]. Their cytotoxicity to tumour cells has been shown to be enhanced *in vitro* by a range of anti-tumour polysaccharides including ß-(1-3) glucans such as Lentinan and TAK[42,43] and acidic polysaccharides from pine cone extracts[44]. Furthermore, there is evidence that H_2O_2 is a direct cytotoxic mediator in the polysaccharide-induced cytotoxicity[42]. *In vivo*, a range of immunomodulatory anti-tumour polysaccharides have been shown to induce PMN activity in mice by increasing the numbers of PMN cells within the tissues[41].

Natural killer (NK) cells are able to kill a wide range of tumour cells *in vitro*[33]. However, the mechanisms by which they are able to recognise and lyse transformed cells in preference to normal cells are not well defined. The binding of NK cells to tumour targets appears to employ cell surface adhesion molecules rather than antigen-specific receptors. In addition, NK activity can be amplified by T cell-secreted lymphokines such as IL-2 and interferons. It has been demonstrated that NK cells may be a first line of defence against transformed cells, and that augmentation of their activity in visceral organs increases the resistance to the growth of cancerous tissues[33]. Other cells that are similar in many respects to NK cells, but which are cytotoxic to a different and often broader spectrum of tumour targets include natural cytotoxic (NC) cells and lymphokine-activated killer (LAK) cells.

The anti-tumour polysaccharide Lentinan has been reported to augment NK activity and this has been suggested as one route by which the anti-tumour activity is mediated[45]. However, the ability of anti-tumour polysaccharides to stimulate NK activity may not always be related to their anti-tumour properties as has been demonstrated in work on "white-type" polysaccharide preparation (WPS) from *Serratia marcescens*[46]. Interestingly, a mechanism by which anti-tumour polysaccharides might stimulate the cytotoxicity of NK cells to tumour cells has been put forward by Mueller and Anderer[24]. They observed that the spontaneous cytotoxicity of human NK and LAK cells against tumour cells could be markedly enhanced by a rhamnogalacturonan (RG) polysaccharide present in preparations from *Viscum album*. As a result of a series of experiments which showed that the enhancement of cytotoxicity could be inhibited (a) by treating the extract with rhamnosidase or polygalacturonase or (b) by acetylated rhamnose and acetylated mannose in a dose-dependent manner, they have proposed a model of synergistic interaction (Figure 1)[23,24,47]. This postulates that the binding of NK and LAK cells to the tumour target cells is enhanced as a result of binding of "rhamnose acetate" of the RG to the NK or LAK cell, and of galacturonic acid to a receptor on the tumour cell. At present, there is little information on the presence of rhamnose acetate in rhamnogalacturonans. It is possible that the acetylated sugars sterically resemble (1-2,4)- and (1-2)-linked rhamnosyl residues found in rhamnogalacturonans.

(ii) Adaptive Immunity. The adaptive immune response is implemented when the defences provided by the innate immune system fail to prevent infection or, in the present context, tumour growth. The main cells involved are macrophages, T cells and B cells. The T cell population is

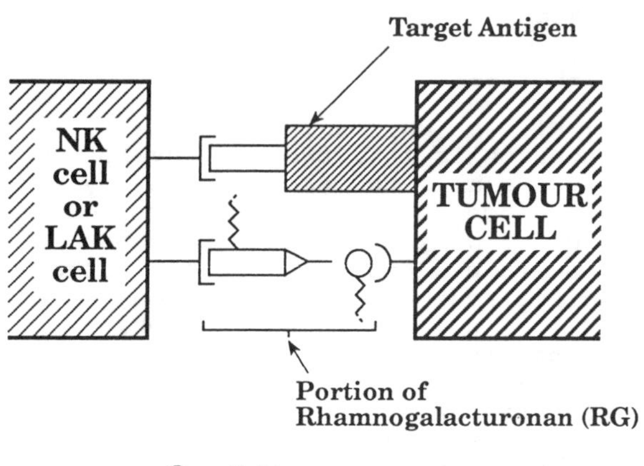

Figure 1 Schematic representation of the interaction between NK and LAK cells with target tumour cells, via rhamnogalacturonan polysaccharides. After Mueller and Anderer[24].

important in orchestrating the adaptive response, hence control of antigenic tumour cells via the direct killing of tumour cells (by cytotoxic T cells) and by activation of other components of the immune system, including those of the innate immune system[33].

Augmentation of the T cell response has been suggested as the mediator of the effects of several anti-tumour polysaccharides. The mode of action of Lentinan has been studied in some detail, mainly in murine model systems, and the polysaccharide has been described as a T cell oriented adjuvant[6] in which macrophages play some part (se above). However it has also been used successfully in clinical trials, significantly extending the life expectancy of patients with advanced and recurrent gastrointestinal cancer when used in combination with other chemotherapy[49]. PSK, has been shown to augment cytotoxic T cell activity in tumour bearing mice after oral or i.p. administration[7], and this has been correlatec with the anti-tumour effect. The host-mediated anti-tumou activity of the polysaccharide NMF-5N (grifolan) from *Grifola frondosa* has also been studied[38] and results suggest that the activity is mediated via effects on both macrophages and T cells.

(iii) Anti-complementary Activity. The complement system consists of a group of plasma and cell membrane proteins which play a major role in the host defence process[33]. Several anti-tumour polysaccharides also exhibi anti-complementary (complement stimulating) activity, particularly those containing (1-3)-linked glucans such a lentinan. The activity includes activation of both the classical and alternative complement pathways and an increase in the C3 splitting activity[6]. However, the relationship between such activity and anti-tumour activity is not clear since many polysaccharides can exhibit anti-complementary activity without anti-tumour activity[1]. Nevertheless, anti-complementary activity would serve to augment any T cell response.

Hence there is great heterogeneity in the range and source of anti-tumour polysaccharides. In addition to functioning as anti-tumour agents in their own right, many have also been shown to act as adjuvants to other cancer treatments such as chemotherapy[49-51], again via stimulation of aspects of the immune system that has been depressed both by the cancer and its treatment. However, although immunomodulatory activity of many anti-tumour polysaccharides has been reported, only in a few cases has it been directly linked to the anti-tumour effect (RGI and NK/LAK cells; see above). In all others, it appears to be an associated property. Furthermore, it is evident that different polysaccharides have different effects on the immune system.

In addition to acting as immunomodulators, some anti-tumour polysaccharides have been found to stimulate the synthesis of collagen from the stroma around capillaries and tissues that are being destroyed by cancer cells[52,53]. These include the bacterial polysaccharide SSM, an arabinomannan, which has been studied in nude (i.e. thyroid deficient) mice and which has been reported to have been used successfully in prolonging the life expectancy of patients suffering from advanced cases of breast cancer[22,54].

3 ANTI-TUMOUR POLYSACCHARIDES FROM PLANT FOODS

As described above, anti-tumour polysaccharides have been obtained from a wide range of sources. Their carbohydrate compositions and structural features are typical of polysaccharides of either exudate gums and mucilages, or cell wall polysaccharides from prokaryotes, fungi, lower and higher plants. The presence of anti-tumour polysaccharides in the cell walls of higher plants suggests that such polymers may also be present in the cell walls of plant organs used as foods. However, if potentially bioactive cell wall polysaccharides are to express their anti-tumour activities, it is likely that they will have to traverse the gastrointestinal tract in soluble form. This is consistent with the observation that by far the majority of herbal remedies involve hot aqueous extracts of medicinal plants, and that the active fractions so far identified are water soluble[2]. Of particular interest, therefore, are the structures of cold- and hot-water soluble anti-tumour pectic polysaccharides from the leaves of *Cassia angustifolia*, the roots of *Angelica acutiloba*, and the cones of *Pinus parviflora* and how these compare with those found in the cell walls of edible plant organs.

Pectic polysaccharides

In general, pectic polysaccharides consist of an α(1-4)-linked, partially methyl-esterified polygalacturonan backbone in which (1-2)-linked rhamnosyl (Rha) residues are interspersed. Side chains consisting of neutral sugars, particularly galactosyl (Gal) and arabinosyl (Ara) residues, are attached to the C-4 of some of the Rha residues. The frequency of the rhamnosyl residues and side chains may vary. Pectic polysaccharides may be classified by virtue of their ease of extraction from the cell wall. About 30 to 40% of the pectic polysaccharides from immature or parenchyma cell walls are readily solubilised by cold water or chelating agents. These polymers are rich in polygalacturonic acid and have a low degree of branching as indicated by a low rha:galA (galacturonic acid) ratio of 1:40 or less[55-58]. However, pectic polysaccharides that require more rigorous treatment such as dilute alkali extraction in the cold exhibit a much greater degree of branching as indicated by a higher Rha:GalA ratio (up to 1:10), and high levels of (1-2,4)-linked Rha; these account for approximately 20% of the cell wall pectic polysaccharides[55,56,59]. Finally, a proportion (30-40%) of the cell wall pectic polysaccharides are highly branched (Rha:galA of up to 1:5[55-59]), and these are not readily extractable by non-degradative methods.

The structures of pectic polysaccharides are not fully resolved. However, studies of pectic polysaccharides from the primary cell walls of sycamore suspension cultured cells have revealed endopolygalacturonase-resistant, highly-branched regions consisting of a backbone of alternating (1-2)-linked Rha and (1-4)-linked GalA residues with side chains attached to C-4 of half of the Rha residues. The structural features of this fraction, named Rhamnogalacturonan I (RG I), are shown in Figure 2[48]. It is likely that structures of this sort are present in cell walls of most higher plants[60] and the frequency of their occurrence within the polygalacturonan moieties determines, to a large extent, the degree of branching of the pectic polysaccharides.

Significantly, structural studies on purified anti-tumour pectic polysaccharides from *Cassia angustifolia* and *Angelica acutiloba* have revealed that these polysaccharides closely resemble RG I (Figure 3a and 3b respectively)[5,19]. They exhibit a backbone consisting of alternating (1-2)-linked Rha and (1-4)-linked GalA, and side chains composed mostly of neutral sugars (mainly Gal) are attached to C-4 of a large proportion of Rha. Thus it is possible that RG-I-type polysaccharides from the organs of fruits and vegetables may also exhibit anti-tumour activity if ingested in a soluble form.

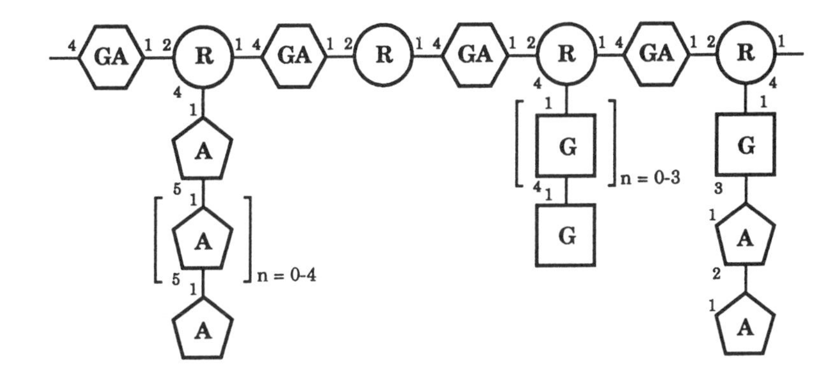

GA D-Galacturonic acid R L-Rhamnose G D-Galactose A L-Arabinose

Figure 2 Selected structural features of Rhamnogalacturonan I (RG I) as characterised[48].

(a)

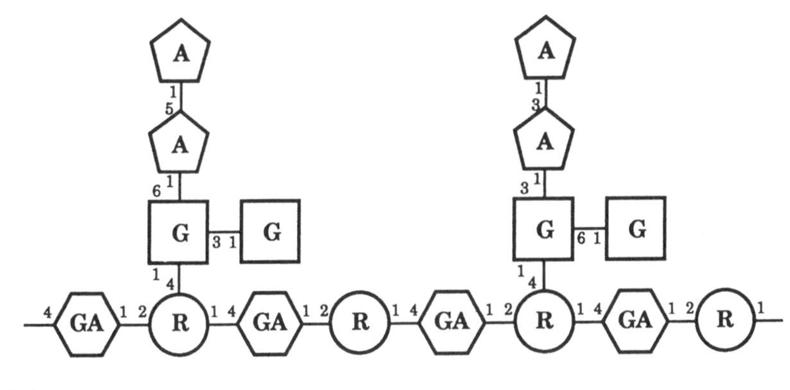

(b)

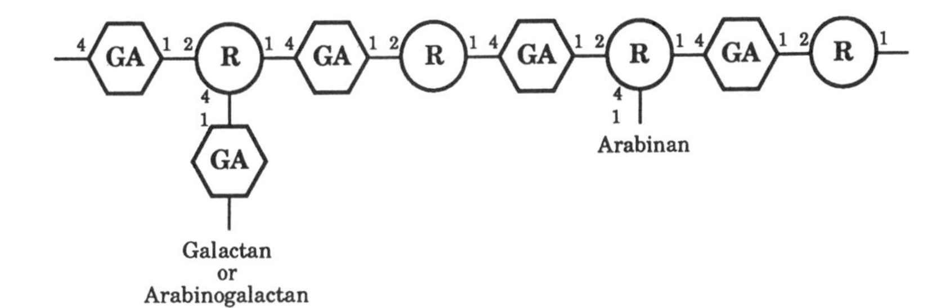

Figure 3 (a) Proposed structural features of the anti-tumour polysaccharide S1A: after Muller et al[5]; (b) a possible partial structural fragment of the anti-tumour polysaccharide AR-4E-2: after Yamada et al[19].

Solubilisation of potential anti-tumour polysaccharides from fruits and vegetables.

Since pectic polysaccharides that contain significant quantities of RG I are branched and are generally cross-linked into the cell wall, they are often cold-water insoluble (see above). However, cooking and processing of vegetables can solubilise such polymers. This is due to heat-catalysed ß-eliminative degradation of the methyl-esterified regions of the polygalacturonan backbone (Figure 4). Such depolymerisation contributes to the solubilisation of pectic polysaccharides of the middle lamella and primary cell wall, facilitating cell separation and associated softening of the vegetable. This is illustrated in the case of cooking of potato, which results in cell separation (Figure 5). Analogous changes occur during fruit ripening, but these are mediated mostly by cell wall degrading enzymes as, for example in tomatoes, in which branched pectic polysaccharides are solubilised[61].

In the case of fresh plant material, soluble RG I-containing polysaccharides will be ingested along with the vegetable or fruit parenchyma. However, many of the RG I-containing pectic polymers solubilised during cooking or processing may be released into the cooking liquor which is usually discarded. It should be remembered that the exploitation of herbal drugs involves ingestion of the hot-water extracts. Therefore, the amount of food-derived soluble RG I-type pectic polysaccharides that are ingested will also be determined by the way in which the anatomy of the vegetable retains the soluble polymers. This is illustrated by the data presented in Table 2[62-65]. The values for RG I-type polysaccharides ingested have been calculated as a function of body weight for a range of fresh and processed vegetables and a ripe fruit. The quantity of RG I has been estimated as 6x the Rha content of the water-soluble pectic polysaccharides isolated from purified cell walls from the fresh and cooked food materials. This estimate is based on the average structural moiety of RG I side chains (Figure 6). However, due to the incomplete release of rhamnose during acid hydrolysis of pectic polysaccharides[66], the values presented may be up to 30% below the correct value and should therefore be regarded as a minimum.

In the case of carrot, cooking results in a decrease in the quantity of RG I ingested. This is due to loss of solubilised pectic polysaccharides into the cooking liquor (results not shown) from the cut surfaces. Pressure-cooked cabbage, however, exhibits a 15-fold increase in the quantity of soluble RG I ingested. This is probably due to the entrapment of solubilised pectic polysaccharides within the cooked cabbage leaf which is covered on each side by a thick, waxy, waterproof cuticle. Ripe pear yields a significant amount of soluble RG I, reflecting the ripening-related solubilisation of pectic

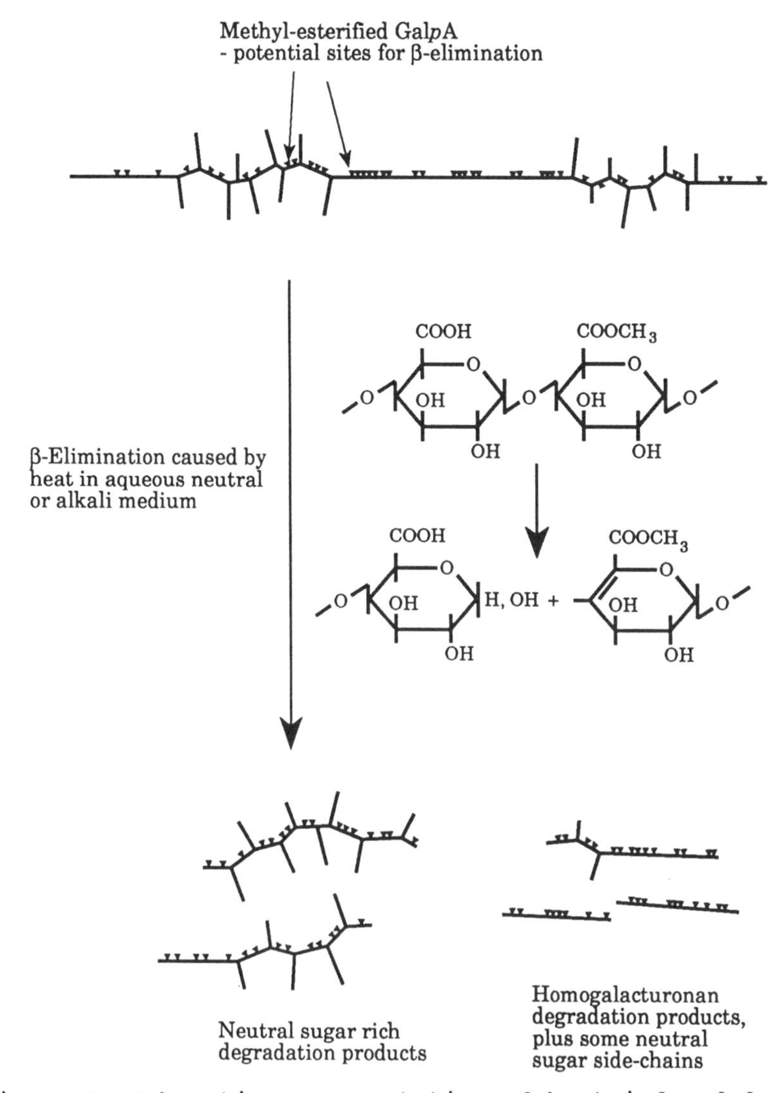

Figure 4 Schematic representation of heat-induced ß-eliminative depolymerisation of pectic polysaccharides.

polysaccharides and the absence of a cooking process that would facilitate the diffusion of such polymers away from the solid tissue.

The results in Table 2 are presented as mg/Kg body weight per typical 75g serving in order to make comparisons with the active doses of anti-tumour polysaccharides shown in Table 1. The results show that an individual of 70 kg body weight consuming six vegetable/fruit portions per day will ingest approximately 2 mg/kg of RG I-type "anti-tumour" polysaccharides in a

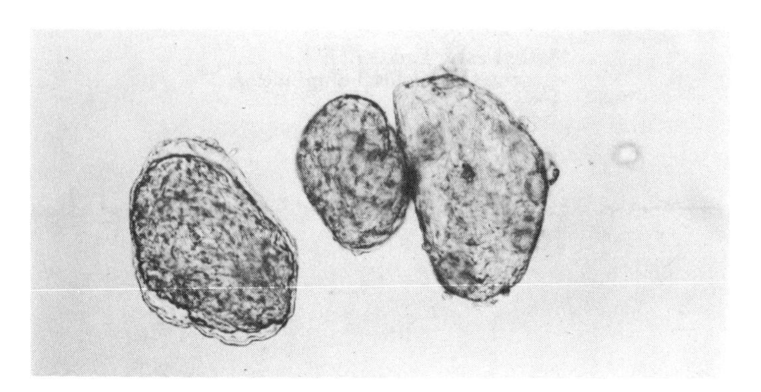

Figure 5 Potato cells that have separated due to cooking.

soluble form. Whilst this is of the same order of magnitude as the effective doses of RG I-type anti-tumour polysaccharides described in Table 1, the polysaccharides are being administered orally as opposed to injection i.p. Unfortunately, there are few studies that make definitive comparisons between oral and i.p. administration. In the case of KGF-C, a water-soluble polysaccharide from kefir grain, the effective doses (i.p. and oral) are broadly similar (between 20 and 200 mg/Kg/day) although the oral doses had to be estimated from the likely daily water consumption by the mice[67]. In contrast, TC-13, a protein-bound polysaccharide extracted from the basidiomycete *Microellabosporia grisea*, is far more effective as an anti-tumour polymer when administered by i.p. injection. Nevertheless, it does exhibit anti-tumour properties when administered orally at a dose of 50 mg/Kg/day[68].

4. ROUTE BY WHICH INGESTED ANTI-TUMOUR POLYSACCHARIDES CAN STIMULATE THE IMMUNE SYSTEM

During digestion of food materials, proteins and starch macromolecules generally undergo considerable degradation by amylases and proteases in the lumen of the gut.

Table 2 Estimated yield of RG I-type polysaccharides from 75g servings of selected fruit and vegetable organs, fresh and cooked

Plant organ	Treatment	RG I (mg/kg)*
Cabbage leaf	Fresh	0.02
Cabbage leaf	Pressure-cooked	0.3
Carrot root	Fresh	0.4
Carrot root	Cooked	0.2
Potato tuber	Cooked	0.2
Pear fruit	Fresh	0.8

* based on a body weight of 70 kg.

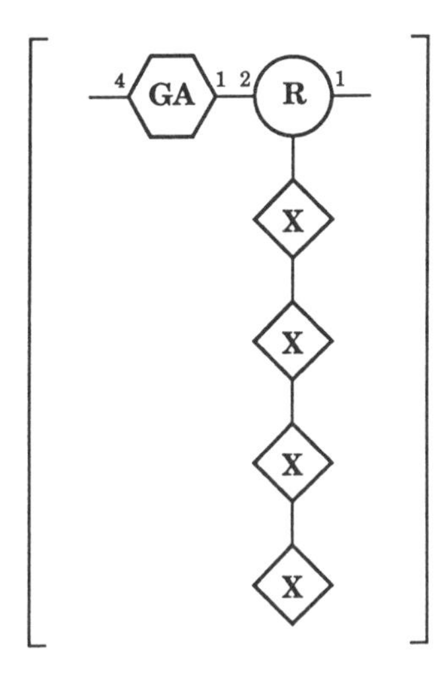

Figure 6 Generalised structure of RG I-type polysaccharides illustrating the ratio of Rha to other glycosidic residues.

Subsequently, the released products (glucose, amino acids and small peptides) are actively transported into the epithelial cells of the small intestinal mucosa whilst some large peptides are absorbed by endopinocytosis and then subject to lysosomal digestion. However, cell wall and related polysaccharides (dietary fibre) are not degraded by enzymes secreted by the human alimentary tract. Accordingly, bioactive anti-tumour polysaccharides will have to be absorbed as intact macromolecules if they are to enter the hepatic portal vein or lymphatic system and come into contact with cells of the immune system - a prerequisite for the manifestation of any immunoregulatory properties. Nonetheless, there is now a considerable body of evidence which indicates that large molecules and even particulates may be absorbed in the small intestine: 1) many workers have demonstrated that the circulation of healthy individuals contains antibodies to many food proteins and their immune complexes[69]; 2) the appearance of intact glycoproteins such as horse-radish peroxidase (HRP) has been followed in the blood and tissues of fish *in vivo*[70,71]; 3) the passage of high molecular weight fragments of protein across isolated animal small intestine has been established; *in vivo* investigations into the permeability of rabbit small intestine as measured by plasma clearance of water soluble molecules have demonstrated that log permeability is proportional to the inverse of log molecular weight (investigated up to a molecular weight of 80 000[72]); 4) there are numerous examples of experiments showing that particles including bacteria and viruses, and inert materials such as carbon in indian ink, can cross the healthy intestine[69]; and finally 5) circumstantial evidence such as the effectiveness both of orally ingested traditional herbal medicines[1,7,10] and orally administered bioactive polysaccharides in clinical use[7] and experimental animals[67,68,73-75] should also be taken into account.

Gastrointestinal absorption of bioactive polysaccharides.

It is likely that orally-ingested anti-tumour polysaccharides would have to be absorbed in the small intestine since they will be degraded rapidly by bacterial fermentation on reaching the colon[76]. The main route of gastrointestinal absorption of digested material is across the epithelium, via either the transcellular or paracellular pathways (Figure 7). The transcellular path encompasses both active uptake and pinocytosis. The paracellular path relies on passive diffusion between the plasmamembranes of adjacent epithelial cells. In traversing the paracellular route, molecules would have to cross the tight junctions[77]. A tight junction consists of a narrow belt that surrounds circumferentially the apical pole of each epithelial cell (Figure 7) where the membranes of the adjacent cells are tightly associated. This prevents the passage of macromolecules: whilst the paracellular route is of considerable importance in fluid and ion transport[69], the transcellular pathway appears to be by far the dominant route for passage of large molecules across the epithelial cells of a healthy intestine as indicated by experiments on the absorption of intact proteins by hamster intestine[78] and rabbit ilium[79]. There is, however, very little work on the absorption of high-molecular weight carbohydrates (see below).

In addition to the epithelial route, it is now apparent that macromolecules may traverse the GI lining by the M-cell route (Figure 8). Evidence for this again stems predominantly from work on the absorption of intact protein molecules. M-cells, (membranous or lymphoepithelial cells) are found in the epidermal layer of the Gut-Associated Lymphoid Tissue (GALT) known as Peyer's patches. The M cells are thought to allow direct access of luminal antigens to the sub-epithelial lymphocytes via pinocytosis, thus facilitating an immune response[69]. Hence, Peyer's patches serve to sample the antigenic components in the lumen of the gut. Indeed, transport of a number of proteins, viruses, and inert particles across the M cells by endopinocytosis has been demonstrated (see references in 69). Such activity would provide a direct route by which anti-tumour polysaccharides could come into contact with cells of the immune system.

There are very few reports on the gastrointestinal absorption of bioactive polysaccharides. However, studies

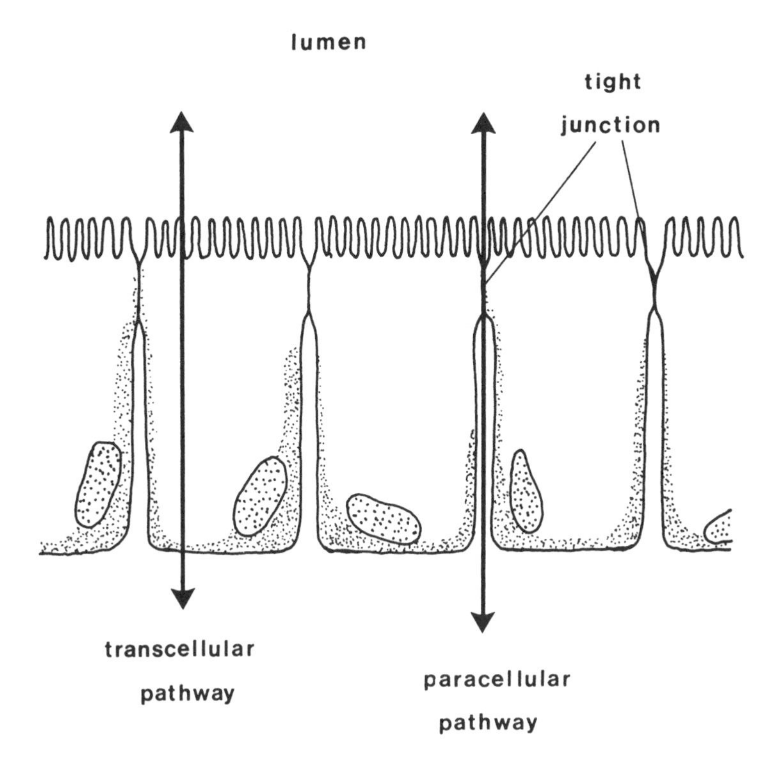

Figure 7 Schematic illustration of the intestinal epithelial barrier.

on 14C and 35S-labelled PSK in rabbits and rats indicated that PSK can be absorbed in its large molecular form, and can exist as such in the blood[7]. More pertinent evidence has come from studies of fluorescence-labelled KS-2 (F-KS), a peptidomannan from *Lentinus edodes* with anti-tumour and interferon-inducing activity. By using the double reciprocal relationship between the fluorescence polarisation value and molecular weight, researchers were able to follow both GI absorption of the molecule and any changes in its size[74]. Orally ingested F-KS was absorbed intact via the hepatic portal vein and intestinal lymphatics. It was also recovered in the urine, but with a reduced molecular weight. Further histological evaluation revealed that F-KS was accumulated in the mesenteric lymph nodes, Peyer's patches, spleen, liver and kidneys, indicating that KS-2 was accessible to the cells of the immune system and the vascular system. A total of 1.25% of F-KS administered was absorbed into the body, and the absorption via the lymphatics was as efficient as that via the portal vein.

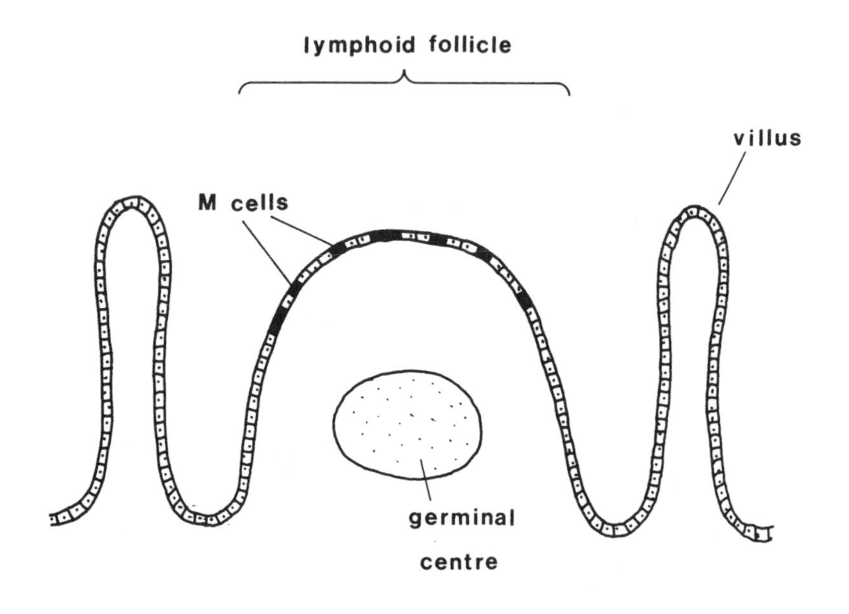

Figure 8 Schematic illustration of a Peyer's Patch.

5. CONCLUSIONS

In this article we have outlined the potential of certain pectic polysaccharides from edible plant organs to provide sources of anti-tumour polysaccharides in the diet. The RG I-type pectic polysaccharides found in the cell walls of plant organs used as foods are structurally comparable to anti-tumour pectic polysaccharides extracted from higher plants. Furthermore, the yield of such polysaccharides from fruits and cooked vegetables in a healthy diet is of the same order of magnitude (as a function of body weight) as the effective doses in anti-tumour assays. Also, there are routes by which such orally-ingested water-soluble polysaccharides can come into contact with cells of the immune system through which their activity is likely to be mediated. In addition to RG I, there are other polysaccharides found in the cell walls of edible plant organs that also closely resemble anti-tumour polysaccharides. Many of these, for example arabinoxylans, mannans and glucomannans, are likely to remain as part of the insoluble part of the cell wall matrix, even after extensive processing. However, there may be other cell wall polysaccharides in addition to those of pectic origin, which may be solubilised. These include, for example, the mixed linkage (1-3)- and (1-4)- linked ß-glucans from cereal endosperm cell walls which are somewhat comparable to anti-tumour polysaccharides such as Lichenan (Table 1). In addition to polysaccharides from the cell walls of edible plant organs, polysaccharides with anti-tumour and other bioactive properties may also be obtained from exudate gums and mucilages. Freely-soluble RG-like polymers (classed as galacturonorhamnans) may be obtained from the exudate gums of Khaya species[80]. However, there is a considerable amount of work to be done before one can confidently attribute anti-cancer properties to the polysaccharides in question.

It is necessary to establish whether or not these potential anti-tumour polysaccharides are able to stimulate the immune system to act against autochthonous tumours, i.e. those that occur spontaneously within the body of the host. Until the mid 1970's, identification of host-mediated anti-tumour polysaccharides employed allogeneic tumours such as Sarcoma 180, that were implanted into the host. It is now accepted that the "anti-tumour activity" exhibited by the effective polysaccharides may have been, in many cases, due to stimulation of the graft rejection mechanisms of the immune system[2]. Since then, efforts have been made to address this and there has been much greater use of assays involving syngeneic tumours (implanted tumours with the same genetic characteristics as the host) and, infrequently, autochthonous tumours. However, even the results of these assays must be treated with caution since syngeneic tumours may "drift" genetically in comparison to their experimental hosts over a period. Furthermore, some autochthonous tumours, particularly those that have been induced by the relatively harsh action of chemical carcinogens, may not always be appropriate models of natural and spontaneously occurring cancer cells. To date, the most rigorously tested polysaccharide is the fungal glucan Lentinan. It has been shown to exhibit marked anti-tumour activity in both syngeneic and autochthonous tumour/host assays and, as discussed, has been successfully used in combination with chemotherapeutic agents in clinical trials in Japan (see above) in the treatment of certain cancers[49]. For the majority of other anti-tumour polysaccharides, however, assays have usually employed either syngeneic and/or allogeneic murine tumours. Often, the allogeneic or syngeneic nature of the assay is not even mentioned, as in the cases of the assays used in testing the anti-tumour activity of the RG I-like polysaccharides from *Cassia angustifolia* and *Angelica acutiloba*, and the acidic polysaccharides from *Pinus parviflora*. In these studies, it appears that the assays employed only allogeneic tumours. Furthermore, as discussed above, the polysaccharides were administered i.p., not orally. Thus, the anti-tumour activities of RG-I and related polysaccharides from plant food material will have to be tested on valid autochthonous tumour systems by oral administration as part of a continued diet if the significance of dietary cell wall polysaccharides in cancer prevention is to be established. What is in no doubt is that many cell wall-derived polysaccharides have the potential to act as immunomodulators.

6 ACKNOWLEDGEMENTS

The authors gratefully acknowledge Drs. E.N.C. Mills, I.T. Johnson and P.W. Needs for useful discussions and Dr. M. Parker for the light micrograph in Figure 5.

7 REFERENCES

1. H. Yamada and H. Kiyohara, Abstracts of Chinese Medicines, 1989, 3, 104.
2. R.L. Whistler, A.A. Bushway and P.R. Singh, Adv. Carbohydr. Chem., 1976, 32, 235.
3. R. Srivastava and K. Kulshreshtha, Phytochem., 1989, 28, 2877.
4. E. Kishida, Y. Sone and A. Misaka, Carbohydr. Res., 1989, 193, 227.
5. B.M. Muller, J. Kraus and G. Franz, Planta-Med., 1989, 55, 536.
6. G. Chihara, J. Hamuro, Y.Y. Maeda, T. Shiio, T. Suga, N. Takasuki and T. Sasaki, Cancer-Detect-Prev-Suppl., 1987, 1, 423.
7. S. Tsukagoshi, Y. Hashimoto, G. Fujii, H. Kobayashi, K. Nomoto and K. Orita, Cancer Treat. Rev., 1984, 11, 131.
8. E. Furasawa and S. Furasawa, Oncology, 1989, 46, 343.
9. E. Furasawa and S. Furasawa, Cancer Lett., 1990, 50,71.
10. H. Sakaagami, M. Ikeda, S. Unten, K. Takeda, J. Murayama, H. Hamada, K. Kimura, N. Komatsu and K. Konno, Anticancer Res., 1987, 7, 1153.
11. G. Aspinal (ed), 'The Polysaccharides, Volume 2', Academic Press, London, 1983.
12. M. McNeill, A.G. Darvill, S.C. Fry and P. Albersheim, Ann.Rev. Biochem., 1984, 53, 625.
13. G. Chihara, Y. Maeda, J. Hamuro, T. Sasaki and F.Fukuoka, Nature, 1969, 222, 687.
14. F. Fukuoka, M. Nakanishi, S. Shibata, Y. Nishikawa, T. Takeda and M. Tanaka, Gann, 1968, 59, 421.
15. S. Suzuki, M. Suzuki, H. Hatsukaiwa, H. Sunayama, T. Suzuki, M. Uchiyama, F. Fukuoka, M. Nakanishi and S. Akiya, Gann, 1969, 60, 273.
16. N. Kumano, Chem. Abs., 1973, 78, 79.
17. W. Nakahara, R. Tokuzen, F. Fukuoka and R.L. Whistler, Nature, 1967, 216, 374.
18. S. Suzuki, T. Saito, M. Uchiyama and S. Akiya, Chem. Pharm. Bull. (Tokyo), 1969, 16, 2032.
19. H. Yamada, K. Komiyana, H. Kiyohara, J.C. Cyong, Y. Hirakawa and Y. Otsuka, Planta Med., 1990, 56, 182
20. T. Kimoto and S. Watanabe, Acta Pathol. Jpn., 1987, 37, 1743.
21. T. Yanagawa, M. Oguro, T. Takagi and K. Takenaga, Gan-To-Kagaku-Ryoho, 1984, 11, 2155.
22. T. Kimoto, Acta Pathol. Jpn., 1987, 37, 1919.
23. E.A. Mueller and F.A. Anderer, Immunopharmacology, 1990, 19, 69.
24. E.A. Mueller and F.A. Anderer, Cancer Res., 1990, 50,

3646.
25. G.H. Algire, F.Y. Legallais and H.D. Parks, J. Nat. Cancer Inst., 1947, 8. 162.
26. G. H. Algire and F.Y. Legallais, J. Nat. Cancer Inst., 1951, 12, 399.
27. I.C. Diller, B. Blauch and L.V. Beck, Cancer res., 1948, 8, 591.
28. M. Belkin, W.G. Hardy, A. Perrault and H, Sato, Cancer Res., 1959, 18, 1050.
29. N. Hasselgreen, J. Cancer, 1938, 34, 280.
30. A. Lazar and D.C. Lazar, J. Nat. Cancer Inst., 1962, 28, 1255.
31. D. Mizano, O. Yoshioka, M. Akamatu and T. Kataoka, Cancer Res., 1968, 28, 1531.
32. R. Tokuzen, Cancer Res., 1971, 31, 1590.
33. D.P. Stites and A.I. Terr, 'Basic and Clinical Immunology', Prentice Hall International (UK) Ltd., London, 1991.
34. E. Furasawa and S. Furasawa, Oncology, 1985, 42, 364.
35. H. Nakajima, Y. Kita, T. Takashi, M. Alasaki, F. Yamaguchi, S. Ozawa, W. Tsukada, S. Abe and D. Mizuno, Gann, 1984, 75,
36. K. Hishinuma, A. Hosono, H. Inaba and S. Kimura, Int. J. Vitam. Nutr. Res., 1990, 60, 288.
37. H. Sakagami, T. Aoki, A. Simpson and S. Tanuma, Anticancer Res., 1991, 11, 993.
38. T. Takeyama, I. Suzuki, N. Ohno, S. Oikawa, K. Sato, M. Ohsawa and T. Yadomae, J. Pharmacobiodyn., 1987, 10, 644.
39. T.L. Gerrard, D.J. Cohen and A.M. Kaplan, J. Natl. Cancer Inst., 1981, 66, 483
40. A.H. Pickaver, N.A. Ratcliffe, A.E. Williams and H. Smith, Nature (New Biol.), 1972, 235, 186.
41. K. Morikawa, Y. Kikuchi, S. Abe, M. Yamazaki and D. Mizuno, Gann, 1984, 75, 370.
42. K. Morikawa, S. Kamegaya, M. Yamazaki and D. Mizuno, Cancer Res., 1985, 45, 3482.
43. K. Morikawa, R. Takeda, M. Yamazaki and D. Mizuno, Cancer Res., 1985, 45, 1496.
44. S. Unten, H. Sakagami and K. Konno, J. Leukoc. Biol., 1989, 45, 168.
45. G. Chihara, Adv. Exp. Med. Biol., 1983, 166, 189.
46. T.W. Evans, T. Keler, P.H. Pham, E. Kovats, A. Aiello, O. Shonekan, H. Friedman and A.G. Johnson, J. Biol. Response Mod., 1988, 7, 296.
47. E.A. Mueller, K. Hamprecht and F.A. Anderer, Immunopharmacology, 1989, 17, 11.
48. J.M. Lau, M. McNeill, A.G. Darvill and P. Albersheim, Carbohydr. Res., 1987, 168, 245.
49. G. Chihara, Y.Y. Maeda, T. Suga and J. Hamuro, Int. J. Immunotherapy, 1989, 5, 145.
50. M. Moriyama, H. Miwa, N. Moriya and K. Orita, Gan-To-Kagaku-Ryoho, 1982, 9, 1102
51. S. Fujimoto, Nippon-Geka-Gakkai-Zasshi, 1989, 90, 1447.
52. T. Kimoto, Cancer Detect. Prev., 1982, 5, 301.
53. T. Kimoto and S. Watanabe, Acta Pathol. Jpn., 1987,

37, 1743.
54. T. Kimoto, S. Watanabe, F. Hyodoh and T. Saito, Cancer Det. Prev., 1988, 11, 173.
55. K. W. Waldron and R.R. Selvendran, Phytochem., 1992, 31, 1931.
56. P. Ryden and R.R. Selvendran, Carb. Res., 1990, 195, 257.
57. R.J. Redgwell and R.R. Selvendran, Carb. Res., 1986, 157, 183.
58. R.J. Redgwell, L.D. Melton and D.J. Brasch, Carb. Res., 1988, 182, 241.
59. P. Ryden and R.R. Selvendran, Biochem. J., 1990, 269, 393.
60. M. O'Neill, P. Albersheim and A. Darvill, Methods in Plant Biochem., 1990, 2, 415.
61. G.B. Seymour, I.J. Colquhoun, M.S. DuPont, K.R. Parsley and R.R. Selvendran, Phytochem., 1990, 29, 725.
62. G. Moates, K.W. Waldron and R.R. Selvendran, Unpublished results.
63. P. Ryden and R.R. Selvendran, Unpublished results.
64. S.G. Ring and R.R. Selvendran, Phytochem., 1981, 20, 2511.
65. M.A. Martin-Cabrejas, K.W. Waldron and R.R. Selvendran, Unpublished results.
66. R.R. Selvendran, J.F. March and S.G. Ring, Analyt. Biochem., 1979, 69, 282.
67. M. Shiomi, K. Sasaki, M. Murofushi and K. Aibara, Jpn. J.Med. Sci. Biol. 1982, 35, 75.
68. M. Kohno, S. Abe, M. Yamazaki and D. Mizuno, Gann, 1982, 73,
69. M.L.G. Gardner, Ann. Rev. Nutr., 1988, 8, 329.
70. E. McLean and R. Ash, Comp. Biochem. Physiol., 1986, 84A, 687
71. E. McLean and R. Ash, Comp. Biochem. Physiol., 1987, 88A, 507
72. C.A. Loehry, A.T.R. Axon, P.J. Hilton, R.C. Hider and B. Creamer, Gut, 1970, 11, 466.
73. M. Murofushi, M. Shiomi and K. Aibara, Jpn. J. Med. Sci. Biol., 1983, 36, 49.
74. A. Yamashita, H. Ohtsuka and H. Maeda, Immunopharmacol., 1983, 5, 209.
75. D. Sabolovic and L. Galoppin, Int. J. Immunopharmacol., 1986, 8, 41.
76. R.R. Selvendran and J. A. Robertson, 'The Chemistry of Dietary Fibre' in 'Dietary Fibre, Chemical and Biological Aspects', Royal Society of Chemistry, London, 1990.
77. J.L. Madara, Am. J. Path., 1990, 137, 1273.
78. D.E. Bockman and W.B. Winborn, Anat. Res., 1966, 155, 603.
79. M. Heyman, R. Ducroc, J-F. Desjeux and J.L Morgat, Am. J. Physiol., 1982, 242, G55.
80. G.O. Aspinall, Adv. Carb. Chem. Biochem., 1969, 24, 333.

ANTI-TUMORIGENIC AND IMMUNOACTIVE PROTEIN AND PEPTIDE FACTORS IN FOODSTUFFS (I)
- ANTI-TUMORIGENIC PROTEIN FROM TRICHOLOMA MATSUTAKE -

Y. Kawamura and M. Ishikawa*

Protein Science Laboratory
National Food Research Institute
Tsukuba, Ibaraki 305 Japan

*Food Research Institute, Momoya Co. Ltd.,
Kasukabe, Saitama Japan

1 INTRODUCTION

Matsutake (*Tricholoma matsutake*) is an edible mushroom called "King of mushroom" in Japan because of its particular fragrance and extremely expensive price. Since at the moment this mushroom has not been able to cultivate artificially, most of the supply comes from natural source, and depends mainly on import.

Some of mushroom, for example, *Lentinus edodes* (Shiitake in Japanese), *Flammulina velutipes* (Enokitake), Coriolus versicolor (Kawaratake) and Agaricus blazei (Himematsutake), contain immunologically active substances such as polysaccharides and protein-bound polysaccharides. These (protein-bound) polysaccharides are extracted from mycelium or fruit body with hot water and were understood to act predominantly as host-mediated immune system stimulators.

In our study of antitumorigenic substances in biological materials, we found that aqueous extract of the fruit body of matsutake mushroom showed selective cytotoxicity against virus-transformed cells. In this paper, we report the selective lethal effect of a proteineous component from matsutake mushroom on SV40-transformed mouse fibroblast. We purified a very strong anti-tumorigenic protein in a homogeneous state.

Experimental Procedures

Materials. Culture mediums, PBS(-), DMEM and MEM were purchased from Nissui Seiyaku. Centriprep-30 and Centricon-30 were obtained from Amicon. DEAE-Toyopearl and TSK gel G3000SW$_{XL}$ were obtained from Tosoh. Phenyl-Superose HR5/5 was obtained from Pharmacia. Dialysis membrane Spectra/Por MWCO25,000 was obtained from Spectram Medical Industry. BSA was obtained from Pierce. All other chemicals were obtained from Nakarai Tesque.

Cell lines and Culture Condition. The Balb/3T3 clone A31 is a cloned mouse cell line developed from

Balb/c mouse embryos (ATCC CCL 163). This line was derived from non-tumorigenic cells and contact-inhibited. SV-T2 is a SV40 virus-transformed Balb/3T3 cell line (ATCC CCL 163.1). Both cell lines were grown in DMEM medium supplemented with 10% calf serum (CS). HeLa is a cell line isolated from a human carcinoma of the cervix (ATCC CCL 2). HeLa S3 is a clonal derivative of the parent HeLa cell (ATCC CCL 2.2). WI-38 VA13 subline 2RA is a SV40 virus-transformed derivative of the human diploid cell line (ATCC CCL 75.1). These cell lines were grown in MEM with non-essential amino acids mixture and supplemented with 10% fetal calf serum. All cell lines were grown at 37°C under 5% CO_2 in a humidified atmosphere.

Assay of antitumor activity. The effect of matsutake components on the proliferation of cells was measured by MTI(3-(4,5-dimethylthiazol-2-yl)-2,5-diphenyl tetrazolium bromide) assay.[1] Each cell was plated at 2.0 x 10^3 cells/well on 96-well plates in 100μl of medium and the plates were incubated for 24 hr under the previous condition. Then to the medium, 10μl of sample solution (dissolved in $PBS^{(-)}$) was added. After incubation for 44 hr, an aliquot of 10μl of MTT solution (5mg/ml $PBS^{(-)}$) was added to the wells and the plates were incubated further for 4 hr. The medium in the wells was removed by aspiration after centrifugation of the plate, and 100μl of acid-isopropanol (0.04N HCl in isopropanol) and 20μl of 3% sodium dodecylsulfate solution were added to each well to dissolve MTT formazan and alcohol-induced insoluble materials, respectively. After a few minutes of mixing, absorbance at 595nm of each 96 well of the plate was read with microplate spectrophotometer, using 655nm as reference wavelength.

Inhibition ratios were calculated by following equation:

$$\text{Inhibition ratio (\%)} = \frac{A-B}{A} \times 100$$

where A is absorbance of control and B is absorbance of treated.

Determination of protein. Protein concentrations were measured by the method of Lowry *et al.*[2] using bovine serum albumin as the standard. In an extensively diluted sample, absorbance at 280nm standardized with BSA was used for the estimation of protein content.

Polyacrylamide gel electrophoresis. The polyacrylamide gel electrophoresis was carried out with a 6.5% gel by the method of Ralmond and Weitranb[3] at 4°C. After electrophoresis, the gel was sliced into 3mm thick slices. The protein in each slice was electroeluted into 50mM Tris, 0.38M Glycine at 4°C, and dialyzed against water. Two dimensional PAGE was carried out with a 6.5% gel, first, native gel in the absence of SDS and second 8% gel in the presence of SDS. SDS-PAGE was carried by the method of Laemmli.[4] The gel was stained by Coomasie Brilliant Blue R-250.

2 RESULTS AND DISCUSSION

Purification Procedure

All purification procedures were carried out at 4°C. Two kilograms of frozen Matsutake (fruit body) were thawed and homogenized in 2 volumes of distilled water in an ice bath. After removing precipitates by centrifugation, the supernatant was brought to 90% saturation with solid ammonium sulfate and kept for 30 min. The precipitates were collected by centrifugation at 10,000 x g for 15 min and dissolved in minimum volume of water. This solution was dialyzed against water using by M.W. 3500 cut off membrane and lyophilized after removing of insoluble materials by centrifugation at 10,000 x g for 15 min. The lyophilized materials were dissolved in 50mM NH_4HCO_3 and fractionated with a Sepharose CL-4B column (2.6 x 87cm). The active fractions were combined and lyophilized. The lyophilized powder was dissolved in 50mM Tris-HCl (pH 7.8) and applied to a DEAE-Toyopearl 650 column (3 x 14.5cm) previously equilibrated with the same buffer. After washing the column with about 400ml of the buffer, elution was carried out with the 1000ml linear gradient of zero to 0.5M NaCl in 50mM Tris-HCl (pH 7.8).

The active fractions obtained from DEAE-Toyopearl 650 chromatography was concentrated by using a centriprep-30 and dialyzed against water. The dialyzed fraction was added by ammonium sulfate at 0.8M, and was centrifuged at 10,000 x rpm for 10 min. The supernatant was applied to a Phenyl-Superose HR5/5 column equilibrated with 0.1M Tris-HCl (pH 7.5) containing 0.8M ammonium sulfate and eluted with a decreasing gradient of 0.8 - 0M ammonium sulfate at a flow rate of 0.15ml/min. Active fractions obtained from Phenyl-Superose FPLC was dialyzed against water, concentrated by using centriprep-30 and centricon-30, and applied to a TSKgel G3000SW_{XL} column (7.8 x 300mm) equilibrated with 0.1M Tris-HCl (pH 7.5) containing 0.3M NaCl. Elution was performed at a flow rate of 0.5ml/min. Active fractions were dialyzed against water and stored at 4°C.

An aliquot of the active fraction from DEAE-Toyopearl 650 chromatography was analyzed by PAGE in the absence of detergent. The gel was sliced into 16 fractions. The activity existed only in slice number 8 (Rm 0.5). As a protein band was observed in the same position with Rm = 0.5, this band was suggested to be responsible for the active protein. The same sample was analyzed by two dimensional electrophoresis. One spot corresponding to the apparent molecular weight of 105 kDa was detected in the second dimensional SDS-PAGE, indicating that this protein was consisted of one kind of polypeptide.

A single peak of activity was eluted at 0.15M ammonium sulfate. When each fraction was analyzed by SDS-PAGE, it was observed that the densitometric determination of 105 kDa protein band paralleled to the antitumor activity. The active fractions obtained from Phenyl-Superose FPLC were dialyzed, concentrated and applied to a TSKgel G3000SW_{XL} HPLC. The activity was eluted as a single peak corresponding to the apparent molecular weight of 210kDa. SDS-PAGE analysis of the fractions from TSKgel G3000SW_{XL} showed that the active fractions contained only the 105kDa protein. From this analysis and two dimensional PAGE, it was suggested that this protein was a homo dimer composed of 105kD protein.

The antitumorigenic protein was purified from the crude extract of matsutake fruit body by the following 5 steps, salting out, gel filtration chromatography, anion exchange chromatography, hydrophobic chromatography and 2nd gel filtration chromatography. The purified protein was homogeneous on the basis of SDS-PAGE analysis and the N-end sequence analysis, and showed the lethal activity with ED_{50} = 8.8ng/ml against a SV40-transformed mouse fibroblast cell line SV-T2 with a slight effect on a non-transformed counterpart, Balb-A31.

We next tested the antitumor activity of the purified protein against not only mouse cell lines but also human tumor cell lines. In preliminary experiments, it had strong cyctotoxic activity against human cell line sand and was also very effective against a primary culture from a uterine cancer from which a malignant type of HPV-18 virus was separated.

The data presented here suggests that this anti-tumorigenic protein may be useful as antitumor drugs.

REFERENCES

1. T. Mosmann, J. Immunol. Methods, 1983, 65, 55.
2. D.H. Lowry, N.J. Rosebrough, A.L. Farr and R.J. Randall, J. Biol., 1951.
3. S.A. Raymond and L. Weitranb, Science, 1959, 30, 711.
4. U.K. Laemmli, Nature, 1970, 227, 680.
5. J.F. Cavins and M. Friedman, Anal. Biochem., 1970, 35, 489.
6. H. Tsugita and T. Uchida, Bio. Industry, 1990, 7, 742.
7. B.A. Bidlingmeyer, S.A. Cohen and T.L. Tarvin, J. Chromatogr., 1984, 336, 93.

ANTI-TUMORIGENIC AND IMMUNOACTIVE PROTEIN AND PEPTIDE FACTORS IN FOODSTUFFS (II)
- ANTI-TUMORIGENIC FACTORS IN RICE BRAN -

Y. Kawamura and M. Muramoto*

Protein Science Laboratory
National Food Research Institute
Tsukuba, Ibaraki 305 Japan

*Food and Life Institute
Japan Tabacco Inc.,
Kanagawa, Japan

1 INTRODUCTION

All biological systems, animal, plant and microorganism, seems to develop any anti-transforming factor, the function of which might be closely related to the protection and/or development of tumor or cancer. In this view, we have been trying to find out anti-transforming or anti-tumorigenic factors in biological materials. Some plants, especially mushrooms, are known to be rich in the biologically active substances such as antibiotics and anti-viral infection and anti-tumorigenic compounds. Here, anti-tumorigenic substances from rice, both of starchy endosperm and bran are studied and isolated by using the specific cytotoxicity against Simian Virus (SV) 40-transformed cell as indicative of anti-tumor (cancer).

Experimental Procedure

Materials. Culture mediums, DMEM and MEM were purchased from Nissui Seiyaku. Centriprep-30 and centricon-30 and 10 were obtained from Amicon. Ultrafiltration membrane YM2 and YC05 were obtained from Amicon. Dialysis membrane Spectra Por MWC025,000, 1000 and 500 from Spectram Medical Industry. Bio-gel P2 and Sephadex G-25 were from LKB/Pharmacia. HPLC column ODS-80TM and TSK gel G3000SW$_{XL}$ were purchased from Tosoh. Proteases, pepsin, trypsin, α-chymotrypsin, and glycosidases, End-β-galactosidase and glucoamylase were from Sigma. All other reagents were from Nakarai Tesque.

Cell lines and Culture Condition. 3T3-Swiss-albino (ATCC CCL92) and SV40 transformed 3T3 were grown in DMEM medium supplemented with 10% calf serum (CS). Hela, Hela S3, and WI-38 VA13 subline 2RA (a SV40-transformed derivative of the human diploid cell line (ATCC CCL 75.1)) were grown in MEM with non-essential amino acid mixture and supplemented with 10% fetal calf serum. All cell lines were cultivated at 37°C under 5% CO_2 in a humidified atmosphere.

Assay of antitumorigenic activity. The antitumorigenic activity of various fractions extracted or separated from rice bran was assayed by measuring cell proliferation with MTT (3-(4,5-dimethylthiazol-2-yl)-2,5-diphenyltetrazolium bromide) assay.[1] Both of transformed and untransformed cell were plated at 2.0 x 10^3 cells/well on 96 well plastic plate in 100μl of medium and were incubated for 24 hr under the condition described above. To the medium, then, 10μl of sample in PBS was added. After 44 hr incubation, an aliquot of 10μl of MTT solution (5mg/ml) in PBS was added to each well and plates were further incubated for 4 hr. The medium in wells was removed by aspiration after centrifugation. Then, 100μl of 0.04N HCl in isopropanol and 20μl of 3% sodium dodecylsulfate solution were added to each well to dissolve MTT formazan and alcohol-induced insoluble matter, respectively. After a few minutes of mixing, the absorbance of each plate was recorded with a microplate spectrophotometer, using a measurement wavelength of 595nm and a reference wavelength of 655nm. Inhibition ratio was calculated by the following equation:

$$\text{Inhibition ratio (\%)} = \frac{A-B}{A} \times 100$$

where A is the absorbance of control and B is that of sample.

Determination of protein. Protein concentration was measured by the method of Lowry *et al.*[2] using bovine serum albumin as the standard.

2 RESULTS AND DISCUSSION

Preparation of Rice Bran Extracts

A fresh prepared rice bran was prepared from the dehulled brown rice. A hundred gram of rice bran was defatted with 500ml of n-Hexane at 30°C, and air-dried. The defatted bran was added by 5 vol (v/w) of 0.001N NaOH and stirred for 4 hr at 4°C. The mixture was neutralized with 1N HCl then centrifuged at 8000g x 40 min. The supernatant was concentrated by evaporation into about 50ml. The concentrates were dialysed against 500ml of distilled water (D.W.) twice, and against 200ml of D.W. once. All of the outer and inner solution was collected. Since the inner solution have some materials insoluble to distilled water, it was centrifuged to obtain the precipitates and the supernatant. The insoluble materials were solubilized with 1N NaCl and centrifuged to get the supernatant. As shown in Figure 1, three fractions were prepared.

Correlation between MTT Assay and Dye-Exclusion Test. To check the reliability of MTT assay as the estimate of the living cell in the present condition, we compared the MTT assay and the dye exclusion assay as

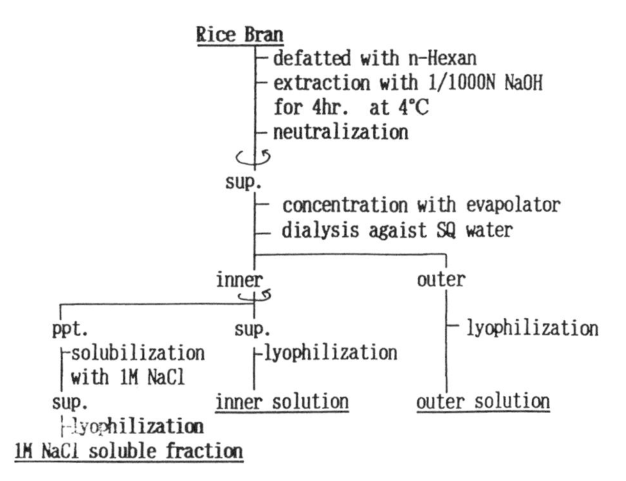

Figure 1

shown in Figure 2. Both assay methods give paralleled lines with 3T3 and SV40-3T3 cells.

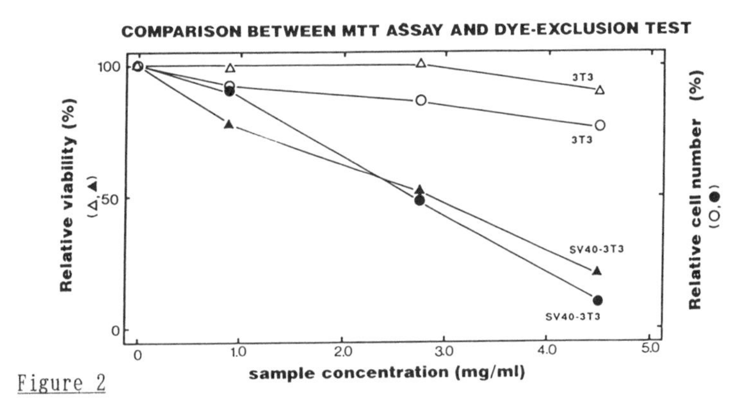

Figure 2

<u>Lethal Activity of Various Extracts</u>. The selective lethal activity against untransformed 3T3 and SV40-transformed 3T3 cell of three fractions of the extracts, 1M NaCl soluble, inner and outer solution, was measured as shown in Figure 3. 1M NaCl soluble fraction showed the nonspecific cytotoxicity to both of 3T3 and SV40-3T3. On the other hand, the inner and outer solution exhibited the selective lethal activity against SV40-3T3. The outer solution was more toxic to SV40-3T3 than inner solution though it was cytotoxic a little to normal 3T3 cells, too. In order to distinguish the toxic substance of the inner solution from the outer solution, we carried out ultrafiltration by using two kinds of membrane YM2 (cut-off mol. wt., 1000) and YC05 (cut-off mol. wt., 500).

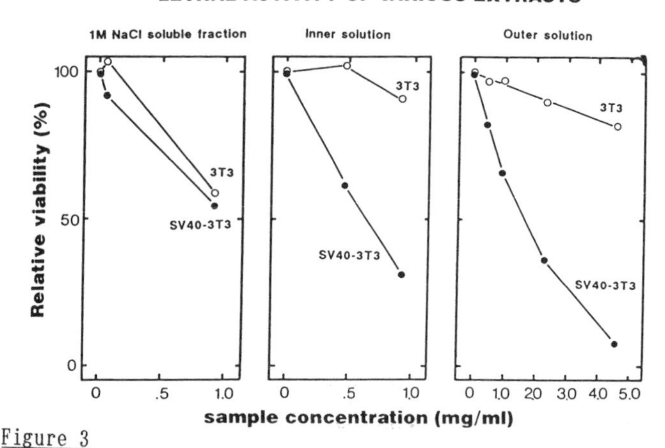

Figure 3

As shown in Figure 4, three fractions except for the fraction below mol. wt. of 500 killed cells, but fractions between mol. wt. of 500 and 1000 seems most selectively cytotoxic against the transformed cells.

These results indicated that the lethal activity observed in the inner solution of the crude extracts after dialysis came from the incomplete dialysis since a 3500 cut-off membrane was used with the first dialysis. Thus, the crude extracts solubilized by 0.002N NaOH were first dialysed completely by using 3500 cut-off membrane for a long time and the outer dialysates were taken. Then, the concentrated dialysates by evaporation were dialysed by using a membrane (cut-off mol. wt., 500) to obtain the inner solution.

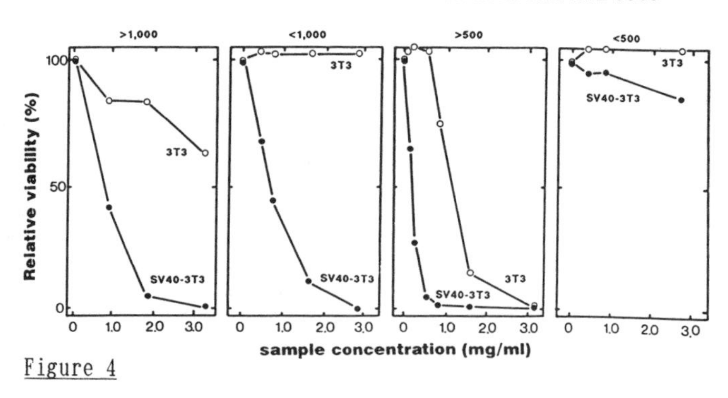

Figure 4

Gel filtration of the inner solution on Bio-Gel P-2. The inner solution from the dialysis by 500 cut-off membrane was freeze-dried. The freeze-dried powder was dissolved in 0.01N acetic acid and applied to a column of Bio-gel P-2 equilibrated with 0.01N acetic acid. The monitoring at 280nm showed many peaks and the determination of phosphorus showed the presence of 2 main peaks. The lethal activity was eluted in two peaks at the position a little later than the void volume.

The positions of both activity peaks did not coincide to those with the absorbance of 280nm and inorganic phosphate (Pi) as shown in Figure 5.

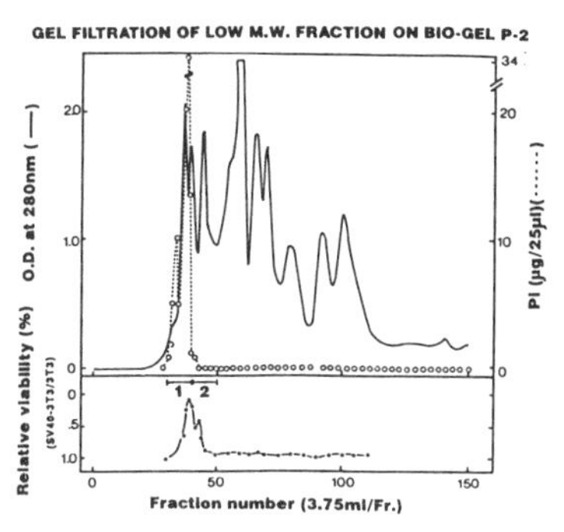

Figure 5

The active fractions were collected and freeze-dried. The profile of the selective lethal activity of both fractions was given in Figure 6. Fraction 1 exhibited the complete selectivity against SV40-transformed 3T3 cells. Between 5.0-2.2 mg/ml of fraction 1, the SV40-transformed cells were killed completely, whereas its normal counterpart was not affected. The lethal activity of fraction 2 was a bit weak compared with fraction 1, but still selectively cytotoxic to the transformed cell. The LD_{50} of fraction 1 and 2 was 1.0 mg/ml and 4.2 mg/ml, respectively.

Reversephase High Performance Liquid Chromatography. The fraction 1, which is more selective and active than the fraction 2, was applied to a HPLC with an ODS column. The lethal activity was eluted in three fractions at relatively low acetonitrile concentration. The most active fraction was collected, concentrated by the freeze-drying, and applied to the second HPLC with an ion exchange column. Elution was carried out with a linear gradient (0-0.4 M) of NaCl. The lethal activity was eluted as a single peak around 0.1 M NaCl.

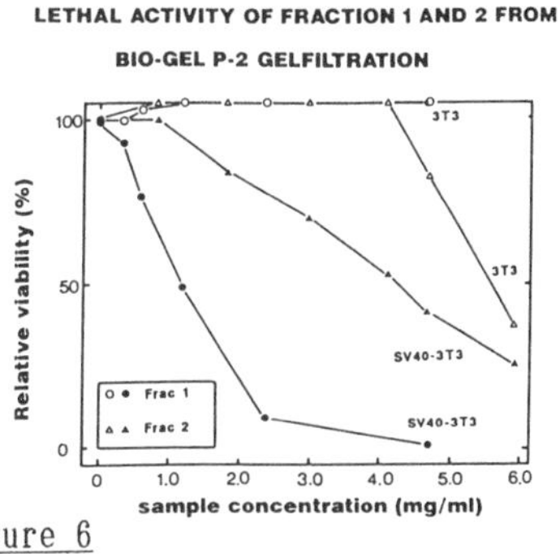

LETHAL ACTIVITY OF FRACTION 1 AND 2 FROM BIO-GEL P-2 GELFILTRATION

Figure 6

The purified sample showed the ED_{50} of 0.9 mg/ml against SV40-transformed 3T3 cell. At this concentration, untransformed normal cells were not killed by the sample at all. Now, the characterization of this compound is in progress.

REFERENCES

1. T. Mosmann, J. Immunol. Methods, 1983, 65, 55.
2. D.H. Lowry, N.J. Rosebrough, A.L. Farr and R.J. Randall, J. Biol. Chem., 1951, 193, 265.

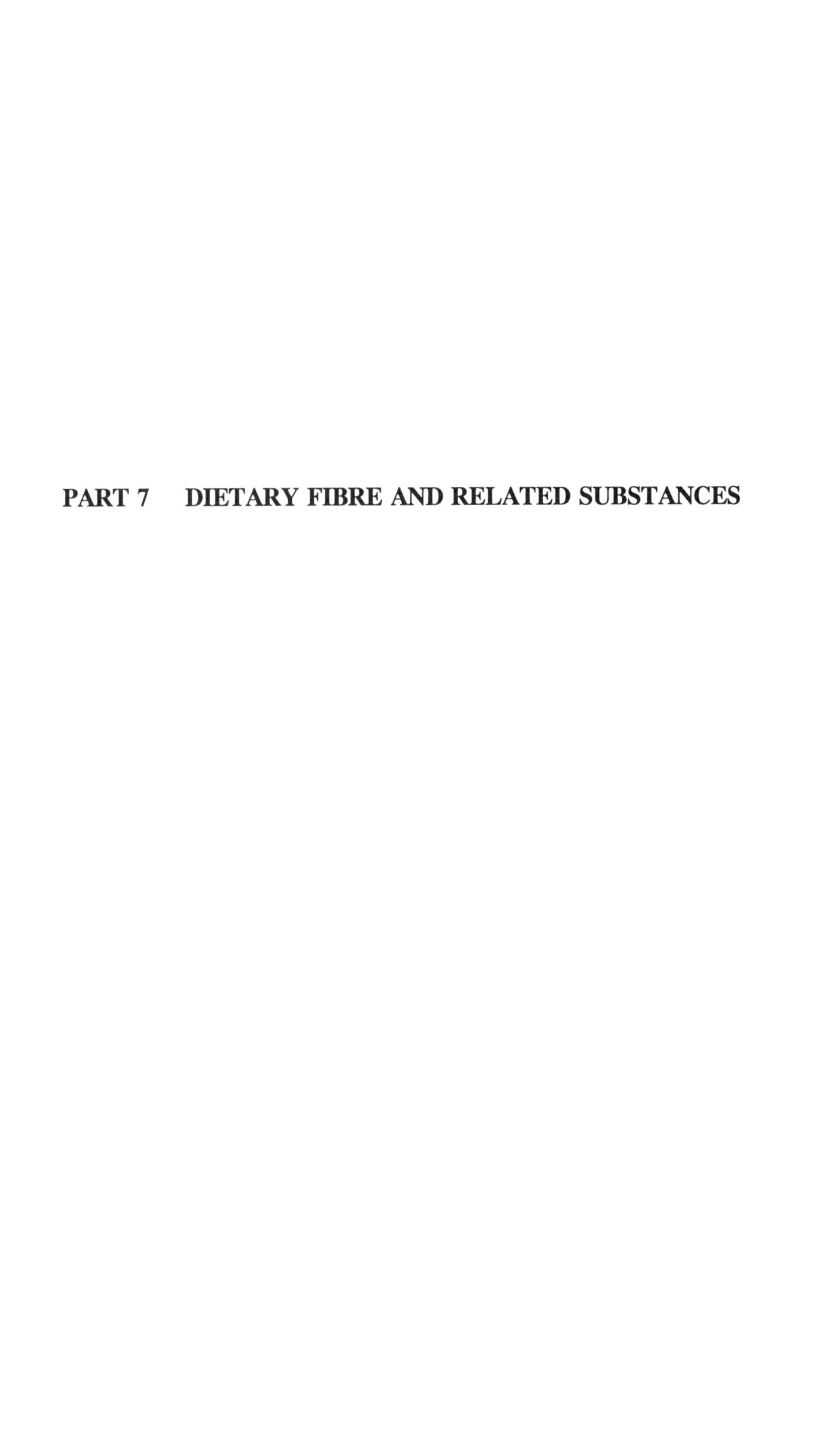

PART 7 DIETARY FIBRE AND RELATED SUBSTANCES

PLANT CELL WALL MATERIAL AND CANCER PROTECTION

S. A. Bingham

Medical Research Council
Dunn Clinical Nutrition Centre
Cambridge CB2 1QL

1 INTRODUCTION

Colorectal cancer is the second most common cancer in western societies, affecting up to 6% men and women by the age of 75. Breast cancer is the most common cancer in women, accounting for 28% of all female cancers in England and Wales. Prostate cancer is becoming more common, and now accounts for 9% of male cancers in England and Wales.[1] Bowel cancer is presently thought to develop by a stepwise accumulation of several mutations, the first of which is the loss of a tumour suppressing gene located on chromosome 5.[2] No direct evidence of the involvement of diet in these changes has so far been shown, but there is a wealth of epidemiological and experimental evidence to suggest that colorectal cancer risk is affected by diet. Hormonal factors, particularly high sex steroid levels, are particularly implicated in breast and prostate cancer, and these may in themselves be influenced by diet.

2 EPIDEMIOLOGY

Risks of most cancers increase markedly with age, but there remains a 7-19 fold range in age standardised levels in different parts of the world for these cancers.[3] Both migrant studies and secular changes in incidence rates show that environmental factors are mainly responsible for these geographical differences. Migrants from low risk areas adopt the colorectal cancer incidence rates of a high risk population within a single generation, for example Japanese migrants to Hawaii, and breast cancer rates within two generations.[3] In Japan itself, there have been striking changes. Whereas rates were low before westernisation, age specific colon cancer rates have increased five fold since 1960,[4] and are fast approaching those recorded in Britain.

Of the many possible environmental risk factors, diet is most strongly associated with these cancer incidence rates, and there are many potential specific dietary factors involved. There is now a persuasive role for the major fraction of cell wall material, non-starch polysaccharides (NSP) in protection against colorectal cancer, and a possible one in protection against breast cancer. The antioxidant micronutrients and carotenoids are becoming increasingly of interest in cancers at all sites,[5] as are the phytoestrogens in breast cancer.[6]

Cross-sectional Studies

Worldwide, intakes of indicators of dietary fibre tend to be higher in countries at low risk of breast and colorectal cancer.[7] Although this inverse association is substantially reduced on controlling for meat and fat consumption[8] three studies within defined Western areas where meat and fat consumption is high, also suggest that NSP intakes are lowest in areas where colorectal cancer occurrence is highest.[4]

Vegetarians have a consistently lower risk for large bowel cancer than omnivores.[9] The comparatively lower breast cancer risk of rural Finns, despite their high intake of fat, has been attributed to the high NSP content of Finnish diets.[7] Hughes has demonstrated a positive association between fibre consumption and menarcheal age. Late menarche is a known protective factor in breast cancer aetiology.[10]

Nevertheless, other dietary factors are involved in addition to fat and meat. For example, age-standardised colorectal cancer rates of the Maoris in New Zealand are approximately half those of New Zealand Whites, and yet intakes of dietary fibre are virtually the same.[11] In South Africa, different racial groups are also at very different risks of bowel cancer, yet recent reports suggest that fibre intakes in these groups are also very similar.[12] Starch intakes in developing communities are known to be higher than in western societies. Like NSP, starch is known to be a substrate for fermentation in the colon, leading to increased faecal weight. Recent studies have confirmed that a high stool weight appears to be protective against colorectal cancer.[13] By modifying hormonal status, phytoestrogens may also be important in protection against breast cancer.[14]

Analytic studies

In general, case control studies show that where it has been measured, fibre has tended to be associated with a reduction in bowel cancer risk. Eleven studies, for example, of 22 have shown that cases reported less 'fibre' than controls, and in only two had they reported eating more. There were no significant differences in nine. Much of this apparent protective effect of fibre is accounted for by the fact that in 12 of 19 studies, cases reported eating smaller amounts of vegetables than controls.[14]

These findings of an apparent protective effect of NSP in colorectal cancer require confirmation with well controlled prospective studies. One study of this type in U.S. nurses has not demonstrated a reduction in colorectal cancer risk in individuals with higher NSP intake,[15] but dietary fibre, from both vegetables and cereals, was protective against colorectal adenoma in a prospective study of American males.[16] The recurrence of adenomas has not been reduced on intervention with bran in Australia.[17] More large prospective and intervention trials are required to establish a definite epidemiological role for NSP in cancer protection. Stool weight should also be measured but few epidemiological studies are likely to attempt this.

The effect of NSP in breast cancer has not been so intensively studied, although meta analyses are reported to show a protective effect of fibre in case control studies after controlling for fat.[7] No protective effect of fibre was reported in the large study of US nurses.[18]

3 ANIMAL STUDIES

The effect of purified sources of dietary fibre on chemically initiated colorectal cancer has been investigated in a large number of studies over the past decade, and the overall findings were collated by the Federation of American Societies for Experimental Biology (FASEB) in 1987.[19] In general, bran appears to have a consistently protective effect against chemical carcinogenesis. Of 17 studies, bran decreased the number of tumours in 13 studies, and increased the number of tumours compared with control levels in only one study. Cellulose also appears protective in six of nine studies, with no significant difference in three. In three of the seven studies, pectin apparently enhanced carcinogenesis, possibly due to the variety of experimental variables in these studies. No consensus was possible for the gums, guar gum and carrageenan.[19]

One study has shown a protective effect of bran against NMU induced mammary carcinoma in animals fed a high fat diet, with no significant effect in animals fed a low fat diet[7].

4 MECHANISMS

The mechanism behind the effect of bran in reducing chemically induced large bowel tumour incidence is likely to vary with different carcinogens used. In humans, some support for the hypothesis that dilution and reduced transit is important comes from studies in which faecal mutagenicity has been consistently reduced by bran supplementation. Fifteen individuals who exhibited high faecal mutagenicity took part in an intervention study whereby fibre intake from whole grain bread was increased by 11g for 4 weeks. Stool bulk increased by 35% and faecal mutagenicity, using the Ames test, decreased by 2.5 to 4.5 fold.[20] The standard Ames test is open to difficulties when used for faecal extract testing, but Venitt, using methods designed to overcome both toxic and nutritive factors in faecal extracts, also found a reduction in faecal mutagenicity with bran, albeit in only one subject in a preliminary study.[21] Kuhnlein et al.,[22] using aqueous faecal extracts, has also shown reductions in faecal mutagenicity with cellulose and with pectin in rats.

Further support or a role for faecal bulk in large bowel cancer protection is suggested by the in vivo monitoring technique of microcapsules.[23] Microcapsules are 100 μ spheres with a semipermeable membrane given by mouth and containing magnetite to allow their recovery from faeces. After diffusion through the outer membrane, mutagens and carcinogens are trapped by covalent links within the contents of the core, and microcapsules containing polyethylene imine (PEI) can be used as surrogates for nitrosation.[23] Studies with humans given microcapsules containing PEI have shown that after transit through the gut, crosslinks between the PEI of the core and PEI of the membrane are formed. Such crosslinks had previously been shown in in vitro studies with known mutagens such as 4-hydroxynonenal.[24] Crosslinks also form during incubation with faecal slurries and are therefore presumed to occur in vivo in the large bowel. Preliminary studies with humans consuming uncontrolled diets show that crosslinking is inversely related to faecal weight.[25] Crosslinking is therefore less likely to occur when faecal contents are diluted, for example by a high NSP or starch diet.

The bacterial metabolite responsible for crosslinking is unknown, but faeces contain a variety of potential crosslinkers and mutagens, including polycyclic hydrocarbons, phenols, N-nitroso compounds, fecapentaenes and heterocyclic amines. Little work on the effect of diet on these has been done, although no relationship between fecapentaene excretion and dietary fibre intake was detected in a questionnaire study, with high excreters less likely to be consuming supplements of vitamin C and E.[26] Fecapentaenes are produced from phospholipids by Bacteroides, the most common species in the human colon.[27]

In breast cancer, one hypothesis is that high fibre diets reduce serum oestrogens by a reduction in faecal glucuronidase and hence increased excretion of inactivated conjugated oestrogens in faeces.[7] However, the effect of fibre with no interference from a change in fat intake on faecal oestrogen and glucuronidase levels has not been investigated. In addition, any changes in glucuronidase concentrations are largely counteracted by the effect of fibre on increasing faecal weight, so that overall levels are either unchanged or increased. The finding of Petrakis et al. however that constipation is associated with greater risk of breast dysplasia does suggest that cell wall material may have a role to play in protection against breast cancer.[28]

5 FERMENTATION

The colon is host to a large and diverse commensal flora of anaerobic bacteria and the major control on the metabolic environment of the flora is via residues entering the large gut from the small bowel. These in turn are determined by dietary intakes, particularly protein and carbohydrate. Carbohydrate entering the large bowel stimulates anaerobic fermentation, leading to the production of short chain fatty acids (SCFA), acetate, propionate and butyrate, gas, and an increase in microbial cell mass. The SCFA produced are absorbed by the intestinal mucosa, where they stimulate sodium absorption and bicarbonate secretion.[29] Fermentation has a number of important consequences in large bowel physiology and possible implications for protection against breast and large bowel cancer.

In in vitro studies for example, high carbohydrate conditions of fermentation increase the rate of breakdown of conjugated lignans found in most high fibre foods, including whole grain cereals, to the unconjugated active form.[29] Few direct investigations of the hormonal effects of lignans have been conducted[6] but one intervention study with the chemically similar isoflavones in soya has shown a direct effect on gonadotrophin release, prolonging the follicular phase and hence the length of the menstrual cycle.[14] Longer menstrual cycles would result in lower lifetime exposure to unopposed oestrogens. Menstrual cycle lengths are longer, isoflavone consumption as soya is higher, and breast cancer risk is lower in Far East populations. At present, there is also no reason to discount a role for phytoestrogens in another hormone dependent cancer, prostate cancer,[1] which has similarly low rates in Far East populations.

As a direct result of fermentation, bacterial cells mass increases, leading to an increase in faecal weight.[31] Cereal fibre, from bran and some resistant starch, has an additional effect because it is only partly fermented and the residual polysaccharides absorb water, also contributing to faecal bulking.[32] With the increase in faecal weight, transit time is reduced and the contents of the large bowel lumen are diluted, which would reduce the time putative mutagens and carcinogens are in contact with the large bowel mucosa, in accordance with Burkitt's original hypothesis.[33] The production of SCFA however may be as important.

Approximately 60, 20 and 20% molar ratios of acetate, propionate and butyrate are formed during fermentation in the human large gut.[29] Molar ratios can, however, be varied in vitro, according to the substrate. In batch cultures of human faecal slurries, 29% of butyrate can be produced from starch, compared with 8, 3 and 2% from an arabinogalactan, a xylan, and pectin.[34] This effect of starch fermentation in increasing butyrate production has also been shown in vivo. Eleven individuals were fed on the glucosidase inhibitor acarbose in order to induce starch malabsorption in the small gut. Molar ratios of butyrate in faeces increased from an average of 21% without starch malabsorption to 30% with malabsorption, a 50% increase. There was no change in the molar ratio of acetate (41%), and a fall in propionate production, from 27 to 21%.[35]

SCFA are absorbed from the large gut, less butyrate being found in the human portal vein.[36] In most species, butyrate is used preferentially to acetate and propionate as a substrate for energy metabolism in the large bowel epithelium.[29] In the isolated human colonocyte, butyrate accounts for about 75% of oxygen consumption, and glucose is able to replace butyrate to a lesser extent in the proximal colon compared with the distal colon. This, together with less ketone-body formation, suggests that butyrate is a major source of energy for the distal colonic mucosa.[37] Acetate was not investigated in these studies, due to an absence of effect in the rat colonocyte.

In the conventional but not germ-free rat, wheat bran and ispaghula significantly enhance epithelial cell proliferation compared with animals fed on fibre-free diets.[38] SCFA, however, directly enhance proliferation rates in both germ-free and conventional rats.[39] Intracolonic infusions of SCFA have also been shown to promote healing in anastomoses of the surgically divided colon of rats.[40] This beneficial effect of SCFA on proliferation and healing is perhaps to be expected, if they are to be considered as nutritional factors for colonic epithelial cells. Excessive cell proliferation is a putative aetiological factor in carcinogenesis, but SCFA at physiological levels are unlikely to promote epithelial proliferation beyond the normal range.[39] High starch diets have been shown to reduce proliferation in mice.[41]

In cultured cell lines, butyrate is a well recognised anti-proliferative agent. At the 1-2 mm level, it acts directly as an inhibitor of DNA synthesis and cell growth, mainly via inhibition of histone deacetylase. Other SCFA are much less active in this respect.[42] The effect is reversible, with a 24 h lag in GI phase before normal growth rates are resumed after removal of butyrate from culture media. Acetylation may be a general mechanism for relaxing DNA, allowing access for repair enzymes; ultra violet radiation damage repair is enhanced and survival increased in human adenocarcinoma cell lines exposed to butyrate for example.[43]

Butyrate is also a known differentiation-inducing agent, reducing cloning efficiency and increasing the expression of membrane glycoproteins such as alkaline phosphatase and carcino-embryonic antigen in some human colorectal cancer cell lines.[44] Other SCFA have little effect compared with butyrate.[44] The effects of butyrate, however, vary amongst different cell lines; in one line derived from familial adenomatous polyposis, butyrate seemed to select for increased malignancy. This effect, however, was not seen in another line derived from a patient with non-inherited, sporadic colon cancer.[45] Very large doses (100-200 mmol/l) of sodium butyrate added to drinking water have been reported to increase chemical carcinogenesis in rats treated with DMH.[46] No effect with tributyrin was shown in a later study.[47] Butyrate may, therefore, be involved in protection against carcinogenesis in the colon and rectum, the only organs in the body exposed to elevated levels. Two small studies have shown lowered faecal butyrate levels of 8 v. 12% total SCFA in patients with colorectal cancer compared with healthy controls.[48,49]

REFERENCES

1. C. Muir, J. Waterhouse, T. Mack, J. Powell and F. Whelan (Eds.), 'Cancer Incidence in Five Continents, 5', IARC Scientific Publication No. 88, 1987.
2. B. Vogelstein, E.R. Fearon, S.R. Hamilton and S.E. Kern, N. Engl. J. Med., 1988, 319, 525.
3. L. Tomatis (Ed.), 'Cancer: Causes, Occurrence and Control', IARC Scientific Publication No. 100, Lyon 1990.
4. S. Bingham, Proc. Nutr. Soc., 1990, 49, 153.
5. D. Thurnham, This Symposium (1993), 109.

6. H. Adlercreutz, This Symposium (1993), 348.
7. D.P. Rose, Nutrition, 1992, 8, 47.
8. G.E. McKeown-Eyssen and E. Bright-See, Nutr. Cancer, 1985, 7, 251.
9. G. Johansson, PhD Thesis, Karolinska Institute, Stockholm, Sweden, 1990.
10. R.E. Hughes, 'Dietary Fibre Perspectives', John Libbey, London, 1990.
11. A.H. Smith, N.E. Pearce and J.G. Joseph, Int. J. Epid., 1985, 14, 79.
12. A.R.P. Walker, B.F. Walker and A.J. Walker. Brit. J. Cancer, 1986, 53, 489.
13. J.H. Cummings, S. Bingham, K. Heaton and M. Eastwood, Gastroenterology, 1992 (in press).
14. A. Cassidy, S. Bingham, J. Carlson and K. Setchell, N. Engl. J. Med., 1992 (submitted).
15. W.C. Willett, M.J. Stampfer, G.A. Colditz, B.A. Rosner and F.E. Spetzer, N. Engl. J. Med., 1990, 323, 1664.
16. E. Giovannucci, M.J. Stampfer, G. Colditz and W.C. Willett, Am. J. Epid., 1990, 132, 783A.
17. R. MacLennan, M. Ward, F. Macrae and M. Wahlqvist, Gastroenterology, 1991, 100, A382.
18. W.C. Willett, G.A. Stampfer, B.A. Colditz et al., N. Engl. J. Med., 1987, 316, 22.
19. S. Pilch (Ed.), 'Physiological Effects and Health Consequences of Dietary Fiber', FASEB, Bethesda, Maryland, USA, 1987.
20. B.S. Reddy, C. Sharma, B. Simi, A. Engle, K. Laakso, P. Puska and R. Korpela, Cancer Res., 1987, 47, 644.
21. S. Venitt, 'Role of the Gut Flora in Toxicity and Cancer', Academic Press, London, 1988, p. 399.
22. U. Kuhnlein, R. Gallagher and H.J. Freeman, Clin. Invest. Med., 1983, 6, 253.
23. I.K. O'Neill, M. Castagnaro, I. Brouet and A.C. Povey, Carcinogenesis, 1987, 8, 1469.
24. A. Ellul, A. Povey and I.K. O'Neill, Carcinogenesis, 1990, 11, 1577.
25. S. Bingham, A. Ellul, J.H. Cummings and I.K. O'Neill, Carcinogenesis, 1992, 13, 683.
26. M.H. Schiffman, Cancer Surveys, 1987, 6, 653.
27. R.L. van Tassel, Piccarielo, D.G.I. Kingston and T.D. Wilkins, Lipids, 1989, 24, 454.
28. N.L. Petrakis and E.B. King, Lancet, 1981, 61, 1203.
29. J.H. Cummings, Gut, 1981, 22, 763.
30. A. Cassidy, PhD Thesis, University of Cambridge, 1991.
31. A.M. Stephen and J.H. Cummings, Nature, 1980, 284, 283.
32. M.I. McBurney, P.J. Horvath, J.L. Jeraci and P.J. Van Soest, Br. J. Nutr. 1985, 53, 17.
33. D.P. Burkitt, Lancet, 1969, ii, 1229.
34. H.N. Englyst, S. Hay and G.T. Marfarlane, FEMS Microbiol. Ecol., 1987, 95, 163.

35. W. Scheppach, C. Fabian, M. Sachs and H. Kasper, Scand. J. Gastroent., 1988, 23, 755.
36. J.H. Cummings, E.W. Pomare, W.J. Branch, C.P.E. Naylor and G.T. Macfarlane, Gut, 1987, 28, 1221.
37. W.E.W. Roediger, Gut, 1980, 21, 793.
38. R.A. Goodlad, B. Ratcliffe, J.P. Fordham and N.A. Wright, Gut, 1989, 30, 820.
39. T. Sakata, Br. J. Nutr., 1987, 58, 95.
40. R.H. Rolandelli, M.J. Koruda, R.G. Settle and J.L. Rombeau, Surgery, 1986, 100, 198.
41. G. Caderni, F. Bianchini, P. Dolara and D. Kriebel, Nutr. Cancer, 1991, 15, 33.
42. J. Kruh, Mol. Cell. Biochem., 1982, 42, 65.
43. P.J. Smith, Carcinogenesis, 1986, 7, 423.
44. R.H. Whitehead, G.P. Young and P.S. Bhathal, Gut, 1986, 27, 1457.
45. R.D. Berry and C. Paraskeva, Carcinogenesis, 1988, 9, 447.
46. H.J. Freeman, Gastroenterology, 1986, 91, 596.
47. E.E. Deschner, J.F. Ruperto, J.R. Lupton and H.L. Newmark, Cancer Letters, 1990, 52, 79.
48. P. Vernia, P. Ciarniello, M. Cittadini, A. Lorenzotti, A. Alessindrini and R. Caprilli, Gastroenterology, 1988, 96, A528.
49. H. Bonnen, M.R. Clausen and P.G. Mortensen, Gastroenterology, 1989, 96, A51.

LIGNANS AND ISOFLAVONOIDS OF DIETARY ORIGIN AND HORMONE-DEPENDENT CANCER

H. Adlercreutz, M.Carson, Y. Mousavi A. Palotie, S. Booms, M. Loukovaara, T.Mäkelä*, K. Wähälä*, G. Brunow* and T. Hase

Department of Clinical Chemistry,University of Helsinki, Meilahti Hospital, SF-00290 Helsinki, Finland
*Department of Chemistry, University of Helsinki, Vuorikatu 20, SF-00100 Helsinki, Finland

1 INTRODUCTION

Hormone-dependent cancers like breast (BC) and prostate cancer (PC) belong to the s.c. Western diseases, which seem to be associated with a diet rich in fat and protein but poor in fiber and complex carbohydrates, particularly whole-grain products and legumes. For more than 10 years we have been interested in the mechanisms by which diet affects the risk of BC, PC and colon cancer (CC).[1,2] This is a brief summary of some studies on the role of lignans and isoflavonoids in human cancer, particularly hormone-dependent cancer.

2 LIGNANS AND ISOFLAVONOIDS IN MAN

In 1979 two cyclically occurring unknown compounds, now called enterolactone (Enl) and enterodiol (End), were detected in urine of the female vervet monkey and women and subsequently identified. They were shown to be diphenols with lignan structure lacking the para-oxygen substitution and differing in this way from plant lignans. They have also been found in other biological materials and in some other animals. In addition, four plant lignans, matairesinol (Mat), lariciresinol (Lar), isolariciresinol (Isolar) and secoisolariciresinol (Sec), and furthermore 7′-hydroxy-Mat and 7′-hydroxy-Enl were identified in human urine by GC-MS (review and structures in.[2,3])

The isoflavonoids are also diphenols and occur in numerous plants and many studies have shown that they have hormonal effects in animals,[4] the most important being the "clover disease". The compound responsible for the disease is equol (Eq), formed by the ruminal bacteria from formononetin (For) present in ingested clover. The literature on the occurrence of the isoflavonoids in animals[4] and in man[2,3,5] has been reviewed. We have identified or detected in human urine the following isoflavonoids: For, methylequol, daidzein (Da), dihydro-Da, O-desmethylangolensin (O-Dma), genistein (Gen), and 3′,7-dihydroxyisoflavan. Eq was identified in human urine independently in two laboratories.[6,7]

3 ORIGIN AND FORMATION OF LIGNANS AND ISOFLAVONOIDS

The mammalian lignans Enl and End are formed from precursors, such as the plant lignans Mat and Sec, which are consumed by man and animals and then structurally modified by intestinal bacteria.[3] The main source of these compounds is whole-grain products, various seeds, fruits and berries.[2,3] Eq and O-Dma are formed by intestinal bacterial action from For and Da present in food stuffs, particularly in soy products (see[8]). The excretion of these compounds is closely associated with fiber intake[2,9] and we suggested that in grain the plant lignans are localized in the aleurone layer[2] containing phytin, polyphenols, enzyme inhibitors and other compounds usually regarded as antinutritional factors.[10] Modern milling techniques usually eliminates this fraction, which does not, with some exceptions, anymore occur in the products supplied to the market for consumption. We have now confirmed by GC-MS techniques the presence of particularly high amounts of lignans in the aleurone layer of barley, rye and wheat grain.

4 EPIDEMIOLOGY OF LIGNANS AND ISOFLAVONOIDS

Urinary lignan excretion was found to be highest in areas with low risk of BC and CC in north-east Finland but lower in the south and particularly low in postmenopausal BC patients in USA.[2,7,9] Lower excretion compared to omnivores and particularly vegetarians were found in young premenopausal BC patients in Finland.[11] However, in Japan with low risk of BC, PC and CC urinary lignan excretion is low, but instead the excretion of isoflavonoids is very high.[8] Furthermore, recent epidemiological studies have shown that subjects consuming soy products are protected with regard to BC,[12] PC[13] and CC (S. Watanabe, personal communication). Japanese men consuming traditional diet and with very low mortality in PC have high urinary isoflavonoid excretion.[8]

5 MECHANISMS OF LIGNAN AND ISOFLAVONOID ACTION AND THEIR ASSOCIATION WITH CANCER

Many plant lignans have been shown to have anticarcinogenic, antiviral, bactericidic and fungicidic activities. The mammalian lignans Enl, End and the isoflavonoids Da, Eq, O-Dma and Gen have all weak estrogenic activity, but definite antiestrogenic activities have also been described.[2,3,5] In the male mouse soy intake inhibited the prostatic dysplasia caused by diethylstilbestrol[14] and soy prevents prostatitis in rats.[15] Enl (in the presence of estradiol) and some isoflavonoids show suppressive effects on BC cells in culture.[16-18] Furthermore, intake of soy, containing isoflavonoids, or linseed containing lignans, inhibit carcinogen-induced breast tumors or early markers of colon carcinogenesis in rats.[19-21] These results are in agreement with the above-mentioned epidemiological studies.

Enterolactone inhibits the aromatase enzyme and competes with the natural substrate androstenedione for the enzyme[2] and may in this way reduce estrogen formation in peripheral and cancer cells. Gen is a specific inhibitor of tyrosine-specific protein kinases and inhibits phosphoinositol turnover and topoisomerase I and II. The enzymes involved play a role for cell proliferation and transformation. Tyrosine kinases are associated with a number of growth factors and have also been associated with oncogene products of the retroviral *src* gene family and is correlated with the ability of retrovirus to transform cells (lit. in[22-25]).

Several plant and mammalian lignans and isoflavonoids compete with estradiol (E2) for the rat uterine nuclear estrogen type II binding site.[26] Gen does not bind to these sites. These sites seem to constitute a component of the genome which regulates estrogen-stimulated uterine growth.[27,28] The most effective with regard to type II site binding of the diphenols found in human urine seem to be Da and Eq, but also some lignans like Mat, Isolar and Enl show competition. It has been suggested that uncontrolled growth and proliferation of malignant cells is directly related not only to the permanent stimulation of nuclear type II binding sites by estrogens or other compounds, but also to very low levels of competitive inhibitors.[27] It seems likely that these phenolic compounds may have a synergistic inhibitory action in this respect.

Both groups of diphenols stimulate SHBG (sex hormone binding globulin) synthesis in the liver and in this way they may reduce the biological effects of sex hormones.[2] An increase in plasma SHBG results in reduction of both the albumin-bound and the free fraction of the sex hormones. The excretion of these compounds in both pre- and postmenopausal Finnish women correlate positively with plasma SHBG.[2,11,26] Furthermore, we found that Enl caused a dose-dependent stimulation of SHBG synthesis in HepG2 cells in culture.[18] Gen and Da (Y. Mousavi, M. Carson and H. Adlercreutz, unpublished) are also strong stimulators of SHBG synthesis in HepG2 cells and definite evidence has now been obtained that Gen has an effect at the mRNA level. (M. Carson *et al.*, unpublished). Since changes in the transcription level of tissue specific genes have been found to be associated with methylation status[29] we have studied the effect of Gen on methylation of the SHBG gene, but found no effect.

Based on the above-mentioned evidence we therefore suggest that the positive associations between urinary lignan and isoflavonoid excretion and plasma SHBG are due to stimulation of SHBG synthesis by these weak estrogens[2] entering the portal circulation in very high amounts. This also would at least partly explain the higher SHBG values seen in vegetarians.[11,30]

The postmenopausal BC patients in Boston had the lowest plasma SHBG[31] and had lower mean excretion of lignans[7] compared to omnivorous and vegetarian controls. Also Eq excretion tended to be lower. The Finnish premenopausal BC subjects had lower SHBG and lower excretion of lignans and isoflavonoids compared to the vegetarians.[11] In many studies low SHBG has been associated with BC (see lit. in[31]).

Enterolactone is rapidly conjugated to a monosulfate (about 90 %)[18,26] and recently we found that circulating Enl monosulfate (MonoS) is a major metabolite in human blood. This is of particular interest in view of the possible important role of estrogen 3-sulfates in BC cell growth.[32] Enl-MonoS could theoretically compete with estrone sulfate (E1S) for the cell sulfatases. We therefore synthesized a mixture of the two Enl-monosulfates. However, we could not see any effect of EnlS on E2 or E1S-stimulated growth of human MCF-7 BC cells. However, as for Enl we found, when the compound was added alone to the cell culture, a weak stimulatory effect on cell proliferation (S. Booms *et al.*, unpublished).

In conclusion, many studies support the view that the lignans and isoflavonoids are strong candidates for a role as protective substances with regard to BC, PC and probably also other types of cancers like CC and solid tumours.

6 REFERENCES

1. H. Adlercreutz, Gastroenterology, 1984, 86, 761.
2. H. Adlercreutz, Scand. J. Clin. Lab. Invest., 1990, 50 (Suppl 201), 3.
3. K. Setchell and H. Adlercreutz, in 'Role of the Gut Flora in Toxicity and Cancer', I. Rowland, Ed., Academic Press, London, 1988, p. 315.
4. K.R. Price and G.R. Fenwick, Food Add. Contam., 1985, 2, 73.
5. H. Adlercreutz, in 'Progress in Diet and Nutrition. Frontiers of Gastrointestinal Research 14', C. Horwitz and P. Rozen, Eds., S. Karger, Basel, 1988, p. 165.
6. M. Axelson, D. Kirk, R. Farrant, G. Cooley, A. Lawson and K. Setchell, Biochem. J., 1982, 201, 353.
7. H. Adlercreutz, T. Fotsis, R. Heikkinen, J. Dwyer, M. Woods, B. Goldin and S. Gorbach, Lancet, 1982, 2, 1295.
8. H. Adlercreutz, H. Honjo, A. Higashi, T. Fotsis, E. Hämäläinen, T. Hasegawa and H. Okada, Am. J. Clin. Nutr., 1991, 54, 1093.
9. H. Adlercreutz, T. Fotsis, C. Bannwart, K. Wähälä, T. Mäkelä, G. Brunow and T. Hase, J. Steroid Biochem., 1986, 25, 791.
10. C. Cantarelli, in 'Nutritional Impact of Food Processing', J.C. Somogyi and H.R. Müller, Eds., Karger, Basel, 1989, vol. 43, p. 31.

11. H. Adlercreutz, K. Höckerstedt, C. Bannwart, E. Hämäläinen, T. Fotsis and S. Bloigu, in ′Progress in Cancer Research and Therapy, Vol. 35: Hormones and Cancer 3′, F. Bresciani, R. King, M. Lippman and J.-P. Raynaud, Eds., Raven Press, New York, 1988 p. 409.
12. H. Lee, L. Gourley, S. Duffy, J. Estève, J. Lee and N. Day, Lancet, 1991, 337, 1197.
13. R. Severson, A. Nomura, J. Grove and G. Stemmerman, Cancer Res., 1989, 49, 1857.
14. S. Mäkelä, L. Pylkkänen, R. Santti and H. Adlercreutz, in ′EURO FOOD TOX III. Proceedings of the Interdisciplinary Conference on Effects of Food on the Immune and Hormonal Systems′, Institute of Toxicology, Swiss Federal Institute of Technology & University of Zürich, CH-8603 Schwerzenbach, Switzerland, 1991 p. 135.
15. O. Sharma, H. Adlercreutz, J. Strandberg, B. Zirkin, D. Coffey and L. Ewing, J. Steroid Biochem. Molec. Biol., 1992, 43, in press.
16. T. Hirano, K. Oka and M. Akiba, Res. Comm. Chem. Path. Pharm., 1989, 64, 69.
17. G. Peterson and S. Barnes, Biochem. Biophys. Res. Comm., 1991, 179, 661.
18. Y. Mousavi and H. Adlercreutz, J. Steroid Biochem. Molec. Biol., 1992, 41, 615.
19. S. Barnes, C. Grubbs and K. Setchell, Breast Cancer Res. Treat., 1988, 12, 128.
20. M. Serraino and L.U. Thompson, Nutr. Cancer, 1992, 17, 153.
21. M. Serraino and L.U. Thompson, Cancer Lett., 1992, 63, 159.
22. T. Akiyama, J. Ishida, S. Nakagawa, H. Ogawara, S.-I. Watanabe, N. Itoh, M. Shibuya and Y. Fukami, J. Biol. Chem., 1987, 262, 5592.
23. M. Makishima, Y. Honma, M. Hozumi, K. Sampi, M. Hattori, K. Umezawa and K. Motoyoshi, Leukemia Res., 1991, 15, 701.
24. K. Higashi and H. Ogawara, J. of Pharmacobio - Dynamics, 1991, 14, S140.
25. K. Kondo, K. Tsuneizumi, T. Watanabe and M. Oishi, Cancer Res., 1991, 51, 5398.
26. H. Adlercreutz, Y. Mousavi, J. Clark, K. Höckerstedt, E. Hämäläinen, K. Wähälä, T. Mäkelä and T. Hase, J. Steroid Biochem. Molec. Biol., 1992, 41, 331.
27. B.M. Markaverich, R.R. Gregory, M.-A. Alejandro, J.H. Clark, G.A. Johnson and B.S. Middleditch, J. Biol. Chem., 1988, 263, 7203.
28. B.M. Markaverich and J.H. Clark, Endocrinology, 1979, 105, 1458.
29. H. Cedar, Cell, 1988, 53, 3.
30. B. Armstrong, J. Brown, H. Clarke, D. Crooke, R. Hähnel, J. Masarei and T. Ratajzak, J. Natl. Cancer Inst., 1981, 67, 761.
31. H. Adlercreutz, E. Hämäläinen, S.L. Gorbach, B.R. Goldin, M.N. Woods and J.T. Dwyer, Am. J. Clin. Nutr., 1989, 49, 433.
32. J.R. Pasqualini, C. Gelly, B.-L. Nguyen and C. Vella, J. Steroid Biochem., 1989, 34, 155.

BILE ACIDS IN A HUMAN MODEL OF COLORECTAL NEOPLASIA

DM Bradburn[1] , IR Rowland[2] , JC Mathers[3] , A Gunn[4] , J Burn[5] , IDA Johnston[1]

Departments of Surgery[1] , Biological and Nutritional Sciences[3] , and Human Genetics[5] Newcastle University, Newcastle upon Tyne. NE2 4HH
Ashington Hospital[4] , West View, Ashington, Northumberland and
BIBRA[2] , Woodmansterne Rd, Carshalton, Surrey SM5 4DS

INTRODUCTION

Familial Adenomatous Polyposis (FAP) is an autosomal dominant genetic condition characterised by the formation of multiple premalignant adenomatous colorectal and duodenal polyps. Affected individuals usually develop colonic polyps in their late teens and one or more of these will undergo malignant transformation within 10-15 years[1].

FAP is a useful model of sporadic colonic cancer (CC). The histological appearance and natural history of the colonic adenomas in FAP are identical to the premalignant lesions in sporadic CC[2]. The genetic defect in FAP (on chromosome 5q22) is the earliest changes in the genetic events of the adenoma carcinoma sequence and is thought to cause a hyperproliferative epithelium[3]. It therefore appears that the propensity to colonic cancer in FAP occurs because they are already "one step along the way" to malignant transformation. It is not unreasonable to suggest that the factors determining the subsequent genetic changes in the adenoma carcinoma sequence are the same in both FAP and CC.

Epidemiological evidence has stressed the importance of diet as a risk factor for colonic neoplasia. It has been proposed that dietary complex carbohydrates are protective whilst a high fat intake has an adverse effect[4]. Fat increases faecal bile acid output, and bile acids are known promoters of CC in animal experiments[5]. In this context, it is interesting to note that abnormal *duodenal*[6] and *faecal*[7] bile acids have been noted in FAP. Changes in bile acid metabolism in FAP may therefore be *additional* to the genetic defect in stimulating the change from normal mucosa to carcinoma.

The pattern of bile acid entering the colon in FAP is not known and a fuller understanding of the steroids entering and leaving the colon in this subject group may allow dietary strategies to be developed to delay the progression of polyposis.

AIMS

1. To determine the amounts and patterns of bile acids arriving at and leaving the

colon in FAP.

2. To examine the effect of colonic polyps on bacterial bile acid metabolism independent of any genetic influence.

MATERIALS AND METHODS

Ileostomy studies. Twelve ileostomists were studied, 6 whose surgery was for FAP, and 6 whose surgery was for ulcerative colitis (UC, controls). No subject had taken antibiotics for 6 weeks prior to the study. Haematological liver function tests were normal, no patient had gallstones or a cholecystectomy and ileal resection was less than 7cm in all cases. Subject details are presented in Table I.

Table I Ileostomy study, subject details.

	sex	age (years)	body mass index (kg/m^2)	duration of ileostomy (years)
FAP	2 male 4 female	mean 43.6 range 27-67	mean 26.7 range 18.0-43.9	mean 8.3 range 5-13
UC	3 male 3 female	mean 50 range 25-80	mean 24.3 range 21.0-30.5	mean 9 range 1-28

Volunteers were admitted to a metabolic unit after an overnight fast (fluids allowed). A known, controlled diet was consumed for 24 hours and ileal effluent was collected 2 hourly and immediately snap frozen. Samples were thawed, pooled, homogenised, freeze dried, and sterols were extracted by established methods[8].

Individual bile acids were measured by HPLC using dexamethasone as an internal standard (25cm x 4.6mm Phase Sep [UK] ODS5 column, eluent [650ml ethanol, 30ml tetrahydrofuran, 320ml water, 3g NaH_2PO_4, 0.29g tetrabutyl ammonium chloride per litre], pH 5.4, flow rate 1ml/minute, UV detector [Gilson] 205nm).

Faecal Studies. Using a combination of DNA markers, ophthalmoscopy and pedigree analysis, individuals undergoing endoscopic screening for FAP were divided into 3 groups as outlined in Table II [9].

No dietary restrictions were imposed and twenty four hour faecal collections were made from all subjects. After homogenising, pH was measured and samples were freeze dried. Bile acids were measured by GLC[8].

Table II Faecal studies, subject details.

group	number	risk of gene carriage	mean age	age range
control	7	< 1%	30.1	9 - 53
FAP gene carriers with no polyps (GCNP)	9	> 98%	25.2	7 - 53
FAP gene carriers with polyps (GCWP)	8	100%	19.9	11-32

Statistics.
Ileostomy data. Differences between groups were examined by ANOVA. Age sex and body mass index were examined as covariate factors.
Faecal data. Data was not normally distributed so were examined by the Mann Whitney test. The null hypotheses tested were:-
1. There is no difference between gene carriers with and without polyps.
2. There is no difference between gene carriers and normal controls.

RESULTS

Abbreviations:- CA =cholic acid, CDCA =chenodeoxycholic acid, prefix T =taurine conjugate, prefix G= glycine conjugate. SED= standard error of the difference of the mean.

There were no differences in ileal wet and dry weights between groups. There were significantly lower 24 hour outputs of TCDCA ($p=0.047$), total taurine amidates ($p=0.092$) and total CDCA amidates ($p=0.088$) in subjects with FAP. Complete results are presented in Table III.

There were no differences in the 24 hour faecal outputs of neutral sterols but the 24 hour output of deoxcholate ($p=0.02$), lithocholate ($p=0.05$) and total bile acids ($p=0.02$) were significantly lower in FAP gene carriers compared to controls. There were no differences comparing FAP gene carriers with and without polyps. Complete results are presented in Table IV.

DISCUSSION

The current data agree with the range of ileal and faecal sterol output which may be calculated from the results of other workers[7 10]. In addition the 24 hour ileal outputs are slightly higher than the faecal outputs consistent with the small amount of bile acid absorption from the colon.

Increased molar ratios of duodenal chenodeoxycholate amidates have been noted in duodenal and gallbladder bile in FAP[6]. If this is reflected in ileal fluid, colonic polyp formation may be influenced. In contrast there were decreased ileal

Table III Ileostomy 24 hour wet and dry weights and sterol outputs.

	UC		FAP		
	mean	range	mean	range	SED
wet weight (g)	409	298 - 600	452	300 - 686	78.8
dry weight (g)	46	39 - 48	50	28 - 64	7.0
ileal output (mmol/day)					
total bile acids	0.730	0.308-1.527	0.381	0.119-0.849	0.2483
TCA	0.068	0.004-0.137	0.056	0.017-0.117	0.0299
TCDCA	0.157	0.052-0.288	0.065	0.029-0.172	0.0402
total taurine amidates	0.225	0.065-0.306	0.122	0.035-0.271	0.0552
GCA	0.190	0.025-0.449	0.115	0.034-0.235	0.0884
GCDCA	0.310	0.012-0.772	0.140	0.053-0.412	0.1307
total glycine amidates	0.500	0.017-1.221	0.261	0.084-0.638	0.2131
total CA amidates	0.259	0.008-0.583	0.172	0.052-0.334	0.1172
total CDCA amidates	0.467	0.140-0.944	0.206	0.071-0.516	0.1363

Table IV 24 hour faecal wet and dry weights and sterol outputs.

	control		no polyps		with polyps	
	median	range	median	range	median	range
wet wt (g)	117	65 - 341	89	53 - 260	79	58 - 210
dry wt (g)	50	17 - 111	26	16 - 51	20	14 - 38
pH	6.37	6.11 - 6.66	6.51	6.07 - 7.10	6.24	5.9 - 7.04
bile acids (μmol/day)						
lithocholate	171	701 - 1014	62	18 - 466	112	9 - 508
deoxycholate	198	138 - 633	37	15 - 366	136	65 - 371
total bile acids	406	219 - 1647	147	32 - 747	288	112 - 879

outputs of taurochenodeoxycholate and total taurine and chenodeoxycholate amidates by FAP subjects in the present studies. This suggests that there is increased recirculation, rather than increased formation of bile acids. Duodenal polyposis in FAP clusters around the ampulla of Vater, implying that bile may be an aetiological factor[11]. Increased recirculation of bile acids in FAP may therefore promote duodenal polyposis.

Increased faecal *concentrations* of primary bile acids have been noted in FAP[7], but we are unaware of other published data for total outputs. We could not detect any primary bile acids in faeces, but the decreased total and individual secondary bile acid outputs in FAP agrees with the results from the ileostomy studies. It is interesting to note that there was not a specific decrease in the output of lithocholate, the chenodeoxycholate metabolite.

In summary, the data do not suggest a primary role for bile acids in colonic polyposis in FAP, but suggests that increased recirculation may augment duodenal polyposis. Duodenal cancer developing from polyps is the commonest extracolonic malignant cause of death in FAP[1]. Dietary bile acid ligands, such as complex carbohydrates decrease the small intestinal absorption of sterols[12] and decrease bile acid recirculation. Further study of the potential value of dietary intervention with such materials in attempts to decrease duodenal cancer in FAP is warranted.

REFERENCES

1. M. Rhodes, D.M. Bradburn, Gut, 1992, 33, 125
2. H.J.R. Bussey, Path Annual, 1979, .14, 61
3. E.R. Fearon, B. Vogelstein, Cell, 1990, 61, 759
4. S.A. Bingham, J Roy Soc Med, 1990, 83, 420
5. B.S. Reddy, Cancer Res, 1981, 41, 3700
6. A.D. Spigelman, R.W. Owen, M.J. Hill, R.K.S. Phillips, Br J Surg, 1991, 78, 321
7. A.L. Watne, H.L. Lai, T. Mance, S. Core, Am J Surg, 1976, 131, 42
8. E. Bailey, A.F.G. Brooks, J Chromatog, 1987, 421, 21
9. J. Burn, P. Chapman, J. Delhanty, C. Wood, F. Lalloo, M.B. Gonzales, K. Tsioupara, W. Church, M. Rhodes, A. Gunn, J Med Genet, 1991, 28, 289
10. I. Bosaeus, B. Sandstrom, H. Andersson, Scand J Gastroenterol 1986, 21, 891
11. A.D. Spigelman, C. Crofton-Sleigh, S. Venitt, R.K.S. Phillips, Br J Surg, 1990, 77, 878
12. I. Bosaeus, N.G. Carlsson, A.S. Sandberg, H. Andersson, Hum Nutr: Clin Nutr, 1986, 40, 429

VARIATIONS OF COLONIC PROLIFERATION, CECAL AND FECAL pH IN RATS FED DIFFERENT CARBOHYDRATES.

Giovanna Caderni, Cristina Luceri and M. Teresa Spagnesi.

Department of Pharmacology,
University of Florence
50134 Florence, Italy.

1 INTRODUCTION

Dietary habits have been associated with the incidence of colon cancer in both experimental and epidemiological studies[1-3].

To explain the correlation between dietary habits and cancer risk it has been suggested that some diets may act as promoters of colonic carcinogenesis, increasing the proliferation of colonic epithelial cells[4,5]. High proliferative activity in the colonic epithelium has been associated with increased risk of colon cancer in humans and experimental animals[6]. Moreover, some studies have suggested that a shift of the proliferative activity from the lower to the upper sections of the crypt, is associated with a higher risk of colon cancer[6].

Some epidemiological and experimental studies also have indicated a correlation between colon cancer risk and colonic pH, suggesting that colon cancer risk is associated with high colonic pH [7,8]. High-fat, high-sugar diets, poor in fibers and complex carbohydrates, are thought to be a risk factor for the development of colon cancer[1-3, 9]. Therefore it seemed interesting to us to study colonic proliferation, cecal and fecal pH in rats fed high-fat diets in which carbohydrates were supplied by sucrose or by starch for 1 month.

2 MATERIALS AND METHODS

Female Sprague Dawley rats weighing about 150 g were used. The animals were fed for a month ad libitum with two isocaloric high-fat diets (23% w/w corn oil) containing sucrose (46% w/w) or corn starch (46% w/w) as a source of carbohydrates. Both the sucrose and the starch diets contained 23% casein, 2% cellulose, 0.3% DL-methionine, 0.2% choline, 4% AIN-76 Mineral Mix and 1.2% AIN-76 Vitamin Mix [10]. There were 12 rats per dietary group.

At the end of the dietary treatment, about 100 mg of feces were freshly collected from individual rats, diluted in 2 ml of saline, homogenized with a glass-Teflon homogenizer and immediately checked for pH with a pH-meter equipped with a glass electrode.

The animals were sacrificed by decapitation, the cecal content was collected from individual animals and the pH immediately determined as described above.

The proliferative activity in the colonic mucosa was assessed by ^{3}H-thymidine incorporation in vitro and autoradiography as previously described [10]. For each rat we determined the labelling index (LI = labelled cells /total of scored cells x 100) and the distribution of the proliferative activity along the crypt. To perform this analysis the crypt was divided in three equal compartments: low, middle and upper, in each of which the LI was measured [6].

3 RESULTS AND DISCUSSION

The results of the determination of cecal and fecal pH in the rats showed (Table 1) that the animals fed the starch diet had significantly lower cecal and fecal pH as compared with the rats fed the sucrose diet.

Table 1. Fecal and cecal pH in rats fed sucrose and starch diets.

	sucrose	starch	P
fecal pH	7.15 ± 0.09	6.79 ± 0.08	0.008
cecal pH	7.20 ± 0.04	7.01 ± 0.05	0.011

Data are means ± SE. P is calculated by the t-test for unpaired samples.

We also determined the proliferative activity of colonic mucosa in the rats fed the two diets and the results indicate that the animals fed the starch diet had a significantly lower proliferation (LI) compared with those fed sucrose (Table 2).

In order to study whether different diets induce variations in the pattern of proliferative activity along the crypt we also analyzed the distribution of the proliferative activity along the crypt. The results of this analysis (Table 2) showed that in the animals fed starch, proliferative activity was decreased mainly in the middle and upper compartments of the crypt (in

Table 2, middle and upper LIs, respectively), thus suggesting a protective role of starch for the colonic mucosa.

Table 2. Proliferative activity of the colonic mucosa of rats fed different diets.

	sucrose	starch	P
LI	5.69 ± 0.74	3.51 ± 0.57	0.03
low LI	11.0 ± 1.82	7.62 ± 1.37	0.16
middle LI	5.04 ± 0.73	2.64 ± 0.47	0.01
upper LI	1.03 ± 0.38	0.22 ± 0.09	0.05

Data are means ± SE. P is calculated by the t-test for unpaired samples.

We then carried out an analysis of the correlations between the proliferative activity in the colon and the fecal and cecal pH in each rat (24 animals); we found a positive correlation between the number of labelled cells per crypt and the cecal pH ($r = 0.49$, $P = 0.01$).

In conclusion, the results of the present paper indicate that rats fed a diet rich in corn starch for one month have lower cecal and fecal pH compared with animals fed a diet in which carbohydrates are supplied by sucrose. We also have demonstrate that the starch-fed rats have lower proliferative activity in the whole crypt and especially in the upper compartments of the crypt. Moreover, the low proliferation in the starch diet is associated with low colonic pH. Therefore, these data might indicate a common underlying mechanism pertaining to both colonic pH and proliferative activity.

A reduction in colonic pH has been suggested to be a protective factor against the development of colon cancer[7,8]. Similarly, a reduction in the proliferative activity in the colonic epithelium and especially in the upper compartments of the crypts has been associated with a low risk of developing colon cancer in both humans and rodents [6]. Therefore these results suggest that dietary starch may be a protective factor against colon carcinogenesis.

ACKNOWLEDGMENTS

This work has been supported by a Grant from "Regione Toscana, Italy".

REFERENCES

1. W. Willet, Nature, 1989, 338,389.
2. W.R. Bruce, Cancer Res., 1987, 47, 4237.
3. D.J.A. Jenkins, A.L. Jenkins, A.V. Rao and L.U. Thompson, Am. J. Gastroenterol., 1986, 81, 931.
4. L.R. Jacobs and J.R. Lupton, Cancer Res., 1986, 46, 1727.
5. G. Caderni, F. Bianchini, P. Dolara and D. Kriebel, Cancer Res., 1989, 49, 1655.
6. M. Lipkin, Cancer Res., 1988, 48, 235.
7. H.L. Newmark and J.R. Lupton, Nutrition and Cancer, 1990, 14, 161.
8. J.R. Thornton, Lancet, 1981, 16, 1081.
9. J.B. Bristol, P.M. Emmet, K.W. Heaton, and R.C.N. Williamson, Br. Med. J., 1985, 291, 1467.
10. G. Caderni, F. Bianchini, A. Mancina, M.T. Spagnesi, and P. Dolara, Cancer Res., 1991, 51, 3721.

INSOLUBLE DIETARY FIBRE RICH FRACTIONS FROM BARLEY PROTECT RATS FROM INTESTINAL CANCERS.

G.H. McIntosh, L. Jorgensen and P. Royle.

CSIRO Division of Human Nutrition, Kintore Avenue, Adelaide, S.A. 5000.

There is increasing experimental evidence that wheat bran (WB) protects humans and experimental rodents from intestinal cancer, particularly when high fat diets are involved. The insoluble dietary fibre (DF) component concentrated in WB is cellulose, which has also been shown to be protective (1). By contrast soluble dietary fibre rich sources e.g. oat bran have been found to be less protective. We found that 5% addition of wheat bran (WB) or barley bran (BB) to a semipurified rodent diet (AIN89) with 20% fat showed 33% fewer rats affected <u>and</u> tumours/rat with WB than BB.

A second study was undertaken to compare three sources of barley DF, commercial barley bran (BB1) outer layer barley bran (BB2) and spent barley grain (SBG)(from brewery) with cellulose (99% pure) and wheat bran (WB), when added at a constant amount of DF (5%) to the rodent diet. Their influence on tumour incidence burden and tumour mass index (TMI) in S-D male rats, induced by 5 weekly doses of DMH (15mg/kg BW) given subcutaneously is shown. Rats were maintained on the diets from weaning until death at 32 weeks of age.

Treatment		Incidence (%)	Tumours/ rat	Tumour Mass Index $\log_{10}$
Cellulose	(10)	80	1.3	1.63
Wheat Bran	(10)	90	1.7	2.11
BB1	(10)	100	2.2	2.23
BB2	(10)	90	1.2	1.77
SBG	(10)	70	1.3	1.20*

Number in parenthesis = no. of rats per treatment.
* SBG significantly different from WB and BB1.
TMI is $\log_{10}$ the sum of areas of all tumours per rat.

As seen SBG was more protective that BB1 or Wheat Bran, the former being a rich source of insoluble DF (lignin and cellulose), the latter being 40% soluble DF (βglucan and arabinoxylan). Wheat bran on the other hand had equivalent levels of insoluble DF, but lacked the hull component of SBG. Although tempting to attribute this beneficial effect to insoluble DF, there are other components in the rich brans which could be protective also (e.g. proteins polyphenolics, terpenoids, protease inhibitors, tocotrienols phytate). It will therefore be important to examine some of these possibilities in future experiments.

1. D.W. Heitman and I.L. Cameron (1990) JNCI 82, 1990.

DIETARY FIBRE AND THE GASTROINTESTINAL EPITHELIUM: DIFFERENTIAL RESPONSE IN THE STOMACH, SMALL INTESTINE AND COLON OF CONVENTIONAL AND GERM-FREE RATS.

B Ratcliffe* , CY Lee, NA Wright, & RA Goodlad.

Imperial Cancer Research Fund,
Histopathology Unit,
35-43 Lincoln's Inn Fields,
London WC2A 3PN.

* Robert Gordon Institute of Technology,
Kepplestone,
Aberdeen.
AB9 2PG

INTRODUCTION

The rates of cell division in the intestinal epithelium can rapidly adjust so that the functional cell mass can adapt to meet changing digestive demands. While several factors influence intestinal adaptation, most can be related to altered food intake, which is one of the best predictors of cell production [1]. The proliferative effects of food can be attributed to the direct or indirect effects of 'luminal nutrition', and this concept can be extended to the distal gut where lack of dietary fibre dramatically decreases cell renewal [2]. Hypoplasia associated with fibre free or elemental diets was originally attributed to a lack of 'bulk'[3], however, the effect has since been shown to be specific to dietary fibre[4] as inert bulk has no effect,[5] which again could be either direct or indirect. Indirect effects of fibre are likely to be mediated via the actions of short chain fatty acids (SCFA's) , which are the end products of hind gut fibre fermentation by the microflora [1], especially as the SCFA's may be the preferential fuel for the colonocytes. Fermentation cannot occur in germ-free rats, which therefore provide an excellent opportunity to dissect out the effects of fibre itself from those of its breakdown products.

Methods

Conventional and germ-free rats [2, 3] were fed a fibre-free, elemental diet (Flexical, Mead Johnson, Slough) with or without a 30% fibre supplement, 1 part Ispaghula (Reckitt & Coleman, Hull) and 9 parts Trifyba (Sanofi, Manchester)[4]. After two weeks on the diets the rats were injected with 1mg/kg of vincristine and killed at timed intervals. The gastrointestinal tract was removed, rinsed, blotted and weighed. Samples from all the regions of the gut were fixed in Carnoy's fluid and stored in 70% alcohol. The tissue was stained with the Feulgen reaction and intestinal and colonic crypts were displayed by microdissection and gently squashed with a coverslip. The number of arrested metaphases in 20 gastric glands, 10 small intestinal crypts, or 20 colonic crypts was counted, plotted against time since injection and the slope of the line gave the crypt cell production rate (CCPR)[5].

Results are presented as the mean ± standard error of the mean. Asterixes are used to denote the results of t-tests versus the respective germ-free group, with * = $p < 0.05$, ** = $p < 0.01$, *** = $p < 0.001$

Results

The water content of the gut of the different groups did not vary, the weights of the regions of the gut are shown in table 1.

Table 1 Gastrointestinal tissue wet weights, expressed as a percentage of total body weight .

	Germ-Free		Conventional		TWAOVA		
	Fibre-free	+ 30% Fibre	Fibre-free	+ 30% Fibre	D	MF	I
Stomach	0.37 ± 0.01	0.47 ± 0.01***	0.39 ± 0.01	0.46 ± 0.01***	§§§	-	§
Small intestine	2.06 ± 0.037	2.14 ± 0.03	1.94 ± 0.03	2.12 ± 0.04**	§§§	-	-
Caecum	0.54 ± 0.023	0.63 ± 0.01	0.28 ± 0.01	0.35 ± 0.01***	§§§	§§§	-
Colon	0.36 ± 0.014	0.56 ± 0.02***	0.34 ± 0.01	0.45 ± 0.02***	§§§	§§§	-

TWAOVA = Two-way analysis of variance, § = p< 0.05, §§ = p< 0.01, §§§ = p< 0.001, D = effect of diet, MF = effect of microflora, I = interaction.

All regions of the gastrointestinal tract were significantly heavier in the fibre supplemented conventional group. In the germ-free group only the stomach and colon weights of the rats were heavier with fibre supplementation. Two-way analysis of variance showed that diet had significant effects on the stomach, small intestine, caecum and colon weights, whilst the microflora only had significant (P< 0.001) effects on the weights of the caecum and colon.

The proliferative activity of the gastric mucosa is shown in fig 1 where fibre stimulated proliferation in both the conventional and the germ-free, with the effect being more marked in the fundus than in the antrum.

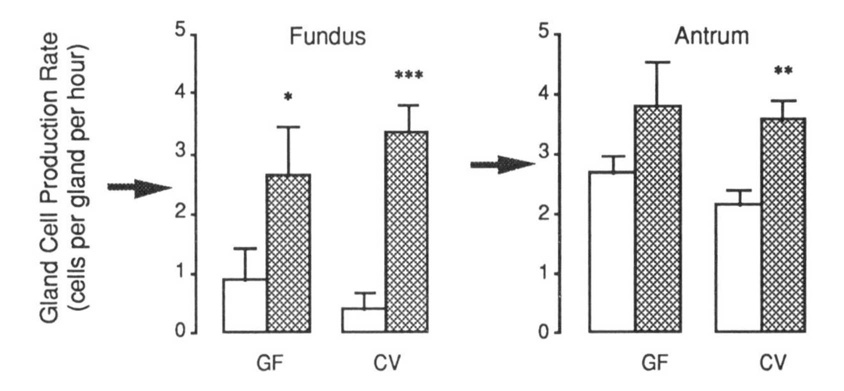

Fig 1 Gland cell production in the stomach. The arrows show the values seen in conventional rats fed a standard chow diet. GF = germ-free, CV = Conventional. Shaded bars = + fibre.

No effect of fibre was noted in the mid small intestine of either group (fig 2), but a proliferative effect of fibre was seen in the distal small intestine where CCPR was increased by 43% when compared to the fibre free group ($p<0.01$).

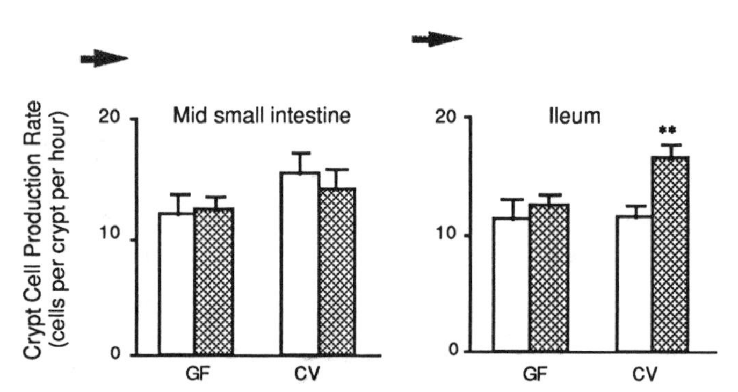

Fig 2 Crypt cell production in the small intestine. The arrows show the values seen in conventional rats fed a standard chow diet. GF = germ-free, CV = Conventional. Shaded bars = + fibre

Fibre had no effect on the CCPR of the colon of germ-free rats (fig 3), but it significantly increased proliferation throughout the colon of the conventional rats. The trophic effect of fibre on the colon of conventional rats was most pronounced in the proximal colon, where the increase was 256%, the increase in the mid colon was 196% whilst in the distal colon the CCPR was 'only' elevated by 97%.

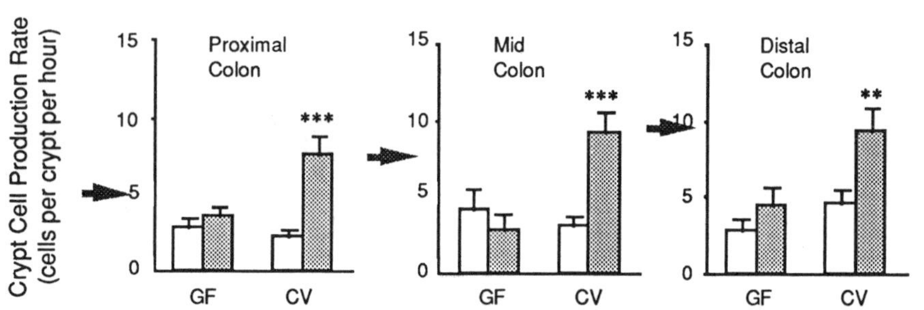

Fig 3 Crypt cell production in the colon. The arrows show the values seen in conventional rats fed a standard chow diet. GF = germ-free, CV = Conventional. Shaded bars = + fibre

Discussion

Fibre can stimulate both the muscle and the mucosa, whilst inert bulk can only stimulate the colonic muscle[5]. The effect on tissue weight was seen in both conventional and germ-free rats, in the present study, suggesting that this is a direct effect, not dependant on fermentation.

When one considers the mucosa it can be seen that there were two distinct types of actions of fibre. In the stomach fibre had a direct effect, as fermentation was not required, whereas in the ileum and colon fibre was only trophic when the microflora was present. This strongly suggests that it is the breakdown products of hind-gut fermentation (short chain fatty acids) that are the trophic agents. Infusion studies would appear to confirm this [6-8] and our infusion studies are reported in another chapter of this book.

The adaptive capabilities of the stomach are less well documented than that of the small bowel or colon, attributable to the technical difficulties in the assessment of gastric proliferation and to the low rates of cell production. Lupton[14] found that fibre supplementation results in expanded proliferative zones in rat gastric mucosa. As this effect was seen in both the conventional and the germ-free rats, the proliferation in stomach could be attributed to its direct effects, perhaps by its abrasion stimulating increased cell loss,[9, 10], however, such an action was not seen in the rest of the gastrointestinal tract.

Because expanded proliferative zones precede and accompany neoplastic transformation, such effects of dietary fibre on the gastric mucosa have potentially negative implications. Furthermore, hyperplasia (including that induced by high fibre diets) can act as a promoter of carcinogenesis in experimental systems[11, 12]. Animal models can be criticised as they often only study the final yield of what is a complex multistage system[13], nonetheless, the present invocation of high fibre diets may need to be reconsidered, especially considering the decline in the incidence of gastric cancer over the last 40-50 years, which would correspond to a similar decline in fibre intake (until recently). Although the proliferative effects reported here were large, the base line of this study was a fibre-free diet, and the increased proliferative rates were not much greater than those seen in chow fed animals.

It should be remembered that these are but a few of the thirty or more actions of fibre, some of which can be attributed to it mechanical and viscous properties, some to its chemical actions, some to its breakdown products, some to the particular properties of plant cell remnant material and some to several other factors associated with a less processed plant based diet.

We have thus demonstrated that dietary fibre has a variety of proliferative effects on the gut. [1] Fibre (and bulk) has a trophic effect on the intestinal muscle. [2] It is also has a trophic role on the gastric epithelium, independent of fermentation. [3] Fibre stimulates proliferation in the ileum and particularly in the colon. This latter effect is entirely dependent on the microflora, and is most prominent at the main sites of short chain fatty acid production.

References

1. Sakata T, Yajima T. Q J exp Physiol 1984, 69. 639.
2. Gustafsson BE. Acta Pathol Microbiol Scand 1948, Suppl LXXIII.
3. Gustafsson BE. Ann Ny Acad Sci 1959, 78. 17.
4. Goodlad RA, Ratcliffe B, Fordham JP, Wright NA. Gut 1989, 30. 820.
5. Goodlad RA, Wright NA. Quantitative studies on epithelial replacement in the gut. In: Titchen TA, ed. *Techniques in life sciences. Digestive physiology.* Ireland: Elsevier Biomedical Press., 1982: p212.
6. Kripke SA, Fox AD, Berman JA, Settle RG, Rombeau JL. J Parenteral and enteral nutrition 1989, 13. 109.
7. Koruda MJ, Rolandelli RH, Settle RG, Zimmaro DM, Romneau JL. Gastroenterology 1988, 95. 715.
8. Sakata T. Br J Nutr 1987, 58. 95.
9. Komai M, Kimura S. J Nutr Sci Vitaminol 1980, 26. 389.
10. Savada D. Med Sci Res 1987, 15. 583.
11. Jacobs LR, Lupton JR. Cancer Res 1986, 46. 1727.
12. Jacobs LR. Prev Med 1987, 16. 566.
13. Fearon ER, Vogelstein B. Cell 1990, 61.

INFLUENCE OF DIETARY FIBERS ON TWO INTESTINAL TRANSFERASES IN RATS INOCULATED WITH A WHOLE HUMAN FAECAL FLORA.

N. ROLAND, L. NUGON-BAUDON, O. SZYLIT

INRA (UEPSD) - Bat. 440
78352 Jouy-en-Josas
FRANCE

1 INTRODUCTION

Several epidemiological surveys have concluded to the "protective" side-effect of dietary fibers, especially in colonic cancer etiology[1-3]. Experimental studies, realized on laboratory animals, indicated that the "protective" effect of fibers towards intestinal carcinogenesis varies with their origin and chemical nature[4-6].
Different hypotheses have been proposed to explain the "protective" side-effect of fibers, most of them insisting on their incidence on the dilution[2] of carcinogens, their adsorption[7] or their metabolism by the intestinal flora[1,8].
Other mechanisms could be involved such as the endogenous Xenobiotic Metabolizing Enzymes (XME) which play a key-role in chemical carcinogenesis[9-11]. Lindeskog showed, in 1987, that diets containing high levels of wheat bran or pectin altered cytochrome P450-dependent enzymes both in the liver and the intestine[10]. Nevertheless, relatively few studies have been realized so far on that issue and, to our knowledge, none are reported on phase II enzymes although they are of tremendous importance in toxics elimination.
The aim of this work was to assay the influence of different dietary fibers on intestinal glutathione-S-transferase (GSH-T) and UDP-glucuronosyl transferase (UDPG-T) specific activities in rats harbouring a human whole faecal flora, isolated from a healthy human donor. This mimicking model has already been used successfully to study the influence of fibers fermentation on nutritional[12] and blood[13] parameters *in vivo*.

2 EXPERIMENTAL

Experimental Diets

Five experimental diets were used and compared to a control diet (Table 1). Each of the experimental diets contained a realistic amount (10%) of one of 5 fibers: wheat bran, oat, cocoa (SOFALIA), inulin (Tirlemontoise

Table 1 composition of diets (% dry matter)

	Control diet	Experimental diets
Fiber	0	10
Mashed potatoes	53.95	43.95
Fish meal	13	13
Soyabean meal	13	13
Corn oil	3	3
Lard	3	3
Cholesterol	0.05	0.05
Sucrose	5	5
Cellulose	7	7
Minerals and vitamins	2	2

sugar-refinery), carrot (ARD). Fibers were chosen for their different chemical structures and properties. All diets were designed to mimick a "human-type" diet with the condition that they respected rodent digestive physiology. All diets were isonitrogenous and isoenergetic. Pelleted diets, packed in double vacuum bags were sterilized by gamma-irradiation at 40 kGy.

Animals: Inoculation and Maintenance

Germ-free adult male Fischer rats aged 10 weeks at the beginning of trials were used. Rats were randomly distributed (3 rats/cage), 6 rats for each experimental diet and 12 rats kept as control group. Animals were housed in Trexler-type isolators fitted with a rapid transfer system (La Calhène, Vélizy, France).
All animals, originating from our breeding unit, were inoculated *per os* (oesophagal tubing) with the whole faecal flora of a healthy adult man, using 1 ml of freshly passed stools 10^{-2} dilution in a liquid medium, pH 7.0, containing 2 g/l casein hydrolysate enzymic (USBC, Cleveland, Ohio), [illegible] g/l yeast extract (Difco), 5 g/l sodium chloride and 1 g/l monopotassium phosphate, prepared in an anaerobic chamber[1[illegible]] and transferred into the isolator in a butyl-rubber stoppered tube.
Animals were fed *ad libitum* and were given sterilized (20 min, 120°C) tap water to drink. Room temperature was 21°C and photoperiods were 12 h. Animal weight was measured once a week for 8 weeks.

Samples Collection

Rats were knocked senseless 8 weeks after inoculation and immediately sacrificed by cervical dislocation. Intestines (small and large) were quickly removed and microsomes were immediately prepared according to the method described by Strobel *et al*[15].

Chemicals

Chemicals were obtained from the following sources: Trizma-hydrochloride, DL-dithiothreitol, phenylmethylsulfonyl fluoride, Folin and Ciocalteu's phenol reagent, glutathione (reduced form), 1-chloro-2,4-dinitrobenzene (grade I), magnesium chloride, chloramphenicol (CAP), sodium salt of uridine 5'-diphosphoglucuronic acid and disodium salt of ethylenediaminetetraacetic acid were from SIGMA. Potassium-sodium tartrate was from MERCK. Albumin (bovine, grade V) was from Touzart & Matignon, France. ^{14}C-CAP labelled in the acetyl moiety with a specific activity of 54 mCi $mmol^{-1}$ was from Amersham, France. Liquid scintillation fluid (Insta-Gel) was from Packard. Isopentyl acetate and copper (II) sulphate were from PROLABO (Paris, France). All other chemicals used were of analytical grade.

Enzyme Assays

Microsomal protein concentrations were determined according to the method of Lowry *et al*[16], using bovine albumin as a standard.
GSH-T activity was assayed according to the spectrophotometric method of Habig *et al*[17] using 1-chloro-2,4-dinitrobenzene.
UDPG-T activity was measured following the radiometric method of Young & Lietman[18] using ^{14}C-CAP.
All assays were performed in triplicate.

Statistical Analysis

Experimental groups were compared to the control diet using the test of Dunnett[19]. Significativity was accepted when $P < 0.05$. Data are expressed as mean ± SEM.

3 RESULTS (Table 2)

Small Intestine

GSH-T specific activity, in the control group, is: 12.10 ± 0.52 nmol/min/mg proteins. It is not modified when either carrot or cocoa fibers are added to the diet. On the contrary, a significant induction of the enzyme specific activity ($P < 0.01$) is observed with wheat bran, oat fiber and inulin (respectively + 41%, + 40%, + 36%).
The mean control value of UDPG-T specific activity is 71.17 ± 7.57 pmol/min/mg proteins. Values obtained with carrot fiber and inulin are increased, although there are no significant differences whatever the diet.

Colon

GSH-T specific activity for the control group is: 7.06 ± 0.54 nmol/min/mg proteins. It is significantly enhanced ($P < 0.05$) when rats are fed the oat fiber diet (+ 40%).

Table 2 GSH-T and UDPG-T specific activity (mean (SEM)), expressed as % of the control values.
(* when $p < 0.05$; ** when $p < 0.01$)

	Small intestine		Colon
	GSH-T	UDPG-T	GSH-T
Control	100.0 (4.3)	100.0 (10.6)	100.0 (7.7)
Wheat bran	141.2 (9.9)**	111.4 (16.1)	66.6 (4.0)
Oat fiber	139.9 (13.2)**	105.0 (20.4)	139.5 (9.4)*
Inulin	135.6 (6.0)**	135.6 (19.2)	88.0 (7.2)
Carrot fiber	117.6 (7.7)	150.0 (17.4)	115.3 (16.4)
Cocoa fiber	108.4 (6.9)	100.8 (10.3)	121.4 (11.9)

Wheat bran has a non-significant depressing effect on the enzyme specific activity (- 33%). The addition of carrot or cocoa fiber or inulin has no influence on colonic GSH-T specific activity.
UDPG-T specific activity was not detectable whatever the diet.

4 DISCUSSION

This work indicates that the addition of realistic amounts of dietary fibers in the diet may alter major intestinal transferases specific activities. This effect depends on the nature of the dietary fiber and the intestinal segment. Alterations of GSH-T are more obvious than those of UDPG-T. In that case, the widely spread values obtained seem to be responsible for the lack of significance.
Among the different fibers that were added to the diet, cocoa fiber has no influence on the enzymes. It seems that only wheat bran and oat fiber are responsible for colonic alterations of GSH-T specific activity (although the decrease observed with wheat bran is not significant with our statistical test). These two fibers are poorly fermentescible and it may be expected that part of them reaches the colonic compartment after going through caecal fermentation. On the contrary, inulin and carrot fiber, very fermentescible, have no effect on the colonic compartment. It is known that they seldom escape metabolism by caecal microflora. Therefore, the next step of that work should be an estimation of caecal XME alterations following an identical experimental design. Another point requires further development: even between the two poorly fermentescible fibers, effects on the GSH-T vary greatly depending on the intestinal localisation: both fibers are responsible for an induction in the small intestine but, if oat fiber still enhances the enzyme specific activity in the colon, wheat bran seems to be responsible for its decrease. All the other alterations observed are increased specific activities.
The alterations observed in the small intestine may surprise since this segment harbours relatively few

bacteria and that fermentation occurs mainly in the large intestine.
Two other hypotheses could explain the "protective" side-effect: a direct effect of fibers on the intestinal wall during their transit or a non-direct effect by metabolites released through fibers fermentation and recycled via the enterohepatic cycle.
To discriminate between these two hypotheses a similar experiment is actually realised on germ-free rats.

REFERENCES

1. D.P. Burkitt, Cancer, 1971, 28, 3.
2. B.S. Reddy, A.R. Hedges, K. Laakso, E.L. Wynder, Cancer, 1978, 42, 2832.
3. J.L. Freudenheim, S. Graham, J.R. Marshall, B.P. Haughey, Am. J. Epidemiol., 1990, 131, 612.
4. B.S. Reddy, H. Mori, M. Nicolais, J. Natl. Cancer Inst., 1981, 66, 553.
5. L.R. Jacobs and J.R. Lupton, Cancer Res., 1986, 46, 1727.
6. J. Roberts-Andersen, T. Mehta, R.B. Wilson, Nutr. Cancer, 1987, 10, 129.
7. R.M. Kay, Am. J. Clin. Nutr., 1978, 31, 562.
8. D.P. Burkitt, J.Natl. Cancer Inst., 1975, 54, 3.
9. P.A. Smith-Barbaro, D. Hanson, B.S. Reddy, J. Nutr., 1981, 111, 789.
10. P. Lindeskog, E. Övervik, T. Hansson, J.A. Gustafsson, Scand. J. Gastroenterol. Suppl., 1987, 129, 258.
11. P. Lindeskog, E. Övervik, L. Nilsson, C.E. Nord, J.A. Gustafsson, Mutat. Res., 1988, 204, 553.
12. C. Dufour-Lescoat, Y. Le Coz, O. Szylit, Sci. Aliments, 1991, 11, 397.
13. C. Andrieux, S. Lory, C. Dufour-Lescoat, R. de Baynast, O. Szylit, Food hydrocoll., 1991, 5, 49.
14. A. Aranki, S.A. Syed, E.B. Kenney, R. Freter, Appl. Microbiol., 1969, 17, 568.
15. H.W. Strobel, W.F. Fang, R.J. Oshinsky, Cancer (suppl.), 1980, 45, 1060.
16. O.H. Lowry, N.J. Rosebrough, A.L. Farr, R.J. Randall, J. Biol. Chem., 1951, 193, 265.
17. W.H. Habig, M.J. Pabst, W.B. Jakoby, J. Biol. Chem., 1974, 249, 7130.
18. W.S. Young and P.S. Lietman, J. Pharmacol. Exp. Ther., 1978, 204, 203.
19. C.W. Dunnett, Biom., 1964, 20, 482.

ACKNOLEDGMENTS

Part of this work was supported by grants from the French Ministry of Agriculture and the Scientific Direction of BSN-France (we wish to thank Dr C. Mercier and Dr J.M. Antoine for their advice).

NITRITE-BINDING PROPERTIES OF DIETARY FIBRES

F. Shahidi and C. Hong

Department of Biochemistry
Memorial University of Newfoundland
St. John's, Newfoundland Canada
A1B 3X9

1 INTRODUCTION

Dietary fibres are defined as plant materials resistant to hydrolysis by the enzymes of the mammalian digestive tract. The most abundant compounds identified as fibre are in plant cell walls. These include structural polysaccharides, structural nonpolysaccharides predominantly lignins, and nonstructural polysaccharides including gums and mucilage. Just as their functions within the plant vary, their effect in foods also depends on their structural identity.[1] It is now widely believed that a diet high in fibre would offer protection against development of colon cancer.[2] However, the mode of action by which dietary fibres may exert their effects is not fully understood.

Plant materials are generally used in emulsified meat products as protein extenders. Preparation of low-fat products may also necessitate the use of plant-based components for appropriate textural status of the final product. These materials and/or their component may also offer additional benefits to processed products, as it might be the case for fibre.

Nitrite is a major ingredient used for preparation of cured meat products. It is responsible for the development of the specific cured flavour and colour of processed meats. By virtue of its strong antioxidant properties in meats, nitrite prevents the formation of warmed-over flavour in cured products. More importantly, nitrite acts as an antimicrobial agent and thus retards the toxin formation by Clostridium botulinum.[3]

Despite all of its desired properties, residual nitrite may undergo reaction with amines and amino acids in meats, or in the stomach, to produce carcinogenic N-nitrosamines.[4,5] To alleviate this potentially serious problem, several approaches have been considered by researchers. Addition of reduced levels of nitrite to meat, use of nitrosamine-blocking agents as well as developing of alternative meat curing systems have been considered.[3] In addition, interaction of nitrite with food components may also affect possible nitrosation of amines and amino acids by residual nitrite.

The objectives of this study were to examine the effects of dietary fibres on the content of analyzable nitrite in aqueous model systems resembling conditions encountered in the stomach and otherwise.

2 MATERIALS AND METHODS

All chemicals used in this study were food- or reagent-grade and were used without any further purification. N-(1-naphthyl)-ethylenediamine dihydrochloride (NED) was purchased from Aldrich Chemical Company (Milwaukee, Wisconsin) and sulphanilamide (SA) was acquired from Fisher Scientific Company (Fair Lawn, New Jersey). Sodium nitrite was obtained from J.T. Baker Chemical Company (Phillipsburg, New Jersey).

Three types of fibre were used in this study. Pea fibre (Centu-Tab) was obtained from Woodstone Foods Ltd. (Portage La Prairie, Manitoba), oat fibre (Better Basics 780 - Advanced white oat fibre) was a product of Williamson Fiber Products, Inc. (Louisville, Kentucky) and flax mucilage was provided by Dr. Stephen Cunnane (Department of Nutritional Studies, University of Toronto, Toronto, Ontario).

Reagents were prepared freshly, each day, according to AOAC procedures with minor modifications.[6] NED (0.2 g) and SA (0.5 g) were dissolved in separate containers in 150 mL of a 15% (v/v) acetic acid solution and were stored in brown glass bottles. A stock solution of sodium nitrite, 1.000 g in a 1 L volumetric flask, was prepared using HPLC-grade water. Serial dilutions were made to obtain test samples.

Fibres were added to model systems at levels 10-100 times the content of nitrite in test solutions. The fibre-nitrite solutions were allowed to stand overnight in 500 mL Erlenmeyer flasks under specified conditions. Free nitrite in the supernatant from each solution was determined, after centrifugation, from absorbance readings of their diazo complex produced between nitrite, NED and SA at 538 nm using a standard calibration curve as reference.[6]

3 RESULTS AND DISCUSSION

The fibres from pea, oat and mucilage from flax reacted with nitrite to varying degrees depending on the pH, the amount of nitrite present as well as the ratio of fibre to nitrite concentration. At room temperature, however, only flax mucilage exerted a significant effect as the concentration of analyzable nitrite in samples was reduced by up to 13.8% (Figure 1).

As the temperature of the solution was increased, the extent of interaction between dietary fibres and nitrite increased. Figure 2 illustrates the enhanced interaction of pea fibre with nitrite at temperatures ranging between 20 and

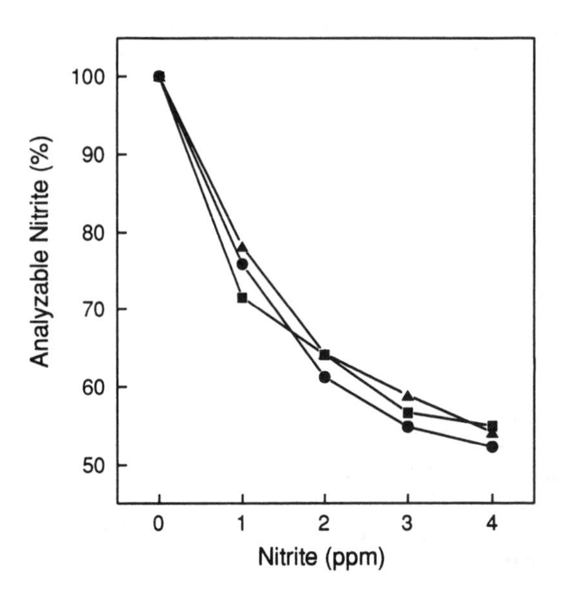

Figure 1 Percentage of analyzable nitrite in aqueous media at 20°C and as affected by pea fibre, ■; oat fibre, ▲ and flax mucilage, ● at a fibre to nitrite ratio (w/w) (R) of 50. Open symbol corresponds to R = 100.

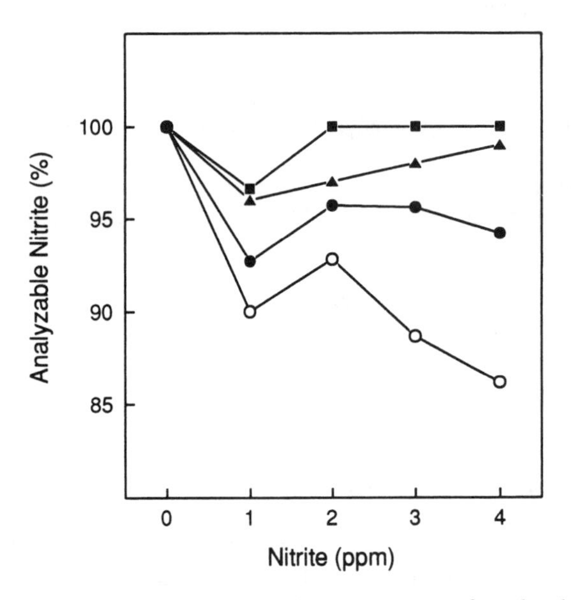

Figure 2 Effect of temperature on the percentage of analyzable nitrite as affected by pea fibre at a fibre to nitrite ratio (w/w) of 50.

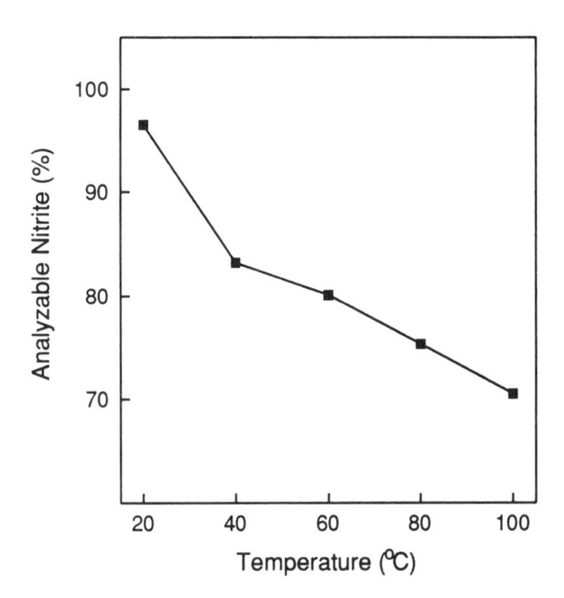

Figure 3 Percentage of analyzable nitrite as affected by pea fibre at a fibre to nitrite ratio (w/w) of 40, ▲; 50, ■; and 100, ●.

100°C. Variation of the interaction of pea fibres with different concentrations of nitrite at 100°C is provided in Figure 3.

The capacity of dietary fibres to react with nitrite is attributable to both the soluble fibres such as those in flax mucilage and to insoluble polymeric materials such as those present in pea and oat fibres. It is known that lignin in fibres can react with nitrite under different conditions.[7,8] The results of this preliminary study have clearly demonstrated the potential of dietary fibres as nitrite scavengers under different conditions. Dietary fibre intake has been associated with protection against colon cancer . A possible reason for such effects may be attributable to the role of dietary fibres in scavenging of nitrite, thus preventing the formation of N-nitrosamines in the gastrointestinal tract.

ACKNOWLEDGEMENTS

This work was supported by the Natural Sciences and Engineering Research Council (NSERC) of Canada.

REFERENCES

1. B.O. Schneeman, Food Technol., 1986, 40(2), 104.
2. H.A. Risch, M. Jain, N.W. Choi, J.G. Fodor, C.J. Pfieffer, G.R., Howe, L.W. Harrison, K.J.P. Craib, and A.B. Miller, Am. J. Epidem., 1985, 122, 947.
3. F. Shahidi and R.B. Pegg, J. Food Chem., 1992, 43, 185.
4. J.I. Gray, J. Milk Food Technol., 1976, 39, 686.
5. N.P. Sen, B. Donaldson, S. Seaman, B. Collins and J.R. Iyenger, Can. Inst. Food Sci. Technol., 1977, 10, A13.
6. AOAC, 15th edition, Association of Official Analytical Chemists, Washington, DC, 1990.
7. C.W. Dence, 'Lignins: Occurrence, Formation, Structure and Reactions', edited by K.V. Sarkanen and C.H. Ludwig, Wiley Interscience, New York, 1971, p. 373.
8. M.A. Rubio, B.A. Pethica, P. Zumun and S.J. Falkehag, 'Dietary Fibres: Chemistry and Nutrition', edited by G.E. Inglett and S.I. Falkehag, Academic Press, London, 1979, p. 251.

WORKSHOP REPORT: NON-STARCH POLYSACCHARIDES (NSP) AND COLORECTAL CANCER: THE CURRENT POSITION

S. Bingham

Dunn Clinical Research Centre
Tennis Court Road
Cambridge
UK

The Workshop was asked to consider first if there is now sufficient evidence to discount a role for NSP in colorectal cancer protection. However, it was felt that NSP probably are important, although one prospective dietary study had not confirmed a reduction in risk in individuals consuming high levels of NSP, and there is a lack of a conclusive mechanism whereby NSP could be protective. Any effect was not due to inert bulking. Possible mechanisms included the effect of the short-chain fatty acid butyrate, produced during fermentation, on cell turnover, but no clear consensus on the role of butyrate has yet emerged. A priority area of research is the study of butyrate and proliferation in humans, but the establishment of 'normal' rates in healthy volunteers and of butyrate production rates *in vivo*, are major problems. Proliferation was to be discussed in more detail in another Workshop.

NSP and other cell wall material also bind putative carcinogens, although little is known of the effect of NSP on their metabolism. The effect of NSP on the immunology of the colon has received little attention, as have its effects on systemic factors such as sex hormone levels which may be important in influencing site-specific sex differences in the colon and rectum, in addition to cancer at other sites. The interaction between NSP and other dietary factors, notably meat and the different classes of fatty acids, also needed further study.

The workshop was in agreement that colorectal cancer risk is inversely related to stool weight though a causal relationship is less certain. Prospective and intervention studies are needed to confirm this on an individual basis, but are unlikely to be conducted in the absence of easily measured biomarkers. NSP has well-documented effects on stool weight, but any food that contains fermentable carbohydrate not digested in the small intestine, such as starch and oligosaccharides, and lactase in lactase-deficient individuals, has an effect on bacterial cell mass and usually therefore stool weight. Starch is relatively abundant in human diets and probably enhances butyrate production *in vivo* and *in vitro*. The hypothesis that starch in its different forms is important in colorectal cancer protection needs to be actively tested in both epidemiological and experimental studies.

PART 8 RESEARCH TECHNIQUE: NEW APPROACHES

TOXICOLOGICAL METHODS TO STUDY MECHANISMS OF NATURALLY OCCURRING ANTICARCINOGENS

Wim.M.F. Jongen, Agrotechnological Research Institute
P.O. Box 17, 6700 AA Wageningen,
The Netherlands

I INTRODUCTION

In the course of this century the role of cancer as a cause of death has become increasingly important. This is not due to an increase in the incidence of specific types of cancer but relates to a reduction in the incidence of other types of diseases. In western societies 1 out of 3 persons gets cancer and 1 out of 4 persons dies of cancer. Epidemiological data show that food plays a major role in the induction of cancer in humans and contributes for ca. 35% in the total incidence with a probability range of 10-70% (1). This range indicates a large uncertainty about the role of specific dietary factors and has resulted in intensive research towards the identification of contributing factors. Since then it has become clear that not only carcinogenic factors are present but that also modulating factors play an important role. Epidemiological data showed that especially the consumption of fruit and vegetables has protective effects against the occurrence of specific types of cancer such as colon cancer. For example, epidemiological data showed that the consumption of cruciferous vegetables is associated with a decrease in the incidence of tumour formation in the gastro-intestinal tract (2). From these vegetables several compounds have been isolated and identified e.g.various breakdown products of glucosinolates which exhibit anticarcinogenic properties in animal experiments (3). To date a large number of naturally occurring compounds are identified which have been shown to possess protective capacity against the induction of cancer in experimental animals following exposure to specific carcinogens.

II THE PROCESS OF CARCINOGENESIS

There is abundant epidemiological and experimental evidence that the process of carcinogenesis is a multistage process in which at least two distinct phases can be recognized; the initiation phase and the promotion phase. Initiation is the genetic event which is considered to be the first step in the onset of carcinogenesis. Although a chemical that can bind covalently with DNA will do so largely at random, only specific lesions will result in genetic alterations that are relevant for the cancer process such as activation of oncogenes (4). The initiation phase comprises two distinct steps, the induction of the molecular lesions and the fixation of these lesions by DNA replication. Promotion is the process whereby an initiated tissue or organ develops focal proliferations of phenotypically altered cells. In its first phase promotion is reversible and promoters appear to act only above a certain threshold level. Promotion can be brought about by aspecific stimuli such as wounding, bacterial infection, cell killing, partial hepatectomy etc. (5). In addition to this aspecific type of effect promotion can be brought about by specific mitogenic stimuli. For example growth factors and hormones can act as promoters and other types of promoters can interfere with growth factor pathways e. g. by influencing receptor affinity and binding sites. In vitro studies have shown that many of these proliferative stimuli are triggered by promoter-membrane interactions. Structural and functional changes in cellular membranes have been reported, activation or inhibition of plasma membrane bound enzymes, modulation of ion transport and transport of small molecules through plasma membranes (6,7,8). One major aim of studies on tumor promotion is to determine what components of a cell society are responsible for maintaining dormancy of initiated cells and as a corollary how tumor promoters interfere with such societal influence to permit clonal expansion. That initiated cells in vivo can remain dormant for extended periods of time is now well established and, some thirteen years ago, it was proposed by Murray and Fitzgerald (9) that these cells may be prevented from clonal expansion by gap junctional intercellular communication (GJIC) with surrounding normal cells and that GJIC may be disturbed by tumor promoters. Among various forms of intercellular communication GJIC is the only form involving direct exchange of ions and low molecular weight molecules(< 1000 daltons) from one cell interior to another. This bi-directional flow occurs through protein channels termed connexons. These connexons constitute a family of proteins and connexon ensembles termed gap junctions are found in most tissues. There is now good evidence that GJIC plays a major role in maintaining tissue homeostasis and cooperativity and important second messenger molecules such as cyclic AMP, Ca^{++} and inositol triphosphate are known to pass through gap junctions. However it is still unknown what is the nature of gap junction permeable suppressive factors that are deemed to exert such suppression.

III TOXICOLOGICAL METHODS TO STUDY MECHANISMS OF MODULATING FACTORS

The concept of a two-stage initiation-promotion carcinogenesis process has been derived originally from experiments on the mouse skin (10). This approach has several unique features. Neither the application of a small dose of an initiating agent to the mouse skin nor the multiple applications of a tumor promoter alone causes tumors. However, many tumors will develop if the tumor promoter is applied after initiation of the skin. Reversing the order of treatment will not result in the appearance of tumors. There is now a large body of data that demonstrates that the two-stage model of initiation and promotion can be extended to other organs as well. Examples are the liver, the colon, the bladder, the lung, the kidney, the pancreas and the thyroid gland (11-14).

In the study of mechanisms of cancer modulating compounds the use of two-stage animal models can provide valuable information with regard to the stage where modulation occurs and whether application of the modulating factor at specific time points in tumor development may lead to different effects as was observed for indole-3-carbinol. When applied in the initiation phase or throughout the experiment, as was done in several studies with rats, it reduced the incidence of tumors (15) but when administered during the promotion phase it acted as a promoter of tumor induction in trout (16).

Parallel to these _in vivo_ developments, a large number of _in vitro_ systems have been developed which are extensively used to study defined endpoints which are relevant for the process of carcinogenesis.

Mutagenicity testing

In the last decades a large number of test systems have been developed and validated for their use in screening for the presence of potential mutagenic compounds in our environment and to examine the type of DNA damage caused by these agents. These assay systems comprise both _in vitro_ systems as well as a number of _in vivo_ systems. The _in vitro_ assays can be divided into two main categories: systems using prokaryotic cells (bacteria) which are able to detect point mutations and small deletions and systems with eukaryotic cells (fungi, yeast, mammalian cells) which are able to detect both point mutations, small deletions and chromosomal aberrations (17).

These _in vitro_ systems can be further subdivided into three main classes, namely those that detect backward mutations, those that detect forward mutations and those that rely on a DNA repair deficiency. Furthermore, test systems using mammalian cells can be divided according to the type of cell culture which is applied namely cultures of primary or mortal cells or cultures of established or immortal cell lines. Primary cells still possess the properties of the same cells in the organism but often require more complex culture conditions. These cells are more suitable for experiments in which the cells are required to have a stable phenotype and genotype similar to that of the in situ cells of origin such as is the case in transformation studies. Established cell lines have already been immortalized and thus differ in several aspects of the cells in the organism. These cells are more convenient to study cell genetics

In considering in vivo systems to study mutagenic potential of chemicals several systems have been developed using various endpoints such as DNA adduct formation, forward mutation and chromosome aberration in somatic and germ cells of insects, fish and various types of rodents such as rat, mouse and hamster.

Test systems for tumor promoters

So far two groups of test systems have been used primarily for in vitro testing of tumor promoters. One group of test models uses irreversible functional and morphological changes (cell transformation) as endpoint whereas the other group uses inhibition of gap junctional intercellular communication as an endpoint.

The use of these assay systems is based on possible theoretical mechanisms of tumor promotion including enhancement of cell transformation, modulation of the neoplastic phenotypes, inhibition of cell differentiation, stimulation of cell proliferation, effects on cellular membranes, modulation of immune response and induction of genetic effects.

Enhancement of cell transformation by tumor promoters forms the basis for several assays using the two-stage protocol. Cells are exposed first to an initiator and then at various time points after exposure to a tumor promoting agent. Endpoints used in these assay systems is morphological transformation defined as altered colony morphology including criss-crossing and piling up of cells.

Other systems such as the mouse epidermal cell line JB6 use growth in soft agar as endpoint. A special feature of this system is that it does not use a two-stage protocol. Exposure to the promoter alone is sufficient for irreversible growth in soft agar. In table 1 an overview is given of the systems that are currently in use.

Table 1 Test systems using cell transformation as end-point

Cell System	Protocol	Assay basis	Reference
BALB/c 3T3 fibroblasts (adult mouse)	two-stage	Focus formation on cell monolayer	Kakunaga (1973)
C3H10T1/2 fibroblasts (mouse embryo)	two-stage	Focus formation on cell monolayer	Mondal et al.(1976)
SHE fibroblasts (Syrian hamster embryo)	two-stage	Focus formation at clonal density	Poiley et al.(1979)
Co-cultures of normal and virally/chemcically transformed 3T3 cells	promoter	Focus formation	Sivak and van Duuren (1970)
JB-6 keratinocytes (newborn mouse skin)	promoter	Anchorage independent growth induction	Colburn (1979)
Adenovirus transformed rat embryo cells	promoter	Anchorage independent growth induction	Fisher et al.(1979)

In the last decade a number of different assay systems have been developed to determine the effects of compounds on gap junctional intercellular communication and to correlate these effects with promoting activity of the compounds. In table 2 an overview is given of the various methodologies applied. For the routine testing of compounds only a limited number of assays has been used such as metabolic cooperation and dye transfer. Assays using metabolic cooperation are based on the transfer of various cellular metabolites which result either in rescue or killing of metabolically deficient cells. Of these the most widely used is based on the enhanced recovery of hypoxanthine-guanine phosphoribosyl transferase (HGPRT) deficient cell mutants from high density cultures of the wild type cells (HGPRT-proficient) in a medium containing a purine analogue as a selective agent. The system uses variants of V79 Chinese hamster cells. However since many tumor promoters display organ specificity, it is difficult to consider the use of fibroblasts representative for all cell types and the possibility of false negatives is one limitation of the assay. Also the lack of adequate biotransformation capability is another limitation (see next section). Some of these limitations may be overcome by the use of dye transfer techniques. The most widely used of these techniques is microinjection of gap junction permeable, membrane impermeable, tracer molecules into single cells followed by monitoring of dye spread to neighbouring cells. One major advantage of the use of micro-injection is that introduction of the dye into cells can be done on any cell type in culture making it possible to study organ specificity of tumor promoters. Additionally, recent developments make it possible to study the effects of compounds on gap junctional intercellular communication at the molecular level and techniques have been developed enabling *in vivo* studies.

Table 2 Methodologies used to study inhibition of gap junctional intercellular communication

Assay method	Cell types	Reference
Metabolic cooperation		
Transfer of 3H labeled nucleotides	Mouse epidermal cells/ Swiss 3T3 cells	Murray and Fitzgerald (1979) (9)
	Chick embryo hepatocytes/ Chinese hamster V79 cells	Jongen et al., (1987) (26)
HGPRT+/HGPRT-	Chinese hamster V79 cells	Yotti et al., (1979)
	Human fibroblasts	Mosser and - Bols, (1982)
	Rat hepatocytes/rat liver epithelial cells	Williams et al.,(1987)
ASS^-/ASL^-	Human fibroblasts/V79 cells	Davidson et al., (1985)
AK^+/AK^-	Chinese hamster V79 cells	Gupta et al., (1985)
Electrical coupling		
	Human amniotic membrane epithelial cells	Enomoto et al.,(1981)
	BALB/c 3T3 cells	Yamasaki et al., (1985)

Table 2, continued

	Skin wounding	Loewenstein and Penn, (1967)
Dye transfer		
Microinjection	Human colon epithelial cell line	Friedman & Steinberg, (1982)
	Mouse epidermal cell line	Fitzgerald et al., (1983)
	Rat myoblasts	Enomoto et al., (1984)
	Chinese hamster V79 cells	Zeilmaker & Yamasaki (1986)
	Hamster tracheal epithelial cells	Rutten et al., (1988)
Photo bleaching		
	Human teratocarcinoma cells	Wade et al., (1986)
Scrape loading	Chinese hamster V79 cells rat glial and glioma cells, rat liver cells, human teratocarcinoma cells, human fibroblasts	El-Fouly et al., (1987)
Gap Junction structure analysis		
Electron-microscope	Chinese hamster V79 cells	Yancey et al., (1982)
	Chick embryo hepatocytes	van der Zandt et al., 1989
	Rat lingual epithelial cells	Tachikawa et al., 1987
	Mouse skin <u>in vivo</u>	Kalimi and - Sirsat, 1984
	Rat liver <u>in vivo</u>	Sugie et al., (1987)
Gap junction molecular analysis		
Gel electrophoresis	Chinese hamster V79 cells	Finbow et al., (1983)
Gap junction antibody	Rat liver <u>in vivo</u>	Traub et al., (1983)
Gap junction gene expression	Rat liver <u>in vivo</u>	Beer et al., (1988) Mesnil et al., (1988)

Abbreviations used: HGPRT, hypoxanthine guanine phosphoribosyl transferase; ASS, argininosuccinate synthetase; ASL, argininosuccinate lyase; AK, adenosine kinase; TPA, 12-O-tetradecanoylphorbol-13-acetate

Many of the in vitro systems for mutagenicity testing have been used extensively in the study of modulating effects of compounds naturally occurring in food plants such as glucosinolates, flavonols, unsaturated fatty acids etc. Modulation of tumor promotion has been studied less extensively. Retinoic acid and quercetin are two examples of compounds which appear to modulate inhibition of intercellular communication by tumor promoters (18,19).

IV ROLE OF BIOTRANSFORMATION

Living organisms are continually exposed to a variety of naturally occurring chemicals. If these compounds are lipophilic they are generally made more hydrophilic by metabolic transformations, mainly oxydations or hydroxylations, and subsequent conjugations to facilitate excretion. This process of metabolic transformation can be divided in two phases. Phase 1 reactions introduce new functional groups into the lipophilic compounds converting them into highly reactive products which can bind covalently to nucleophilic molecules. Phase 2 metabolism comprises synthetic reactions with small endogenous molecules that are coupled to functional groups originally present or introduced by phase 1 metabolism.

The ability of carcinogens to exert their effects depends largely upon the balance between activating and deactivating enzymes. Any change in this balance will result in a change in the biological effect. Many compounds, naturally occurring in the human diet modulate the biotransformation of several carcinogens, resulting in reduced tumor incidence (20). This implies compounds which inhibit the formation of electrophilic intermediates by acting as inducers of alternative pathways as well as compounds which change the balance between activating and deactivating enzyme systems.

The liver is the organ predominantly involved in the biotransformation of many xenobiotics. For practical purposes, in the majority of in vitro studies liver homogenates or subcellular fractions have been used to mimic in vivo metabolism. The use of this kind of preparations has several disadvantages. Due to homogenization and fractionation of cells the balance between activating and deactivating enzyme systems is disturbed. Especially conjugation reactions, which are located in different cellular compartments are much less operative (21). This kind of disadvantage may be overcome by the use of intact cells as metabolizing system. Isolated hepatocytes resemble in their structural and biochemical properties the in vivo situation much more closely than subcellular fractions (22). When freshly isolated hepatocytes are cultured they show a rapid decline in their capacity for biotransformation. Especially the various isozymes of the cytochrome P450 family show a rapid loss of activity. To overcome this problem several methods have been applied like addition of hormones, addition of enzyme inducers and co-culture with epithelial cells or on extracellular membranes. Although some of these methods were partially successful in retaining the total cytochrome P450 activity, selective changes were observed in the pattern of different cytochrome P450 isozymes (23). In contrast to parenchymal cells isolated from mammalian liver, chick-embryo hepatocytes maintain their initial levels of cytochrome P450 enzyme activities in vitro for at least 3 days (24). Moreover, induction with known enzyme inducers such as phenobarbital, 3-methylcholanthrene or Aroclor 1254 resulted in more than two-fold increase in cytochrome P450 content (25). Also when this system was used to study modulating effects of dietary components such as several indole compounds and the synthetic flavonol ß-naphthoflavone treatment of cultured chick-embryo hepatocytes with these compounds, resulted in increases in activities of both phase 1 and phase 2 enzyme systems. In the next section examples will be given of studies on the mechanisms of modulation of benzo(a)pyrene (B(a)P) mediated mutagenicity by some of these compounds.

V A CO-CULTURE SYSTEM TO STUDY MECHANISMS OF MODULATING COMPOUNDS

The system consists of two cell types, primary chick-embryo hepatocytes and V79 Chinese hamster cells. Primary chick-embryo hepatocytes are isolated from 15-day old chick embryos and cultured for 24h. After treatment for a specific time with the modulating compound, the compound is removed and V79 cells are added. 2 h later the mutagen is added and the cells are exposed. In case that simultaneous treatment is wanted the modulating compound is added together with the mutagen. After exposure the cells are dissociated and the V79 cells are used for determination of changes in the genetic endpoints such as plating on microscopic slides for SCE determination or in Petri dishes for measurement of HGPRT- mutants (26).

Following this type of approach detailed studies were carried out to investigate the mechanisms underlying observed protective effects of various modulating compounds on B(a)P mediated mutagenicity (27,28). Treatment with indole-3-carbinol and ß-naphthoflavone resulted in increases in cytochrome P450 associated enzyme activities. When metabolite formation of B(a)P was studied, large increases were observed in the amounts of specific metabolites. However no shift was found in the ratios between the various metabolites when compared with metabolite formation following treatment with the carcinogen 3-methylcholanthrene. Especially formation of the proximate mutagenic and carcinogenic metabolite B(a)P-7,8-dihydrodiol did not differ between the three compounds. This indicates that induction of cytochrome P450 associated enzyme activity as such is not an indicator for modulating capacity. However pretreatment with I3C and ß-naphthoflavone followed by exposure to B(a)P resulted in decreased mutagenic effects.

Experiments with subcellular fractions showed that the mechanisms underlying these protective effects were different for the respective compounds. In the case of I3C the protective effects results from a changed balance of the enzyme systems involved in the I3C biotransformation process. There is an overall increase in the rate of metabolism but the increases in conjugating enzyme activity compensate for the increases in cytochrome P450 associated enzyme activities. In the case of ß-naphthoflavone the available data strongly suggest that the inhibitory effects cannot be ascribed to the inducing capabilities of the compound but instead seem to be due to the formation of an intracellular pool of ß-naphthoflavone which acts as a competitive inhibitor for B(a)P metabolism.

VI PROBLEMS ASSOCIATED WITH THE STUDY OF CANCER MODULATING COMPOUNDS

Selection of mutagen/carcinogen

In an effort to fight cancer in humans, already in 1982 the National Research Council in the USA recommended increased consumption of cruciferous vegetables (29). At that stage the exact mechanism of the protective effect was not known. Later on the identity of several active principles were identified as breakdown products of glucosinolates and it was shown that the probable explanation for the observed protective effects is the induction of enzymes of the biotransformation system. Treatment with the isolated compounds or the vegetables followed by exposure to known carcinogens caused a shift in the balance between activating and conjugating enzyme systems favouring conjugation and resulting in a decrease of the biological activity of the carcinogen. This is an important observation since the majority of known carcinogens are not carcinogenic per se but have to be activated by enzymes of the biotransformation system to become biologically active. This has also important consequences for the conclusions which can be drawn from this type of experiment. Bioactivation of carcinogens from different chemical classes occur through different biochemical pathways and in the case of halogenated compounds can be brought about also by conjugating enzymes (30). In the case of the brassica compounds exposure to carcinogens, which are activated by conjugating systems, will lead to increased effects instead of reduced effects. Apparently the outcome of this type of study depends largely on the choice of the carcinogen to which the animals are exposed. In table 3 an example is given of the effects of pretreatment with indole-3-carbinol, one of the breakdown products of glucobrassicin on the mutagenic effects of compounds from different chemical classes. Mutagenicity was determined by measurement of the number of sister chromatid exchanges. Using a co-culture system consisting of primary chick-embryo hepatocytes and V79 Chinese hamster cells it was shown that in the case of benzo(a) pyrene and dimethylnitrosamine pretreatment with indole-3-carbinol resulted in decreased biological activity whereas in the case of dibromoethane pretreatment resulted in enhanced mutagenic effects.

Table 3 Modulating effects of indole-3-carbinol pretreatment on SCE induction by mutagens from different chemical classes

Exposure			SCEs/chromosome		
Compound (%)	Time (h.)	Dose (μg/ml)	Without	With	Change
B(a)P	24	7.5	1.46±0.08	1.07±0.06	-33%
DMNA	4	1500	0.91±0.04	0.48±0.07	-46%
2-AA	4	25.0	0.81±0.10	0.87±0.02	__
DBE	4	5.3	1.11±0.05	1.45±0.06	+40%
EMS	24	100	1.04±0.04	1.02±0.03	__
Control	24	0	0.27±0.02	0.28±0.03	__

B(a)P= benzo(a)pyrene; DMNA= dimethylnitrosamine; 2-AA= 2-aminoanthracene; DBE= dibromoethane; EMS=ethylmethanesulfonate. Experiments were performed using a co-culture system of primary chick-embryo hepatocytes and V79 Chinese hamster cells (Data taken from Jongen et al., 1989).

Quantification of modulating effects

When the effects of modulating factors on the biological activity of mutagens and carcinogens are studied, quantification of mutagenicity is an important aspect in the interpretation of the results. In a previous section of this paper the use of intact cells as a more representative metabolizing system for testing has been advocated. When co-culture systems are used transport of reactive intermediates from the metabolizing cells into the recipient cells can take place via two routes namely via the culture medium and via cell-to-cell contact where gap junctions act as gates.
This phenomenon is known as metabolic cooperation. The existence of functional gap junctions between homologous and heterologous cells has been shown to occur. The existence of metabolic cooperation between metabolizing cell and recipient cell allows the transport of reactive intermediates through gap junctions. If a compound or its metabolites inhibits metabolic cooperation this will result in reduced mutagenic effects in the recipient cells. Especially if modulating factors are examined for their potential to modulate biotransformation of model compounds and at the same time these factors inhibit metabolic cooperation this may lead

to wrong conclusions. Inhibition of metabolic cooperation is considered to be a tumor promoting factor whereas in this type of study this property will result in reduced mutagenic effects in the recipient cells. For example if the well known tumor promoter TPA is added to a co-culture system consisting of primary chick-embryo hepatocytes and V79 Chinese hamster cells benzo(a)pyrene mediated mutagenicity is reduced with at least 50% (31).

Interaction with other dietary components

Another problem especially associated with in vitro testing of anticarcinogenic compounds is that in most studies only single pure compounds are tested whereas when human consumption occurs the presence of the food matrix usually will influence the capacity of compounds to act as inducers of cancer or as cancer preventive agents.
Several studies have shown that indole compounds can be chemically nitrosated resulting in direct acting mutagenic N-nitroso compounds and that when these N-nitroso compounds were administered to the forestomach of rats in vivo they induced preneoplastic lesions in this organ(32). Since these compounds occur in the human diet at significant concentrations, these findings suggested the discovery of a potential human risk associated with the consumption of vegetables containing these compounds. However studies towards the chemical stability of the nitrosated indole compounds showed that an equilibrium exists between the nitrosated indole compound and the presence of free nitrite. Mutagenic activity could only be observed if considerable amounts of free nitrite were present (33). This raised questions about the relevance of these findings. Tiedink et al.,(34) showed that mutagenic activity could be observed when vegetable extracts were treated with nitrite. However, involvement of indole compounds in this activity could be excluded.

VII CONCLUSIONS

A major aim of research towards identification of protective factors in the diet is: (1) to come to dietary advice with regard to human consumption based on detailed knowledge of the mechanims and (2) to provide plant breeders and growers with relevant information on how to improve the quality of existing crops and set priorities in the development of new crops with respect to the presence of these factors.

Generally , it should be emphasized that the knowledge, at present available, on potential protective capacity of dietary components is in many instances still fragmentary and far from sufficient to result in dietary advices.

VIII REFERENCE

1. Doll, R and Peto, R., (1981); JNCI, 66, 1192.
2. Graham, S, (1983), Cancer Res., 43, 24095
3. Wattenberg, L.W. and Loub, W.D., (1978) Cancer Res., 38, 14105
4. Yarden, Y., et al., (1986), Nature, 323, 226
5. Slaga, T., (1984) Acta Pharmacol. Toxicol., 55,

(suppl.) 107
6. Yamasaki, H., (1984), In: Mechanisms of tumor promotion Vol. IV, CRC press inc., 1
7. Mufson, R.A., (1984), ibid, 109
8. Trosko, J.E. and Chang C.C., (1984), ibid., 119
9. Murray, A.W. and Fitzgerald, D.J., (1979), Biochem. Biophys. Res. Commun., 91, 395
10. Berenblum, I., (1954), Cancer Res., 14, 471
11. Peraino, C. et al., (1973) Cancer Res., 33, 2701
12. Narisawa, T. et al., (1974), JNCI, 53, 1093
13. Colburn, N.H. et al., (1980) Teratog: Carcinog. Mutag.1, 87
14. Witschi, H.P. and Lock, S., (1979), Toxicol. Appl. Pharmacol., 50, 391
15. Pence, B.C. et al., (1986), JNCI, 77, 269
16. IARC, (1986), Long-term and short-term assays for carcinogens, Vol. 83
17. Rutten, A.A.J.J.L. et al., (1988) Carcinogenesis, 9, 315
18 Wärngard, L. et al., (1987) Carcinogenesis, 8, 1201
19. Wattenberg, L.W., (1983), Cancer Res., Suppl. 41, 2991
20. Wright, A.S., (1980), Mutation Res., 75, 215
21. Moldeus, P., (1987), In: Drug Metabolism: from molecules to man, Taylor and Francis, London, 309
22. Wortelboer, H.M. et al., (1990), Biochem. Pharmacol, 40, 2525
23. Althaus, F.R. et al., (1979), J. Biol. Chem., 25, 2148
24. Topp, R.J. and van Bladeren, P.J. (1986), Arch. Toxicol, 59, 150
25. Jongen, W.M.F. et al., (1987), Toxic. in vitro, 1, 105
26. Jongen, W.M.F. et al., (1989), Toxic. in vitro, 3, 207
27. Jongen, W.M.F. et al., (1988), Mutation Res., 202, 155
28. National Research Council, (1982), Drug, Nutrition and Cancer, 15
29. Van Bladeren, P.J. et al., (1980), Biochem. Pharmacol, 29, 2975
30. Jongen, W.M.F. et al., (1986), Mutation Res., 159, 133
31. Wakabayashi, K., (1985), Mutagenesis, 1, 423 and (1991), personal communication
32. Tiedink, H.G.M. et al., (1989), Fd. Chem. Toxic., 27, 723
33. Tiedink, H.G.M. et al., (1990), Mutation Res., 232, 199

Note: Bibliographics of references mentioned in the various tables may be obtained from the author upon request

ISOLATION AND IDENTIFICATION OF PUTATIVE CARCINOGENS AND ANTICARCINOGENS FROM DIETARY AND FAECAL SAMPLES BY SUPERCRITICAL FLUID EXTRACTION AND HPLC.

A.D'Odorico[1*], I.T. Gilmore[2], A. Morris[2], A.J. Young[1] and R.F. Bilton[1].
[1] School of Biomolecular Sciences, Liverpool John Moores University, Byrom St., Liverpool L3 3AF U.K. [2] Gastroenterology Unit, Royal Liverpool University Hospital, Prescott St. Liverpool L7 8XP U.K.[*Present address: Institute of Internal Medicine, Padua Medical School, Italy]

1. INTRODUCTION

Colorectal cancer (CRC) is one of the major neoplastic diseases of the developed countries of Western Europe and North America. There is strong epidemiological and experimental evidence to suggest that the incidence of CRC is related to the consumption of high fat/red meat, low fibre diets. Such diets also tend to be deficient in the antioxidant vitamins A, C and E and carotenoids. Traditional extraction techniques of biological material can be lengthy and will often lead to the production of artifacts or even the degradation of sensitive compounds. Supercritical fluid extraction (SFE) has shown great potential in environmental analyses, but its use has not been evaluated for the integrated analysis of vitamins, carotenoids and bile acids, all of which may be of importance in the aetiology of CRC[1,2,3].

2. MATERIALS AND METHODS

Plasma and faecal materials were obtained from a healthy male subject on a balanced diet, rich in fruit and vegetables. Lyophilised faecal samples were extracted using an ISCO 100D single-pump SFE at 7500 psi at 31 °C and a flow rate of 2.0 ml/min. Plasma samples (1.0 ml) were adsorbed onto a large excess (14 g) of anhydrous Na_2SO_4 and extracted as above.
Following extraction, samples were dried and stored at -20°c prior to analysis. Pigment profiles of faecal and plasma samples were obtained using reversed-phase HPLC. Carotenoids were resolved on a 5 μ Spherisorb ODS2 column (250 x 4.6 mm) using a solvent gradient of 0-100% ethyl-acetate in acetonitrile/water (9/1 v/v)over 25 min at 1.0 ml/min. A HP1040 diode-array detector was used to monitor absorption spectra on-line.

3. RESULTS AND DISCUSSION

Supercritical fluid extraction

Extraction of small quantities of lyophilised faecal material with supercritical CO_2 alone is not satisfactory. Two main problems were encountered. Firstly, exposure to supercritical fluids caused compaction of the faecal material at the bottom of the extraction tube, making quantitative extraction particularly difficult. This was overcome by evenly dispersing the faecal material in an excess of anhydrous Na_2SO_4. Secondly, the solubility of carotenoids and some of the other, more polar, components of faecal material is poor in CO_2 alone and compounds will elute over a wide range of temperature and pressure. Static extraction was therefore performed in the presence of modifiers such as toluene or benzene. The use of these modifiers resulted in the elution of the carotenoids and the K vitamins as a concentrated fraction. Highly polar compounds such as the bile acids could only be extracted with the addition of methanol. Temperature and, especially, pressure were also found to have a considerable effect on the overall efficiency of extraction, thus extraction in CO_2 at 2000 psi was not effective in eluting any pigments from faecal material and the pressure had to be raised to 7500 psi for the elution of the carotenes and carotene-epoxides. The addition of toluene further resulted in the elution of the chlorophylls and the remaining xanthophylls. Careful manipulation of temperature, pressure and use of the modifiers provide the opportunity for the fractionation of a complex mixture of compounds for subsequent separate analysis.

Faecal material

The HPLC analysis of carotenoids extracted from faecal material from a healthy individual using supercritical CO_2 is shown in Fig.1. The major pigments detected were lutein, lycopene, α- and ß-carotene together with substantial quantities of analogues of chlorophylls *a* and *b* in which the soret peak λmax was reduced and their R_T was increased. The mass spectra of these compounds have yet to be determined. In addition to these compounds, a number of other carotenoids have been observed, namely violaxanthin and it's 5,8-epoxide furanoid derivative aurochrome (produced by the acid conditions in the stomach), zeaxanthin, monohydroxylycopene and phytoene. Again, due to the acidic conditions, no traces of either neoxanthin (the other main green-leaf carotenoid) or its furanoid derivative, neochrome were detected in the faeces, although neoxanthin was almost certainly originally present in the diet in green vegetables. A number of polar carotenoids found in both faecal and plasma samples have been provisionally identified as ketocarotenoids (ε,ε-carotene-3,3′-dione, 3′-hydroxy-ε,ε-caroten-3-one and 3-hydroxy-ß,ε-caroten-3′-one). These are possible oxidation products of the common dietary carotenoids, lutein and zeaxanthin and have been reported in egg yolk[5].

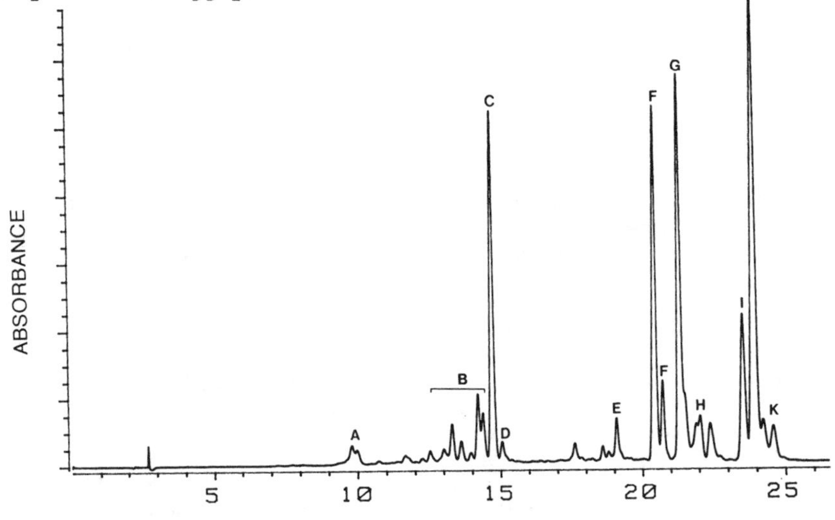

Figure 1. Reversed-phase HPLC of pigments (monitored at 447 nm) extracted from human faeces using SFE. Peak identifications: A. violaxanthin and aurochrome; B. mixture of ketocarotenoids (see text); C. lutein; D. zeaxanthin; E. monohydroxylycopene; F.'chlorophyll *a*'; G. lycopene; H. 'chlorophyll *b*', I. α-carotene, J. all-*trans*-ß-carotene, K. *cis*-isomers of ß-carotene.

Although the pigment profile shown in Fig. 1 is typical of faecal material, the pigments found in the faeces obviously reflect the dietary intake of an individual. Thus a number of other profiles have been observed for the same individual, and have shown particular variation in the levels of ß-carotene, lycopene and lutein.

Plasma carotenoids

The HPLC analysis of carotenoids from plasma following SFE is shown in Fig. 2. The pigment profile is quite different to that obtained from faecal material as a number of potential carotenoid metabolites are present and the chlorophylls are completely absent as these are not absorbed through the gut wall. High levels of α- and ß-carotene, lycopene (3 geometrical isomers), and lutein are present. ß-Cryptoxanthin is also found in high amounts, together with two compounds tentatively identified as 2′,3′-anhydrolutein and 3,4-anhydrolutein, which are very rarely found in dietary sources and are possible artifacts formed as a result of enzymatic dehydration of lutein or de-esterification of lutein acyl esters (see Khachik et al. [4]). The possible significance, if any, of the presence of these carotenoids and the ketocarotenoids described earlier is not known.

Other components which can be extracted with supercritical CO_2 and readily resolved on this chromatographic system include the acyclic carotenoid biosynthetic intermediates phytoene, phytofluene and ζ-carotene which are common components of many vegetables, together with α- and γ-tocopherol and retinol.

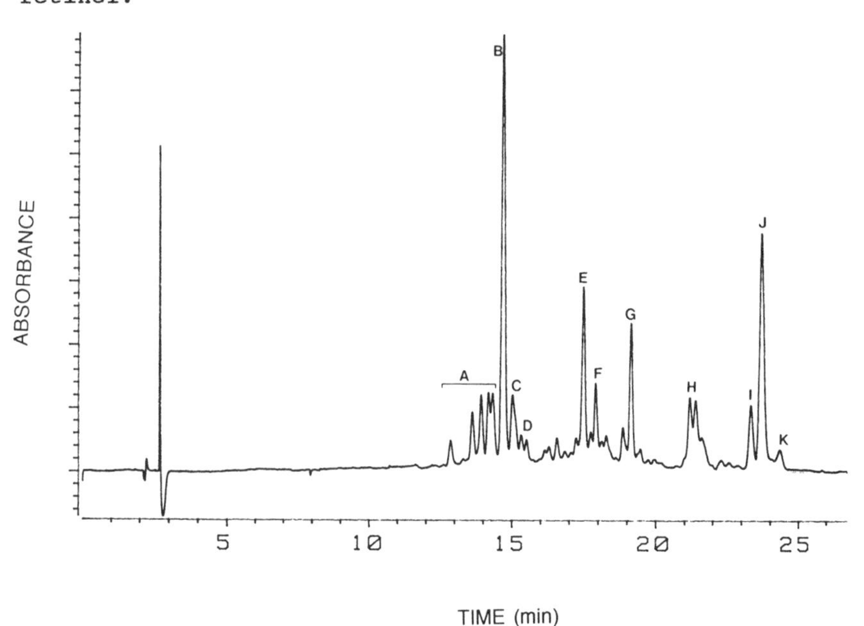

Figure 2. Reversed-phase HPLC of carotenoids (monitored at 447 nm) extracted from human plasma using SFE. Peak identifications: A. mixture of ketocarotenoids (see text); B. lutein; C. zeaxanthin; D. *cis*-isomers of lutein; E. 2′3′-anhydrolutein; F. 3,4-anhydrolutein, G. ß-cryptoxanthin; H. lycopene; I. α-carotene, J. all-*trans*-ß-carotene, K. *cis*-isomers of ß-carotene.

4.CONCLUSIONS

As an alternative to conventional extraction of faecal and other materials, SFE has a number of advantages. It can provide a rapid and relatively cheap method of extraction for a range of compounds for which traditional methods may necessitate a range of different methodologies. Perhaps the most important feature of SFE is that it facilitates minimal exposure of samples and isolated compounds to oxidative conditions, allowing the analysis of sensitive compounds. This is especially true for carotenoids which are especially prone to the production of artifacts.
The data presented in this report are limited to the HPLC analysis of pigments extracted using SFE. However, supercritical technologies are at their most powerful when a coupled SFE/SFC system is used, permitting on-line extraction and analysis of carotenoids and other compounds under optimum conditions, thus minimising degradation and the production of artifacts through *cis/trans* isomerisation etc. Preliminary experiments with the SFC of carotenoids are promising, and an SFE/SFC programme is currently underway.

5. ACKNOWLEDGEMENTS

The authors would like to thank The Royal Society and the Liverpool Cancer Charity for equipment funding to support this programme.

6. REFERENCES

1. Babbs, C.F. Free Radicals in Biology and Medicine,1990, *8*, 191-200.
2. Golding, J., M. Paterson and L.J. Kinlen. Br. J. Cancer, 1990, *62*, 304-308.
3. Mathews-Roth, M.M. Pure Appl. Chem., 1991, *63*, 147-155.
4. Khachik, F., G.R.Beecher and M.D. Goli. Pure Appl. Chem.,1991, *63*, 71-80.
5. Matsuno, T.,T. Hirono,Y. Ikuno, T. Maoka, M. Shimizu and T. Komori. Comp. Biochem. Physiol., 1986, *84B*, 477-481.

CELL PROLIFERATION AND MORPHOMETRY IN ENDOSCOPIC BIOPSIES

RA Goodlad, S Levi*, CY Lee, & NA Wright.

Imperial Cancer Research Fund,
Histopathology Unit,
35-43 Lincoln's Inn Fields,
London WC2A 3PN.

* Gastroenterology Department,
Royal Postgraduate Medical School,
DuCane Road,
London W12 ONN.

INTRODUCTION

Accurate assessment of cell turnover in man may prove to be invaluable for the understanding of a wide variety of physiological and disease processes, especially when one considers the association between proliferation and carcinogenesis. The gastrointestinal epithelium is particularly well suited for proliferative studies, as turnover rates are rapid, and the anatomical divisions between the reproductive and functional compartments are well defined[1].

Several methods are available for the determination of cell proliferation in the intestine of animals, but these either depend on labelling of dividing cells with nucleotide analogues, or on the arrest of cells entering mitosis[2]. Ethical considerations constrain the use of these very useful techniques in man. Nevertheless, one technique, the microdissection technique[3-5], in which bulk stained tissue is carefully teased apart under a dissection microscope, can be applied to human biopsy samples to quantify intestinal epithelial cell proliferation in man.

We have applied such a technique to a range of human gastrointestinal biopsies obtained at endoscopy. Mitoses per gastric gland or intestinal crypt were counted and the area of these compartments was traced using a drawing tube, as area measurements have the best correlation with direct counts of cell number[6]. The technique was validated by comparing results gathered using microdissection with data from the same animals that had been quantified in depth previously using well-established kinetic methods.

Methods

Animal tissue from our misoprostol experiments, which had been previously assayed by well established, tritiated thymidine-based techniques[7-9], was re-evaluated by the microdissection technique. Dogs were given a high dose of the prostaglandin analogue, misoprostol, for 77 days and then their dividing cells were labelled with tritiated thymidine and the number and position of labelled cells in autoradiographs scored.

The human part of this study was approved by the RPMS ethical committee. Biopsies were fixed in Carnoy's fluid for 4 hours and then stored in 70%

ethanol before analysis. The tissue was bulk stained with the Feulgen reaction, microdissected, and the number of mitoses per gland or crypt determined, as was the area.
Fifteen to twenty glands or crypts were quantified from each biopsy. Only distinct late prophases, metaphases, anaphases and telophases were counted. The outline of the gastric gland or duodenal crypts was traced using a drawing tube (see fig 1) and these tracings were later digitised to determine area.

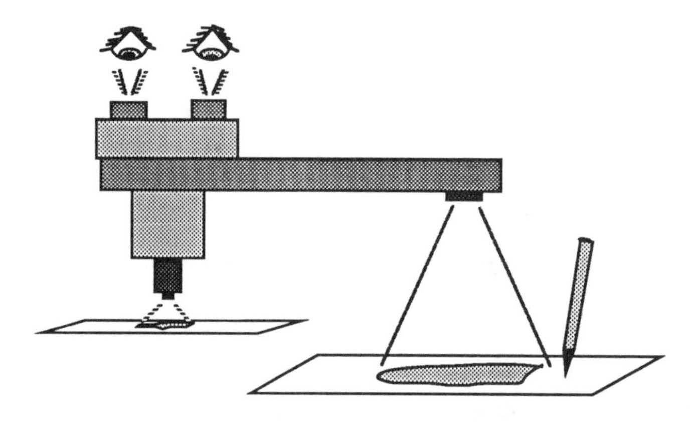

Figure 1. Diagram of the drawing tube. An image of the pencil is optically projected into the microscope's field of view to trace the object of interest.

Results The microdissection technique could readily be applied to tissue from the stomach, small intestine, colon and rectum. Less than half a biopsy usually gave enough tissue for quantification. The length of the glands and crypts was approximately the same, but the diameter and hence the area varied as shown in Table 1. There was a marked proximo-distal gradient in mitotic activity and area. There was a significant correlation ($p<0.001$, $r=0.90$) between mitoses per gland or crypt and area.

Table 1 The number of mitotic figures per gland or per crypt and the respective areas for these. The results are the mean (±SEM) n = 5

Site	Mitoses per gland or crypt		Area (mm^2) per gland or crypt	
	mean	±	mean	±
Fundus	0.8	0.08	0.018	0.003
Body	1.2	0.10	0.020	0.001
Antrum Lesser	4.6	0.38	0.029	0.002
Duodenum 1	5.2	0.43	0.028	0.002
Duodenum 2	4.5	0.61	0.024	0.002
Jejunum	5.9	0.58	0.020	0.001
Terminal Ileum	6.7	1.10	0.036	0.010
Caecum	14.2	0.93	0.060	0.003
Transverse Colon	12.2	1.08	0.057	0.000
Rectum	8.1	1.84	0.058	0.015

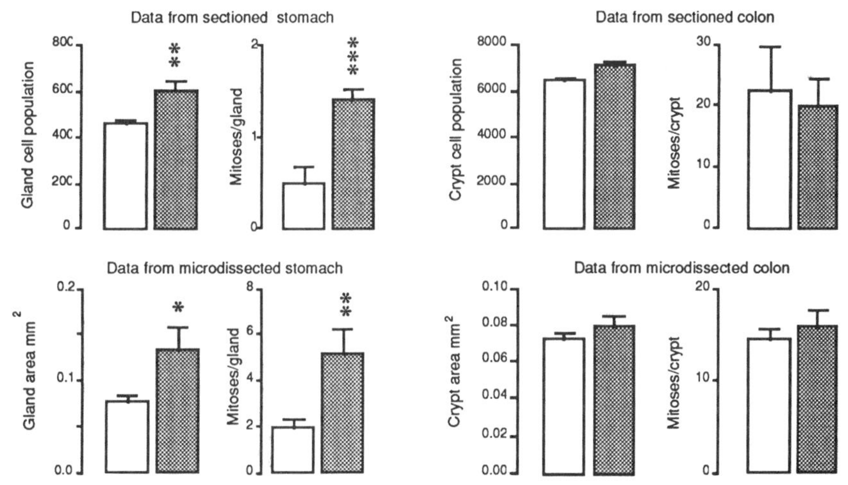

Fig 2. The effects of 77 days treatment on the section based and on the microdissection based measures.

The data from the misoprostol studies are shown in fig 2.The response of the stomach of the test group was very similar using both methods, as were the results from the colon, in which the data from the sectioned material showed more variability, presumably as far less mitoses were scored. The number of mitoses per crypt column in section was 1.0 ± 0.1 whilst the number of mitoses seen in a microdissected crypt was 15.0 ±1.1, thus 15.7 ± 2.4 more mitoses were seen in a microdissected crypt. In order to count the same number of mitoses as seen in 30 microdissected crypts one would need to score 450 crypt sections.

There was a significant correlation between cell population (derived from sections) and crypt area ($R = 0.78$, $P > 0.005$).

Discussion

The microdissection method gave similar results of proliferation and crypt cell mass to that obtained in the same tissue by autoradiography-based techniques, but in less than one sixth of the time taken to score the autoradiographs. In addition the precision of measure was much greater. Several groups have advocated the use of *in vitro* methods for the assessment of biopsies. We do not favour these as they are very labour intensive, can only be applied to a few patients at a time, and require immediate treatment of the biopsy. More importantly they are severely limited by trauma of biopsy, problems of diffusion (the birth rate at the edge of a cultured explant may be twice that seen at the centre[10]) and changes in intracellular nucleotide pool sizes[11]. In addition, the proliferative activity varies considerably with time after biopsy, being considerably reduced a few hours after biopsy[12]. Some methods allow the biopsy several hours to stabilise from the trauma, but this will also remove many of those factors involved in the regulation of cell proliferation[13].

Most proliferative indices are a ratio of dividing to non-dividing cells, so that if compartment size alters, indices may be confounded[7]. Thus well oriented, axially sectioned, glands and crypts must be studied in longitudinal and transverse section, so that the crypt can be reconstructed. Very few such crypts can be obtained in a small biopsy. In addition, mitotic figures migrate towards the crypt lumen, thus axially sections will overestimate proliferation by 30-40%, necessitating the determination of Tannock's correction factor[14]. One great advantage of the technique is that many more mitotic figures are seen, as indicated below in fig 3. In the dog colon this ratio was 15:1, in the rat it was approximately 8:1.

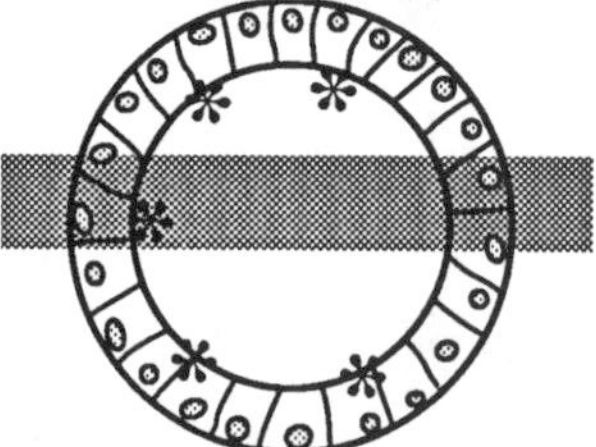

Fig 3. Diagram of a crypt in transverse section, *'s represent mitotic figures and the shaded bar a histological section.

The scoring is relatively rapid, as only mitotic figures need be scored, not the interphase cells. The investigation of whole crypts can also be applied to the exploration of the process of crypt duplication (by fissuring and bifurcating), the 'crypt cycle', which is analogous to the cell cycle[15]. The ease of use, the requirement of less than half a biopsy sample (which can be stored for years), and the ability to score every mitotic figure present, without concern over stereological artifacts, makes this method the one of choice for almost all applications concerned with proliferative effects in human gastrointestinal tissue. We have now successfully applied this technique in several studies[15-19].

REFERENCES

1. Goodlad RA. Dig Dis. 1989, 7, 169.

2. Goodlad RA, Wright NA. Quantitative studies on epithelial replacement in the gut. In: TA T, ed. *Techniques in the life sciences: Techniques in digestive physiology.* Ireland: Elsevier Biomedical Press, 1982: 212/1-212/21.

3. Wimber DR, Lamerton L. Radiat Res 1963, 18, 137.

4. Clarke RM. J Anat 1970, 107, 519.

5. Ferguson A, Sutherland A, MacDonald TT, Allan F. J Clin Pathol 1977, 30, 1068.

6. Hasan M, Ferguson A. J Clin Pathol 1981, 34, 1181.

7. Goodlad RA, Madgwick AJA, Moffatt MR, Levin S, Allen JL, Wright NA. Gut 1989, 30, 316.

8. Goodlad RA, Madgwick AJA, Moffatt MR, Levin S, Allen JL, Wright NA. Gastroenterology 1990, 96, 1.

9. Goodlad RA, Mandir N, Levin S, Allen JL, Wright NA. Gastroenterology 1991, 101, 1229.

10. Finney KJ, Ince P, Appleton DR, Sunter JP, Watson AJ. J Anat 1986, 149, 177.

11. Maurer HR. Cell tiss kinet 1981, 14, 111.

12. Appleton GVN, Wheeler EE, Al-Mufti R, Challacombe DN, Williamson RCN. Gut 1988, 29, 1544.

13. Goodlad RA, Wright NA. Bailliere's Clinical Gastroenterology 1990, 4, 97.

14. Tannock IF. Expl Cell Res 1967, 47, 345.

15. Cheng H, Bjerknes M, Amar J, Gardiner G. Anat Rec 1986, 216, 44.

16. Levi S, Goodlad RA, Lee CY, Stamp G, Walport MJ, Wright NA, et al. Lancet 1990, 336, 840.

17. Goodlad RA, Lee CY, Levin S, Wright NA. Experimental Physiol 1991, 76, 561.

18. Sullivan PB, Brueton MJ, Tabara Z, Goodlad RA, Lee CY, Wright NA. Lancet 1991, 338, 53.

19. Levi S, Goodlad RA, Stamp G, Lee CY, Walport MJ, Wright NA, et al. Gastroenterology 1992, 102, 1605.

DETECTION OF ABNORMAL MUCOSAL CELL REPLICATION IN HUMANS: A SIMPLE TECHNIQUE

J.A. Matthew[1], J.D.Pell[1], A. Prior[2], H.J. Kennedy[2], I.W. Fellows[2], J.M. Gee[1] and I.T. Johnson[1]

[1]AFRC Institute of Food Research, Norwich Research Park, Colney, Norwich.
[2]Norfolk and Norwich Hospital, Brunswick Road, Norwich.

1 INTRODUCTION

The initiation and promotion of colorectal tumours occurs over a prolonged period during which there is an accumulation of genetic abnormalities in the rapidly proliferating crypt cells. Human subjects whose dietary habits are associated with a low risk of colorectal cancer tend to have a relatively quiescent colorectal mucosa (1). In contrast, a high rate of mucosal cell proliferation associated with inflammatory bowel disease is a risk factor for neoplasia (2). Moreover the distribution of dividing cells within the crypts is itself a diagnostic parameter which can be used to identify the early stages of neoplastic change (3).

In order to explore the relationship between dietary factors and colorectal carcinogenesis, a reliable technique for the measurement of mucosal cytokinetics is needed, that can be applied to relatively large samples of human subjects. In this paper we report on a simple method for the assessment of cytokinetic parameters. The technique has been validated by comparison with the mitotic arrest technique using rats, and then applied to human intestinal biopsies obtained during routine diagnostic endoscopy. The detection of changes in proliferative indices characteristic of chronic ulcerative colitis (UC) is described.

2 MATERIALS AND METHODS

Animals and diets

Forty male Wistar strain rats (140-150g) were divided into 4 groups of 10 and housed singly in wire-bottomed cages in an animal house with controlled temperature, humidity and light/dark cycle (12h light/ 12h dark). A dietary strategy was used to vary the rate of mucosal cell proliferation at 3 different sites along the alimentary tract. Two groups of 10 rats received a nutritionally complete semisynthetic diet containing insoluble cellulose (10g/100g); the other groups received similar diets in which cellulose was replaced with the viscous polysaccharide guar gum. Both diets contained corn oil (8g/100g). After 14 d of ad libitum feeding, food was withdrawn at 09.00 h. All animals in one pair of guar-and cellulose-fed groups were given an intra-peritoneal injection of vincristine sulphate, deeply anaesthetised with phenobarbitol and killed at approximately 12 min intervals over 2h. The other pair of groups was killed similarly but received no vincristine sulphate. For each animal the abdomen was opened with a ventral midline incision, the alimentary tract was removed and samples of tissue (10 mm) were taken from the jejunum (10% of small intestinal length), the ileum (95% of small intestinal length) and the caecum, and transferred to fixative.

Human subjects

Colonic and rectal biopsies were obtained from patients undergoing colonoscopy for a variety of clinical indications. The study was approved by the Norwich Health Authority Ethical Committee, and informed consent was obtained from patients prior to the colonoscopy session. The clinical history of each patient was available from hospital records, and a diagnosis was made on the basis of endoscopy and diagnostic histology where appropriate. In addition to the biopsies obtained for clinical purposes, two additional samples were obtained from flat mucosa in the transverse colon and the rectum of each patient and transferred immediately to fixative (ethanol:acetic acid; 75:25). Patients with ulcerative colitis (UC) were defined as those with a confirmed history of the disease but for whom no evidence of current inflammation or dysplasia was found, and those with some evidence of low grade inflammation but no evidence of dysplasia. Adenoma patients were those from whom a polyp was removed at endoscopy, either at the current session or on a previous occasion.

Measurement of crypt cell production

The crypt cell production rate was assessed by the mitotic arrest technique in groups of animals treated with vincristine sulphate (4). Briefly, the tissue was dehydrated and stained in bulk, small clumps of crypts were isolated, flattened beneath a coverslip and examined under the compound microscope. The number of dividing nuclei blocked in metaphase was determined in 10 crypts from each site. The crypt cell proliferation rate was calculated from the slope of the regression line obtained by plotting the number of blocked metaphases against time of exposure to vincristine.

In human biopsies, and in the rat tissue not exposed to the antimitotic drug, the cytokinetic parameters were assessed by a modified version of the technique described by Goodlad et al (5). Crypts were isolated and examined as before, and the numbers of dividing cells were estimated by counting all nuclei in prophase, metaphase, anaphase or telophase. For human tissue, the length of each crypt was estimated by comparison with an eyepiece graticule, and the position of each dividing cell was noted. The data for 10 crypts from each biopsy were entered on a computerised database, using software designed for the purpose. Each crypt was divided automatically into quintiles and the number of cell divisions occurring in each of 5 zones was calculated. The diagnostic classifications of patients were not known to the histologist. The significance of differences between means was estimated using Student's t-test for unpaired data.

3 RESULTS AND DISCUSSION

The metaphase-arrest technique is a well established method of estimating the rate of mucosal cell crypt cell proliferation (4), which gives an absolute measure of cell production (cell divisions per crypt/unit time). It has a number of advantages over other methods of assessing cell proliferation, in that there is no need for in vitro incubation, nor for conventional histology and autoradiography. Several potential sources of error are thus avoided. However the toxicity of antimitotic drugs has precluded the use of this technique in humans, except in a few studies with cancer patients (6). In the present study we used diet to vary the rate of crypt cell proliferation in rats and compared the cytokinetic parameters obtained by each method. The CCPR ranged from 4.9 divisions per crypt/h in the caecum of rats fed cellulose to 20.2 divisions per crypt/h in the ileum of rats fed guar gum. There was an excellent correlation between CCPR and observed mitoses/crypt when the results were compared by linear regression ($r = 0.98$; $P <0.001$). These results are consistent with the findings of Goodlad et al (5), and confirm that the direct summation of mitoses in microdissected crypts gives a sensitive and reproducible estimate of mitotic activity.

Human colonic biopsies can be readily microdissected and examined under the compound microscope in the same way as animal tissue. In the present study we compared the total numbers and spatial distribution of mitoses in 17 patients with UC and 14 with colorectal polyps. The total numbers of mitoses in each compartment, in both sets of patients are illustrated in Fig 1A and B. Crypts from patients with colitis contained higher numbers of dividing cells in compartments 3 ($p< 0.05$), 4 and 5 ($p<0.01$). In Fig 1B the numbers of dividing cells in each compartment are expressed as a percentage of the total for the whole crypt. This data confirms that the distribution of dividing cells in the tissue obtained from patients with colitis is shifted significantly. The curve for UC crypts is, in effect, rotated so that the proportion in compartment 2 is significantly lower than that for patients with polyps ($p< 0.05$), whilst the proportion in compartments 4 and 5 is significantly increased ($p<0.01$).

Patients with chronic UC are known to be at increased risk of developing colorectal carcinoma (1). Although the mechanism underlying this relationship is not entirely clear, the abnormal cell proliferation associated with chronic inflammatory disease appears to be a risk factor. In a recent study Biasco et al (7) used the thymidine labelling index to demonstrate that in patients with UC the proliferative zone is shifted toward the surface of the mucosa, when compared to normal subjects and patients with adenoma. Our present results are consistent with this report.

The technique described here is inexpensive and fast, and can be applied to stored tissue. It is therefore ideally suited to large scale experimental studies concerned with the relationship between diet and colorectal disease. It may also be well suited to clinical use where the prime consideration is to identify patients at particular risk of neoplasia. The underlying variation in the distribution of dividing cells along the crypt is relatively low, so that abnormal tissue, with a large number of dividing cells in the compartments nearest the mucosal surface, can be quickly and easily identified by comparison with a reference population.

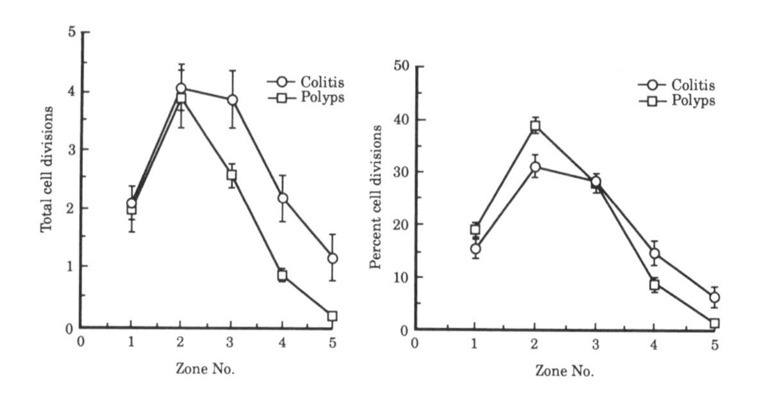

Figure 1 Total numbers (A) and spatial distribution (B) of dividing cells in crypts obtained from UC and adenoma patients.

4 ACKNOWLEDGEMENTS

The authors are grateful to Dr. G.C. Barker and Mrs. R. Thorpe of IFRN for software development and data logging respectively.

5 REFERENCES

1. J.H. Butt, J.E. Lennard Jones and J.K. Ritchie, Med. Clin. North Am. 1980, 64, 1203.
2. M. Lipkin, K. Uehara, S. Winawer, A. Sanchez, C. Bauer, R. Phillips, H.T. Lynch, W.A. Blattner, J.F. Fraumeni Jr., Cancer Lett. 1985, 26, 139.
3. M. Ponz de Leon, L. Roncucci, P. Di Donata, L. Tassi, O. Smerieri, M.G. Amorico, G. Malagoli, D. DeMaria, A. Antonioli, N.J. Chahin, M. Perini, G. Rigo, G. Barberini, A. Manenti, G. Biasco and L. Barbara, Cancer Res. 1988, 48, 4121.
4. N. Wright and M. Alison, In: The Biology of Epithelial Cell Populations Vol.1, pp. 97-202, Clarendon Press 1984, Oxford, UK.
5. R.A. Goodlad, S. Levi, C.Y Lee, N. Mandir, H. Hodgson and N.A. Wright, Gastroenterol., 1991, 101, 1235.
6. N.A. Wright, D.R. Britton, G. Bone and D.R. Appleton, Cell Tissue Kinet. 1977, 10, 429.
7. G. Biasco, G.M. Paganelli, M. Miglioli, S. Brillanti, G. Di Febo, G. Gizzi, M. Ponz de Leon, M. Campieri and L. Barbara, Cancer Res, 1990, 50, 1156.

RAPID DETECTION OF INDUCERS OF ENZYMES THAT PROTECT AGAINST CARCINOGENS

Hans J. Prochaska*, Annette B. Santamaria#, and Paul Talalay#

*Molecular Pharmacology and Therapeutics Program
Memorial Sloan-Kettering Cancer Center
New York, New York 10021 USA

#Department of Pharmacology and Molecular Sciences
The Johns Hopkins School of Medicine
Baltimore, Maryland 21205 USA

1 INTRODUCTION

Although agents that prevent cancer may interrupt the neoplastic process via a variety of mechanisms[1,2], many recognized anticarcinogens exert their protective effects by inducing electrophile-processing Phase II enzymes[3,4]. Over the last 15 years our research has been guided by the postulate that Phase II enzyme inducers protect against the development of cancer[5]. Indeed, potential anticarcinogens of clinical interest such as oltipraz [5-(2-pyrazinyl)-4-methyl-1,2-dithiole-3-thione] were correctly predicted to be anticarcinogens based solely on their ability to induce Phase II enzymes[6,7].

Since the systematic screening for compounds that induce Phase II enzymes *in vivo* is time-consuming and expensive, we became interested in a simple *in vitro* system to evaluate and screen for Phase II enzyme inducers. In this chapter, we describe a direct assay of Phase II enzyme-inducer activity in cells grown in microtiter plates[8]. Moreover, activity can be conveniently assayed in vegetable extracts. Remarkably, vegetables that have been shown to protect against cancer are active in our system[9]. As described elsewhere in this monograph, the assay has permitted the isolation of the major inducer of Phase II enzymes from broccoli[10].

2 THE ASSAY FOR INDUCTIVE ACTIVITY

NAD(P)H:(Quinone-acceptor) Oxidoreductase (QR) as a Marker Enzyme

QR is a cytosolic, dicoumarol inhibitable, FAD-dependent protein that catalyzes the obligatory two-electron reduction of a wide variety of quinones by NAD(P)H. It is expressed in virtually all tissues, and is exceedingly responsive to induction by a large number of xenobiotics[11].

Although a compelling case can be made that QR can protect against quinone-mediated cytotoxicity[12], it is clear that its elevation by anticarcinogens is coordinate with other protective enzymes such as glutathione *S*-transferases and UDP-glucuronosyltransferases. Our confidence that QR is a marker of the general elevation of other Phase II enzymes has been bolstered by the demonstration that the 5'-flanking regions of QR and the Ya subunit of glutathione *S*-transferase are similar[13-16].

Hepa 1c1c7 Cells as a Model Cell Line to Test Inducer Activity

The complexities and expense involved with screening for anticarcinogens *in vivo* motivated us to develop an *in vitro* model for Phase II enzyme induction. We found that the Hepa 1c1c7 murine hepatoma cell line possessed an easily measurable and highly inducible QR activity, and was responsive to most compounds that were active in rodents[17]. This cell line[18] and its mutant subclones[19,20] have been crucial in identifying the molecular mechanisms by which the Ah (Aryl hydrocarbon) receptor activates the transcription of aryl hydrocarbon hydroxylase in response to planar aromatic hydrocarbons. Accordingly, with these cell lines, we developed a model for the regulation of Phase II enzymes by xenobiotics[21,22]. Recent molecular evidence has verified our earlier proposals[13-16].

The microtiter plate assay. Since the Hepa 1c1c7 cell line is responsive to the same compounds which are active in rodents, we had proposed it would be useful in screening for presumptive anticarcinogens by virtue of inductive activity[17]. Although the *in vitro* assay is considerably more rapid than screening compounds for inductive activity in rodents, the assay of QR specific activity in conventional tissue culture plates was time-consuming and cumbersome (e.g., scraping the plates, homogenizing, centrifuging to collect cytosol, assaying the fractions for QR activity and protein content).

These complexities are largely avoided by growing and assaying the Hepa 1c1c7 cells directly in microtiter wells[8]. The procedure is simple: (a) cells are plated in duplicate sets of microtiter plates; (b) cells are re-fed media containing inducing agents dissolved in 0.1 % dimethylsulfoxide or 0.2 % acetonitrile; (c) after cells are grown for an additional 24-48 h, one set of plates is lysed with 50 μl/well of digitonin and the QR activity is assayed by adding 200 μl/well of a cocktail containing bovine serum albumin, Tween 20, FAD, glucose 6-phosphate, $NADP^+$, glucose-6-phosphate dehydrogenase, MTT [3-(4,5-dimethyl-2-yl)-2,5-diphenyltetrazolium bromide], and menadione dissolved in Tris buffer. Before kinetic microtiter plate readers were available, the reaction was stopped at 5 min by addition of dicoumarol, after which the absorbance of the formazan dye is measured (610 nm); (d) the second set of plates is stained in a vat containing crystal violet, destained in tap water, and the retained dye is solubilized with 0.5% sodium dodecyl sulfate in 50 % ethanol and is measured (610 nm). The data from the MTT assay reflects QR activity; that of the crystal violet assay reflects cell mass or total protein. The latter assay provides gratuitous information of the cytotoxicity of the compounds tested. Since the data were obtained from a duplicate set of plates, the computation of the specific activity can be easily made using commercially-available spreadsheet programs. Moreover, it is easy to carry out serial dilutions in these plates, and it is therefore convenient to obtain dose-response curves of many samples (e.g., the fractions from a chromatographic procedure).

Although a number of methods for measuring QR activity exist, we decided to adapt the MTT method[23] for staining QR activity in gels for our microtiter assay (see Figure 1). We measure the blue color that is produced when MTT is reduced by the hydroquinone product of the QR reaction, menadiol, to form the formazan dye and menadione. An NADPH generating-system is used as the source of reduced nicotinamide nucleotide, since significant MTT reduction can occur directly through NADH-dependent dehydrogenases. Since both substrates are regenerated, the rate of MTT reduction is linearly proportional to the amount of QR assayed up to optical density changes of 0.5 per minute. Thus, cells with high and low levels of QR are easily and accurately measured. Finally, dicoumarol can assess whether the reduction of MTT is due to QR since it is a specific and potent inhibitor of this enzyme.

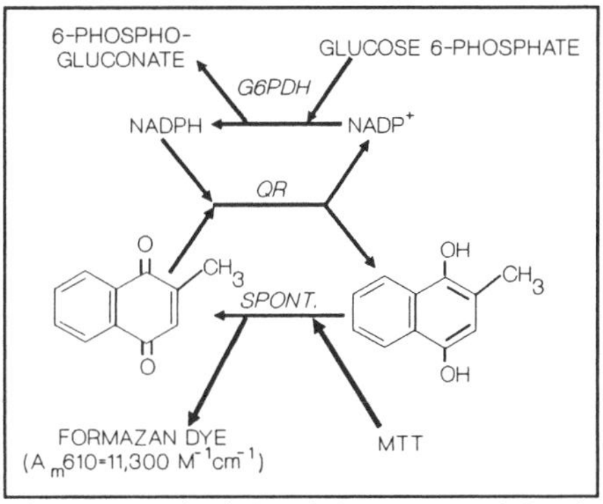

Figure 1 Principle of the Assay of QR in Microtiter Wells.

The model has allowed us to survey many compounds and has permitted the identification of novel inducers[24,25]. Moreover, this system has allowed us to screen a large number of vegetable extracts.

3 VEGETABLES AS ENZYME INDUCERS

We obtained a large number of diverse organically-grown produce and tested them for inducer-activity[9]. Samples were homogenized in 2 vol/wt deionized and distilled water, lyophilized and stored at -20°C until analyzed. We found that the lyophilized products lost activity when standing at room temperature for long periods of time. The lyophilized powders were extracted for 6-24 h with 35 vol/wt of acetonitrile, filtered, and dried on a vacuum centrifuge. Residues were dissolved in acetonitrile and the suspensions were placed in media (0.2 % final concentration) and fed to the Hepa 1c1c7 cells as described above. The only modification made to the procedure described by Prochaska and Santamaria[8] was to heat the fetal calf serum for 1 h at 56°C in the presence of 2 % (wt/vol) activated charcoal. This treatment of fetal calf serum rendered the Hepa cells more susceptible to inducers and decreased the basal QR activity, thus increasing the ratio of inducer-treated cells to controls.

Our survey of vegetables has been published elsewhere[9], but some of our results are summarized in Figure 2. Members of the families Cruciferae and Liliaceae potently induced QR activity, whereas members of Solanaceae were inactive. Intriguingly, the former families, not the latter have been implicated as reducing cancer risk in man (see references cited in Prochaska *et al.*[9]). Moreover, dietary supplementation of cruciferous vegetables has been shown to prevent carcinogen-induced malignancy in rodents[1,26]. Based on our data, and the ease with which the data could be collected, an effort to characterize the active inducer(s) in vegetables is being undertaken. The successful isolation of the major inducer in broccoli[10] is described elsewhere in this volume.

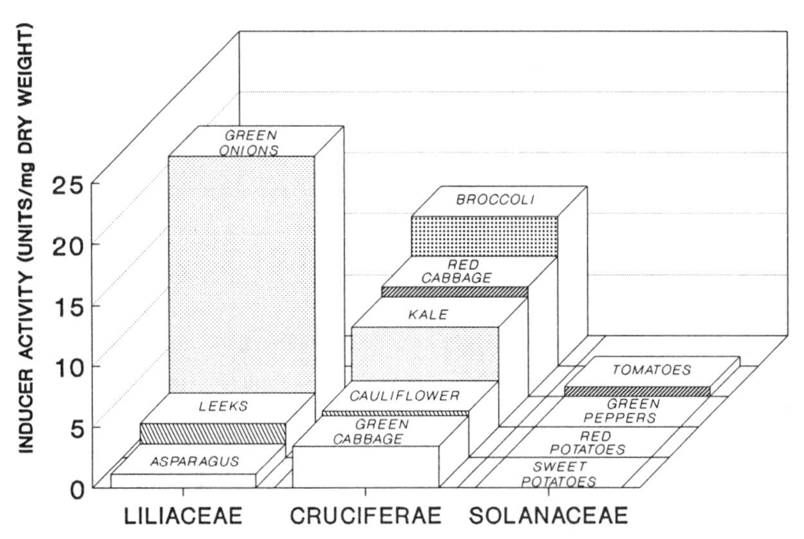

Figure 2 Potency of induction of QR in Hepa 1c1c7 murine hepatoma cells by samples from three families of commonly-consumed vegetables. Extracts were prepared as described in the text. One unit of inducer activity is defined as the amount of extract required to double the QR specific activity of Hepa 1c1c7 cells growing in a microtiter well containing 150 μl of medium. Data for Liliaceae and Solanaceae are from Table 1 whereas data for Cruciferae are means obtained from Table 2 of Prochaska *et al.*[9]

4 CONCLUSIONS

Persuasive evidence has been accumulated that a compound may possess anticarcinogenic potential *if* it can elevate the levels of Phase II enzymes. Although some Phase II enzyme inducers are carcinogens, many are not. Moreover, carcinogens can act as *anti*carcinogens under the appropriate experimental circumstances. It is clear that Phase II enzyme inducers as a group possess significant biological activity. Since foods that humans consume possess inducer activity, it is important to identify and characterize these components. The novel microtiter assay may be the most practical method for these purposes. It is hoped that data generated with this assay will permit the development of rational guidelines for prevention of cancer in man.

* * * *

Acknowledgements. These studies were supported by grants from the National Cancer Institute (PO1 CA 44530) and from the American Institute for Cancer Research. H.J.P. was supported by the National Cancer Institute Training Grant CA 09243 during the course of these studies, and is a recipient of an American Cancer Society Junior Faculty Research Award (JFRA-422).

REFERENCES

1. L.W. Wattenberg, Cancer Res., 1983, 43, 2448s.
2. L.W. Wattenberg, Cancer Res., 1985, 45, 1.
3. P. Talalay, M.J. De Long and H.J. Prochaska, "Cancer Biology and Therapeutics", edited by J.G. Cory and A. Szentivani, Plenum Press, New York, 1987, p. 197.
4. P. Talalay, Adv. Enzyme Regul., 1989, 28, 237.
5. C. Huggins and J. Pataki, Proc. Natl. Acad. Sci., 1965, 53, 791.
6. S.S. Ansher, P. Dolan and E. Bueding, Hepatology, 1983, 3, 932.
7. L.W. Wattenberg and E. Bueding, Carcinogenesis, 1986, 7, 1379.
8. H.J. Prochaska and A.B. Santamaria, Anal. Biochem., 1988, 169, 328.
9. H.J. Prochaska, A.B. Santamaria and P. Talalay, Proc. Natl. Acad. Sci., 1992, 89, 2394.
10. Y.S. Zhang, P. Talalay, C.G. Cho and G.H. Posner, Proc. Natl. Acad. Sci., 1992, 89, 2399.
11. L. Ernster, R.W. Eastabrook, P. Hochstein and S. Orrenius (editors), Chemica Scripta, 1987, 27A, 1.
12. H.J. Prochaska and P. Talalay, "Oxidative Stress:Oxidants and Antioxidants", edited by H. Sies, Academic Press, London, 1991, p. 195.
13. R.S. Friling, A. Bensimon, Y. Tichauer and V. Daniel, Proc. Natl. Acad. Sci., 1990, 87, 6258.
14. T.H. Rushmore and C.B. Pickett, J. Biol. Chem., 1990, 265, 14648.
15. T.H. Rushmore, M.R. Morton and C.B. Pickett, J. Biol. Chem., 1991, 266, 11632.
16. L.V. Favreau and C.B. Pickett, J. Biol. Chem., 1991, 266, 4556.
17. M.J. De Long, H.J. Prochaska and P. Talalay, Proc. Natl. Acad. Sci., 1986, 83, 787.
18. O. Hankinson, Proc. Natl. Acad. Sci., 1979, 76, 373.
19. O. Hankinson, R.D. Anderson, B.W. Birren, F. Sander, M. Negishi and D.W. Nebert, J. Biol. Chem., 1985, 260, 1790.
20. A.G. Miller, D. Israel and J.P. Whitlock,Jr., J. Biol. Chem., 1982, 258, 3523.
21. H.J. Prochaska, M.J. De Long and P. Talalay, Proc. Natl. Acad. Sci., 1985, 82, 8232.
22. H.J. Prochaska and P. Talalay, Cancer Res., 1988, 48, 4776.
23. B. Höjeberg, K. Blomberg, S. Stenberg and C. Lind, Arch. Biochem. Biophys., 1981, 207, 205.
24. P. Talalay, M.J. De Long and H.J. Prochaska, Proc. Natl. Acad. Sci., 1988, 85, 8261.
25. S.R. Spencer, L. Xue, E.M. Klenz and P. Talalay, Biochem. J., 1991, 273, 711.
26. J.N. Boyd, J.G. Babish and G.S. Stoewsand, Fd. Chem. Toxicol., 1982, 20, 47.

ISOLATION AND IDENTIFICATION OF THE PRINCIPAL INDUCER OF ANTICARCINOGENIC PROTECTIVE ENZYMES FROM BROCCOLI

Y. Zhang and P. Talalay
Department of Pharmacology and Molecular Sciences
The Johns Hopkins University School of Medicine
Baltimore, Maryland 21205, U.S.A.

C.-G. Cho and G.H. Posner
Department of Chemistry
The Johns Hopkins University School of Arts and Sciences
Baltimore, Maryland 21218, U.S.A.

1 INTRODUCTION

Epidemiological studies in man indicate that increased consumption of vegetables lowers the risk of malignancy.[1,2] The mechanisms responsible for protection are multiple, complex, and incompletely understood. Feeding of vegetables, or of many of their minor chemical constituents, protects rodents against chemical carcinogenesis.[3,4] Such treatment also elevates the activities of Phase II detoxication enzymes (e.g., NAD(P)H:quinone reductase, glutathione transferases, and glucuronosyltransferases) in the tissues of these animals. Many lines of evidence strongly support the belief that enhancement of Phase II enzymes that inactivate electrophiles is a major mechanism responsible for protection against the toxic and neoplastic effects of carcinogens.[5,6]

Measurement of NAD(P)H:quinone reductase (QR) activity in Hepa 1c1c7 murine hepatoma cells in culture provides a reliable, rapid and economical method for the detection and quantitative assessment of inducer activity.[7,8] When these assays are carried out on cells grown in 96-well microtiter plates, considerable economy and efficiency is achieved.[9,10] By use of mutant cells defective in cytochrome P-450 induction, this system can also make the important distinction between <u>bifunctional</u> inducers that stimulate the synthesis of both Phase I (cytochromes P-450) and Phase II enzymes, and <u>monofunctional</u> inducers that elevate Phase II enzymes, selectively.[11] Monofunctional inducers are unlikely to activate carcinogens and are therefore more desirable as chemoprotectors.

Recently, the Hepa 1c1c7 cell system has been used to survey organic solvent extracts of a variety of commonly consumed vegetables for QR inducer activity.[10] Crucifers, and specifically those of the genus <u>Brassica</u>, were found to be especially rich in inducer activity. Among vegetables belonging to the species <u>Brassica oleracea</u>

(broccoli, brussels sprouts, cabbage, cauliflower, kale and kohlrabi), several varieties of broccoli were found to be rich sources of inducer activity. We selected a sample of SAGA broccoli for detailed elucidation of the chemical nature of enzyme inducer(s).[12]

2 RESULTS AND DISCUSSION

Isolation of the Inducer from SAGA Broccoli. When acetonitrile extracts of lyophilized samples of SAGA broccoli were subjected to preparative scale reverse phase HPLC (in a methanol/water gradient), more than 70% of the applied inducer activity was eluted in a single region of the chromatogram. The most active fractions obtained from several chromatographies were pooled and further purified on preparative TLC plates developed with acetonitrile. The inducer activity was associated with a single band which was then subjected to reverse phase HPLC (in a water/acetonitrile gradient). All of the applied inducer activity was eluted in a single peak which was homogeneous on analytical TLC.

Identification of Inducer. The identity of the inducer was established by spectroscopic methods and confirmed by synthesis[12] to be (-)-1-isothiocyanato-(4*R*)-(methylsulfinyl)butane which is known as sulforaphane:

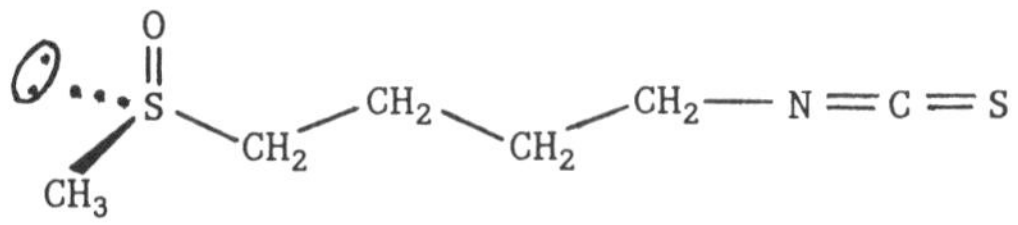

$$CH_3-S(=O)-CH_2-CH_2-CH_2-CH_2-N=C=S$$

Sulforaphane was first isolated from hoary cress and some other plants, but its abundance in these plants is not known. However, the glucosinolates of sulforaphane and its closely-related olefin, sulforaphene [4-isothiocyanato-(1*R*)-(methylsulfinyl)-1-(*E*)-butene], have been detected in the seeds of a large number of plants.[13] In some seeds the quantities of these glucosinolates are substantial. Many aliphatic isothiocyanates containing terminal methylthio groups at the oxidation state of sulfide, sulfoxide, or sulfone and varying in chain lengths have been isolated from plants, largely as their glucosinolates.

Inducer Potency of Sulforaphane and its Structural Analogues in Cultured Cells. The concentration of sulforaphane required to double (CD) the QR activity in the murine hepatoma cells under standard conditions was 0.16-0.20 μM. This is a revised and lower value than previously reported,[12] and is based on more extensive determinations with several synthetic samples. Since synthetic (*R*,*S*)-sulforaphane and the isolated (*R*)-sulforaphane gave closely similar CD values, the inducer potency is unaffected by the chirality of the sulfoxide group. Synthetic analogues of sulforaphane differing in the state of oxidation of sulfur and the number of

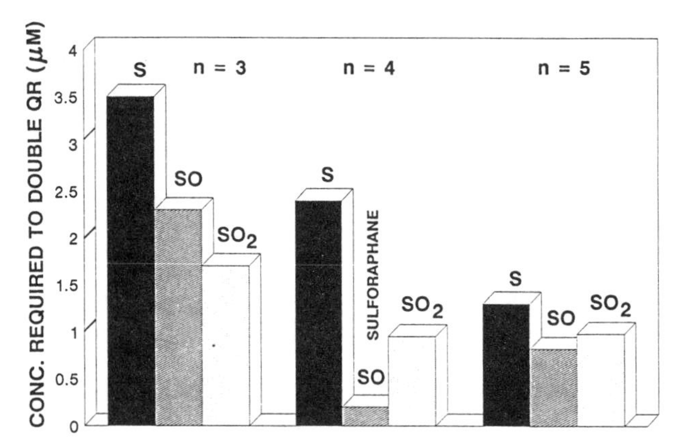

Figure 1. Potency of induction of quinone reductase (QR) in Hepa 1c1c7 murine hepatoma cells by sulforaphane [CH_3-SO-$(CH_2)_4$-NCS] and analogues differing in the state of oxidation of the sulfur atom (-S-, -SO-, or -SO_2) of the methylthio group and the number of methylene groups (n = 3, 4, or 5) bridging the methylthio and isothiocyanate groups. The values shown are the concentrations of compound required to double (CD values) the quinone reductase specific activities under standard assay conditions.[9,10] The CD value for sulforaphane is 0.16-0.20 µM.

methylene groups bridging the isothiocyanate and the methylthio groups were synthesized and their inducer potencies compared to that of sulforaphane. The results (Figure 1) show that sulforaphane is remarkably potent. Indeed, it is the most potent monofunctional inducer so far identified.[5] The sulfoxides and sulfones are more potent than the sulfides, and compounds with 4 or 5 methylene groups are more potent than those containing only 3 methylene groups. Comparison of sulfoxides and sulfones shows that their relative potencies depend on the chain lengths.

Induction of Quinone Reductase and Glutathione Transferase Activities in Mouse Organs. The ability of synthetic (R,S)-sulforaphane, erucin (CH_3-S-$(CH_2)_4$-NCS) and erysolin (CH_3-SO_2-$(CH_2)_4$-NCS) to induce quinone reductase in various organs of female CD-1 mice has been determined according to a standard protocol.[14] The sulfoxide (sulforaphane) and its sulfide analogue (erucin), in doses of 15 µmol per day administered by gavage for 5 days, raised the specific activities of both enzymes in the cytosols of several organs by 1.6- to 3.1-fold. The sulfone was considerably more toxic, but even doses of 5 µmole daily for 5 days elevated the specific enzyme activities in several tissues. The results for sulforaphane are shown in Figure 2.[12]

Is Sulforaphane the Principal Inducer of Phase II Enzymes in SAGA Broccoli? Several observations suggest

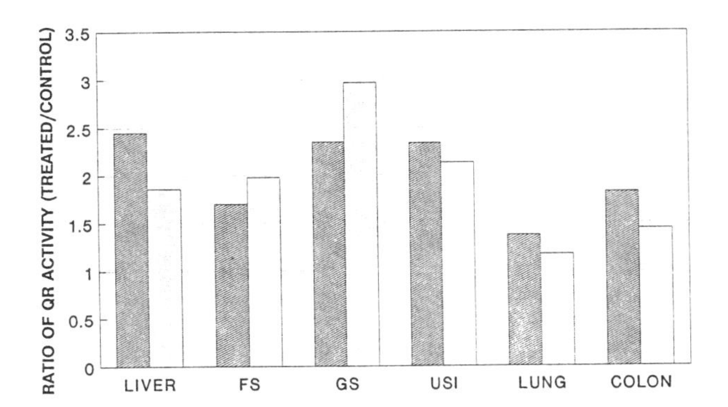

Figure 2. Induction of quinone reductase [hatched] and glutathione transferase (measured with 1-chloro-2,4-dinitrobenzene) [stippled] in cytosols obtained from liver, forestomach, (FS), glandular stomach (GS), upper small intestine (USI), lung and colon of female CD-1 mice treated with 15 μmol daily doses of sulforaphane for 5 days. The ratios of the specific enzyme activities of treated to control animals (4-5 per group) are shown in the bars.[12]

that most of the inducer activity for Phase II enzymes extractable from SAGA broccoli can be attributed to its sulforaphane content. (1) The isolation procedure gave a high yield and more than 70% of the initial inducer activity was confined to a single peak of the initial HPLC. The peak fractions also contained the great majority of the isothiocyanate eluted from the column.[12,15] Furthermore, the inducer activity in these fractions was recovered in high yield in the final compound. (2) In an independent method of isolation, lyophilized SAGA broccoli was subjected to high vacuum sublimation. The sublimate was found to contain comparable inducer activity to that isolated in the conventional way. Sulforaphane was isolated from the sublimate and its structure confirmed by NMR. Moreover, comparison of the isothiocyanate content of the sublimate measured by cyclocondensation with 1,2-benzenedithiol[15] and of inducer activity indicated good agreement if the inducer was assigned a CD value of 0.17 μM (in agreement with the measured value for sulforaphane). (3) Since volatile isothiocyanates or other inducers might escape detection by these methods, a sample of fresh SAGA broccoli that had not been lyophilized was extracted with methanol or a methanol/acetonitrile mixture. The extract was assayed for isothiocyanate content and for inducer activity. About 80% of the inducer activity could be accounted for by the isothiocyanate content, if it was assumed that the isothiocyanate was a single compound with CD = 0.16 μM, again in agreement with the value determined experimentally for sulforaphane. All of the evidence suggests, therefore that sulforaphane is the principal inducer of Phase II enzymes extractable from SAGA broccoli.

3 SUMMARY

Induction of Phase II detoxication enzymes is a major mechanism for protection against the toxic and neoplastic effects of carcinogens. By monitoring quinone reductase activity in Hepa 1c1c7 murine hepatoma cells we have found that most of the inducer activity of extracts of SAGA broccoli can be accounted for by a single isothiocyanate; sulforaphane [(-)-1-isothiocyanato-(4R)-(methylsulfinyl) butane]. Sulforaphane is an exceedingly potent monofunctional inducer. Several structural analogues, differing from sulforaphane in the oxidation state of the sulfur of the methylthio group and the number of methylene groups linking the methylthio and isothiocyanate functions are also inducers, but are all significantly less potent.

Acknowledgements.These studies were supported by a U.S. Public health Service Grant (P01 CA44530) awarded by the National Cancer Institute, Department of Health and Human Services.

REFERENCES

1. National Research Council, "Diet, Nutrition and Cancer," 1982, National Acad. Sci., Washington.
2. National Research Council, "Diet and Health," 1989, National Acad. Sci. Press, Washington.
3. L.W. Wattenberg, Cancer Res. Suppl.,1983, 43, 2448s.
4. L.W. Wattenberg, Cancer Res., 1985, 45, 1.
5. P.Talalay, M.J. De Long and H.J. Prochaska, Proc. Natl. Acad. Sci. USA, 1988, 85, 8261.
6. P. Talalay, Adv. Enzyme Regulat., 1989, 28, 237.
7. H. J. Prochaska, M.J. De Long and P. Talalay, Proc. Natl. Acad. Sci. USA, 1985, 82, 8232.
8. M.J. De Long, H.J. Prochaska and P. Talalay, Proc. Natl. Acad. Sci. USA, 1986, 83, 787.
9. H.J. Prochaska and A.B. Santamaria, Anal. Biochem., 1988, 169, 328.
10. H.J. Prochaska, A.B. Santamaria and P. Talalay, Proc. Natl. Acad. Sci. USA, 1992, 89, 2394.
11. H.J. Prochaska and P. Talalay, Cancer Res., 1988, 48, 4776.
12. Y. Zhang, P. Talalay, C.-G. Cho and G.H. Posner, Proc. Natl. Acad. Sci. USA, 1992, 89, 2399.
13. M.E. Daxenbichler, G.F. Spencer, D.G. Carlson, G.B. Rose, A.M. Brinker and R.G. Powell, Phytochemistry, 1991, 30, 2623.
14. M.J. De Long, H.J. Prochaska and P. Talalay, Cancer Res., 1985, 45, 546.
15. Y. Zhang, C.G. Cho, G.H. Posner and P. Talalay, Anal. Biochem., 1992, 205, 100.

QUANTITATION OF ISOTHIOCYANATES BY CYCLOCONDENSATION WITH 1,2-BENZENEDITHIOL

Y. Zhang,* C.-G. Cho,+ G.H. Posner,+ and P. Talalay*

*Department of Pharmacology and Molecular Sciences, The Johns Hopkins University School of Medicine, Baltimore, Maryland 21205, U.S.A. and

+Department of Chemistry, The Johns Hopkins University School of Arts and Sciences, Baltimore, Maryland 21218, U.S.A.

1 INTRODUCTION

A wide variety of isothiocyanates and their glucosinolate (thioglucoside N-hydroxysulfate) precursors are present in plants and their seeds.[1-3] These substances are commonly accompanied by the enzyme myrosinase (thioglucoside glucohydrolase; EC 3.2.3.1) which is released upon plant injury and hydrolyses glucosinolates, principally as follows:

$$R{-}C(S{-}C_6H_{11}O_5){=}NOSO_3^- + H_2O \xrightarrow{\text{Myrosinase}} R{-}N{=}C{=}S + HSO_4^- + C_6H_{12}O_6$$

Glucosinolate $\qquad$ Isothiocyanate $\qquad$ Glucose

Depending upon reaction conditions (e.g., pH) and the chemical structure of the glucosinolates, other products may also be formed (e.g., thiocyanates, nitriles, oxazolidinethiones).[4]

Since isothiocyanates and glucosinolates display a variety of biological, toxicological and therapeutic activities, measurement of their quantities, particularly in plants consumed by man is important.[2,4] Isothiocyanates are responsible for odors and flavors of plants and for the sharp taste of condiments such as horseradish and mustard. Some isothiocyanates are goitrogens. They also have antifungal and antibacterial activities. Recently, considerable interest has been focused on the role of isothiocyanates as inducers of detoxication enzymes in animal tissues,[5-7] and the associated protective effects of isothiocyanates and glucosinolates against chemical carcinogenesis.[5,8-10] For these reasons, a simple generic method for the sensitive and specific measurement of organic isothiocyanates was developed.[11]

2 RESULTS AND DISCUSSION

Principle of Method

The reaction of monothiols with many organic isothiocyanates leads to the rapid formation of relatively unstable thiocarbamates which have UV spectra that are not significantly more useful than the parent isothiocyanates for spectroscopic analyses. However when isothiocyanates react with vicinal dithiols, the UV spectral changes are more complex. The thiocarbamate formed by the addition of the first thiol group to the highly electrophilic carbon atom of the NCS group is susceptible to attack by the second thiol group. The ensuing cyclization leads to the formation of a trithiocarbonate and the expulsion of the nitrogen of the R-NCS group as the corresponding amine[11,12]. Reaction of isothiocyanates with an excess of 1,2-benzenedithiol (**1**) under mild conditions results in the stoichiometric formation of 1,3-benzodithiole-2-thione (**2**) which has highly favorable UV spectroscopic properties (λ_{max} 365 nm; a_m 23,000 $M^{-1}cm^{-1}$) for analytical purposes:

R—N=C=S + HS SH (**1**) ⟶ S=C S S (**2**) + $R—NH_2$

Most of the work in developing the analytical system was done with 1,2-benzenedithiol as reagent. Similar results have been obtained with 3,4-dimercaptotoluene which has the advantage of being a solid with a less offensive odor.

Standard Assay System. Based on this reaction, a standard assay system for isothiocyanates was developed. The reaction mixture contained in a final volume of 2.0 ml: 900 μl of 100 mM potassium phosphate buffer (pH 8.5), 900 μl of methanol, 100 μl of the isothiocyanate (1 - 100 nmol) to be determined in methanol or water, and 100 μl of 80 mM 1,2-benzenedithiol in methanol which was added last to initiate the reaction. The reaction mixtures were heated at 65°C for 60 min, and their absorbances were measured at 365 nm and corrected for appropriate blanks (reagents and solutions analyzed).

Chemical Specificity and Rates of Reaction of Isothiocyanates. As might be expected on the basis of the chemical mechanism, the reaction is specific for isothiocyanates. No change in absorption at 365 nm was observed in the standard system when 10 μM concentrations of KCN, KOCN, KSCN, C_6H_5COCN, $C_6H_5CH_2CN$, $C_6H_5CH_2NCO$ or $C_6H_5CH_2SCN$ were tested. Similarly several oxazolidinethiones and one glucosinolate (sinigrin; allyl glucosinolate) were completely unreactive.

All organic isothiocyanates tested including a variety of alkyl, arylalkyl, cyclohexyl, and phenyl isothiocyanates were fully reactive, except tert-butyl and other tertiary isothiocyanates.

The rates of reaction of various isothiocyanates were temperature-dependent and varied considerably. Thus under standard assay conditions phenyl-NCS reacted more rapidly than propyl-NCS, which in turn underwent cyclocondensation more rapidly than cyclohexyl-NCS. All isothiocyanates tested reacted quantitatively within the standard 60 min heating period at 65°C.

Applications

Identical linear calibration curves have been obtained over a wide range of concentrations from 2.5 to 100 nmol of propyl-NCS or phenyl-NCS, in the standard 2.0-ml assay system. Five-fold increases in sensitivity can be achieved by reducing the reaction volumes.

Measurement of Isothiocyanate Content of Chromatographic Fractions of Plant Extracts. Fractions of acetonitrile extracts of lyophilized broccoli obtained by reverse phase HPLC can be conveniently and rapidly analyzed for total isothiocyanate content by cyclocondensation with 1,2-benzenedithiol. The application of this procedure is illustrated in Figure 1 as reported by Zhang et al.[11] The peak fractions varied in isothiocyanate content from 6.39 nmol/ml to 1.09 μmol/ml. Recovery of added internal standards to these fractions was quantitative.

Measurement of Isothiocyanates in Crude Plant Extracts. Isothiocyanates are often present in rather low concenrations in crude aqueous or organic solvent extracts of plants, which may also have relatively high UV absorptions at 365 nm. The direct measurement of 1,3-benzodithiole-2-thiones may be difficult. Under these circumstances, a simple reverse phase HPLC procedure (Whatman Partisil 10-ODS2; isocratic elution with 80% methanol: 20% water) can be used to separate and quantitate the reaction product.

Measurement of Myrosinase Activity. The release of isothiocyanates from glucosinolates by the action of myrosinase can also be monitored by the cyclocondensation reaction. Other methods for assaying myrosinase activity are available. Monitoring of the liberation of glucose from glucosinolates lacks specificity, whereas measurement of the decline of UV absorption at 227 nm of sinigrin is difficult to apply when the activities of myrosinase are low. The present method does not have these limitations.

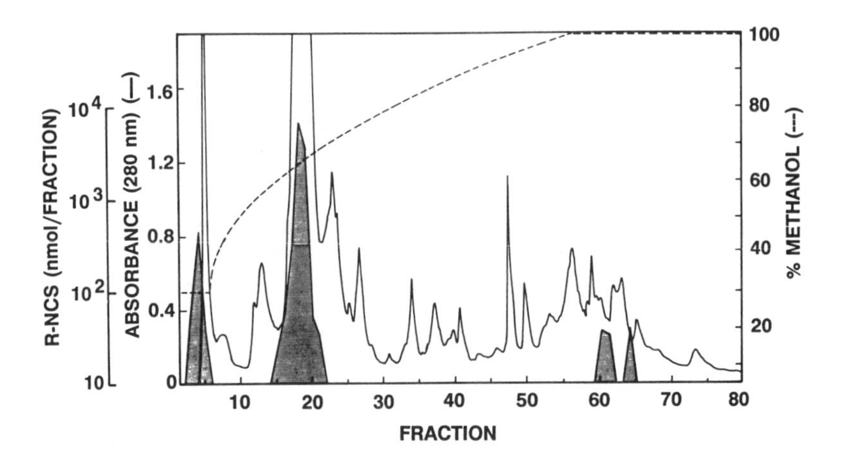

Figure 1 Reverse phase HPLC of acetonitrile extract of lyophilized broccoli. About 80 mg of extracted material was applied to a 1 x 50-cm preparative column and eluted with a gradient from methanol/water (30/70, by vol) to 100% methanol at a flow rate of 3 ml/min. The absorbance at 280 nm was monitored and 6.0-ml fractions were collected. Appropriate aliquots of each fraction were analyzed for isothiocyanate content by reaction with 1,2-benzenedithiol in the standard assay system. A total of 11 μmol of isothiocyanate was obtained in four regions of the chromatogram: Fractions 3-5, 535 nmol; Fractions 15-21, 10.4 μmol; Fractions 60-61, 72.4 nmol; and Fraction 64, 38.3 nmol. Note that the scale for isothiocyanates is logarithmic. (From Zhang et al.[11], with permission).

3 SUMMARY

Reaction of isothiocyanates with an excess of 1,2-benzenedithiol under mild conditions results in the quantitative formation of 1,3-benzodithiole-2-thione, which has favorable spectroscopic properties (λ_{max} 365 nm; a_m 23,000 $M^{-1}cm^{-1}$) for analytical purposes. Aliphatic, cycloaliphatic, and aromatic, but not tertiary isothiocyanates react quantitatively. Thiocyanates, cyanates, isocyanates, cyanides, and related compounds do not interfere with the assays. The method has been used to quantitate the isothiocyanate content of plant extracts and of chromatographic fractions obtained from such extracts, and for the assay of myrosinase (thioglucoside glucohydrolase; EC 3.2.3.1) activity.

Acknowledgements. These studies were supported by a U.S. Public Health Service Grant (P01 CA44530) awarded by the National Cancer Institute, Department of Health and Human Services.

REFERENCES

1. A. Kjaer, Fortschr. Chem. Org. Naturst., 1960, 18, 122.
2. G.R. Fenwick, R.K. Heaney and W.J. Mullin, CRC Crit. Rev. Food Sci. Nutr., 1983, 18, 123.
3. M.E. Daxenbichler, G.F. Spencer, D.G. Carlson, G.B. Rose, A.M. Brinker and R.G. Powell, Phytochemistry, 1991, 30, 2623.
4. H.L. Tookey, C.H. VanEtten and M.E. Daxenbichler, in: "Toxic Constituents of Plant Foodstuffs," (I.E. Liener, ed.), Academic Press, New York, 2nd Ed. 1980, pp. 103.
5. V.L. Sparnins, P.L. Venegas and L.W. Wattenberg, J. Natl. Cancer Inst., 1982, 68, 493.
6. P. Talalay, M.J. De Long and H.J. Prochaska, Proc. Natl. Acad. Sci. USA, 1988, 85, 2261.
7. Y. Zhang, P. Talalay, C.-G. Cho and G.H. Posner, Proc. Natl. Acad. Sci. USA, 1992, 89, 2399.
8. L.W. Wattenberg, A.B. Hanley, G. Barany, V.L. Sparnins, L.K.T. Lam and G.R. Fenwick, in: "Diet, Nutrition and Cancer" (Y. Hayashi et al., eds.), Japan Sci. Soc. Press, Tokyo/VNU Sci. Press, Utrecht, 1986, pp. 193.
9. L.W. Wattenberg, Cancer Res. 1985, 45, 1.
10. M.A. Morse, S.G. Amin, S.S. Hecht and F.-L. Chung, Cancer Res. 1989, 49, 2894.
11. Y. Zhang, C.-G. Cho, G.H. Posner and P. Talalay, Anal. Biochem., 1992, 205, 100.
12. C.-G. Cho and G.H. Posner, Tetrahedron Lett., 1992, 33, 3599.

THE BIOLOGICAL ASSAY OF NATURAL MUTAGENS USING THE P53 GENE

C. E. Couet, A. B. Hanley, S. Macdonald and L. Mayes

M.A.F.F. Food Science Laboratory
Norwich Research Park
Colney
Norwich NR4 7UQ

Natural toxicants comprise a significant and recognised hazard to health through their ingestion in foods and metabolism. The widespread occurrence of toxic principles in foods makes it important to target those which present the greatest risk.

A range of natural toxicants exhibit their toxic effect by binding to DNA thereby inducing errors in the replication and/or translation of the primary genetic material. Under certain circumstances the result of these mutational events can be the induction of the carcinogenic process leading to tumour formation. The link between adduct formation and cancer has been firmly established however the precise nature of that link and the factors which determine whether a given mutation will initiate a carcinogenic event are much less clear. Recent studies have implicated specific genes with the onset of tumour growth. One such gene is p53. Adduct formation at specific highly conserved regions of p53 has been found in a number of human cancers including some which are thought to be a result of ingestion of environmental carcinogens e.g. aflatoxins, N-nitroso compounds. The potential of p53 alterations as a biological assay method for natural carcinogens has been suggested. In order to adequately determine the usefulness of p53 as a predictive screen it is first of all necessary to discover if specific binding occurs in a suitable test system. The second step in the process is to determine if the binding of natural carcinogens follows a defined and predictable pattern and if so whether the structure of the mutagen will give any indication of the likelihood of exposure resulting in tumour formation. The preliminary studies outlined here describe an attempt to carry out the first stage of this process by investigating the specificity of binding of pyrrolizidine alkaloids[1] to a specific part of the sequence of the p53 gene.

Pyrrolizidine alkaloids occur in herbal remedies which contain comfrey (*Symphytum* spp.) and certain other plants. They are potent hepatotoxins and ingestion results in a condition known as veno-occlusive disease. In addition, the alkaloids are activated *in vivo* by P-450 type enzymes to give a pyrrolic intermediate which readily binds to DNA and is considered to induce cancer formation. A prerequisite for the formation of the pyrrole is the occurrence of a double bond between C-1 and C-2 of the base portion of the molecule. It follows therefore that alkaloids which lack this feature are unable to be activated to species which will form adducts with DNA.

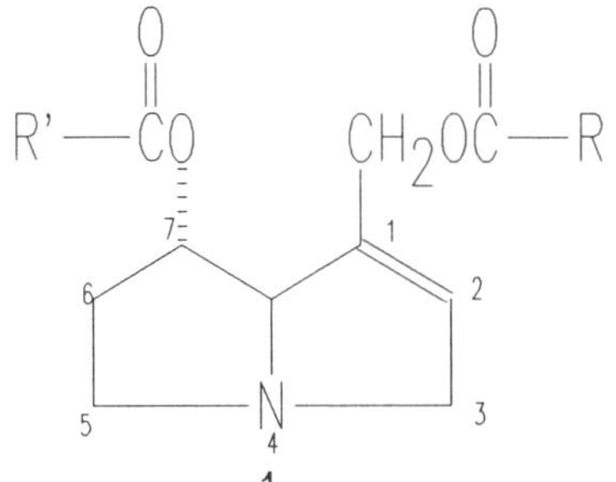

1

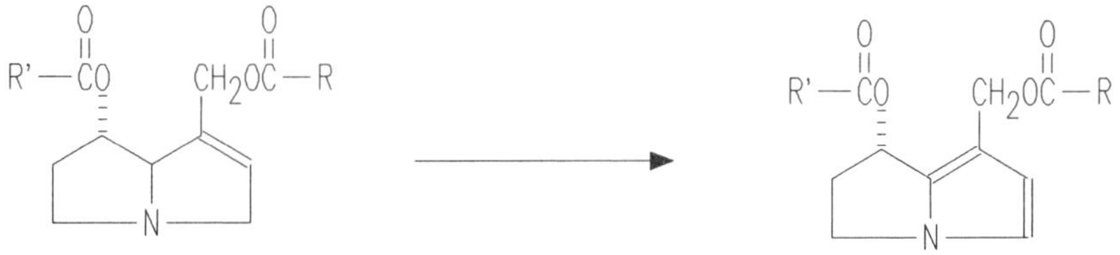

A range of pyrrolizidine alkaloids were activated using rat liver microsomes. Unfortunately, the yield of activated product was low probably because of the low level of P-450 type enzymes present in the preparation. Both chemical and enzymic activation were assessed as potential methods for production of metabolites, however, they proved to be incompatible with the cell cultures being used. A second source of activating enzymes was investigated - the mesocarp of avocado. A preparation from this source proved to be highly active in the metabolism of a range of pyrrolizidine alkaloids and hence was used in all subsequent studies.

The next stage in the process is the assay of the cell culture system for the section of the p53 gene of interest. A number of mutations have been detected in exon 7 of the gene and in particular at position 3 of codon 249. Both G-C and G-T transversions have been detected in tumor samples. Each of these mutations will result in the loss of a Pal I restriction site and this was the basis of the bioassay method. Two primers were constructed which were external to exon 7 - 5' - CTTGCCACAGGTCTCCCCAA-3' and the corresponding primer at the other end of the exon 5' -AGGGGTCAGCGGCAAGCAGA-3'.

These primers were used to probe DNA extracted from a human Chang liver cell line. A fragment of the expected size was isolated (236 base pairs) which contained a single Pal I site (GGCC) approximately mid way through the exon.

The Chang liver cells were challenged with three different pyrrolizidine alkaloids in an activating system which included avocado-derived P-450 enzymes. DNA isolation was carried out by pcr using the primers prepared previously and the isolated DNA checked by agarose gel electrophoresis. In all cases a fragment of the expected size was isolated. The DNA was then restricted with Pal I and run on a gel. A small amount of unrestricted DNA appeared to be present in those samples which had been incubated with the pyrrolizidine alkaloids although quantification was not possible. The restricted samples were amplified using pcr once again and analysed by gel electrophoresis. Those samples which had been incubated with the pyrrolizidine alkaloids contained a band of about 230 base pairs suggesting that the restriction site had been lost in some of the challenged cells.

Some work remains to be done to confirm these findings and to optimise the conditions, however, it would appear that mutations in one particular region of the p53 gene may provide some predictive information concerning the binding of carcinogens to DNA. The mechanism of binding and activation, the sequence of these events and how this relates to specificity of binding are also of interest.

WORKSHOP REPORT: RESEARCH TECHNIQUES - IN VIVO METHODOLOGIES

Dr Okezie I. Aruoma

Pharmacology Group
University of London King's College
Manresa Road
London
SW3 6LX
UK

The aim of the workshop was to address research techniques currently available, or becoming available, that would facilitate progress in our understanding of the multifactorial mechanisms involved in cancer. Cancer is one of the degenerative diseases of old age, although exogenous factors such as smoking in humans, alcohol and dietary factors may substantially influence it. Thus the relevance of various methodologies in food and toxicological research were discussed.

Discussions emanating from the conference as a whole suggest that foods, especially fruits and vegetables may afford protection against cancers of the epithelial cells. Indeed, all dietary components have to become available for them to have physiologically meaningful effects *in vivo*. The workshop argued that the characterization and quantification of the various components (carotenoids, retinols, tocopherols) in serum and in foods would facilitate a better interpretation of epidemiological studies. The role of lipid peroxidation (the free radical reaction upon lipids) and cancer was extensively discussed in the conference. It is not surprising that the detection and measurement of lipid peroxidation is often cited as evidence in support of the involvement of free radical reactions in toxicology and in human disease. It would be necessary to understand how lipid peroxidation of cellular importance relate to mechanisms of cell damage including oxidation of proteins, inactivation of enzymes, loss of ionic homeostasis and damage to genetic material. Lipid peroxidation damages cells directly by attacking membrane structures and indirectly by releasing reactive products. Oxidation to lipoproteins is implicated in atherogenesis.

Due to the variety of topics discussed at the workshop, it has been possible only to comment briefly on each of the contributions, and where further information is required, readers are invited to peruse the related chapters in this volume.

<u>*In vivo* markers of free radical reactions</u>

Free radicals and other reactive oxygen species (ROS) are constantly formed in the human body and have been implicated in human diseases such as cancer, rheumatoid, malaria, atherosclerosis and in autoimmune deficiency syndrome (AIDS). It remains to be fully established whether oxidative stress makes a significant contribution to the pathology of a given disease or whether it is merely an epiphenomenon. Specific assays applicable to human patients would greatly contribute to progress in our understanding of the role played by free radicals in normal physiology and in human diseases. Although many of the ROS can serve useful physiological functions, they can be toxic when generated in excess and this toxicity is often aggravated by the presence of ions of such transition metals as iron and copper. There is a need to develop *in vivo* markers for assessing free radical reactions. Methods involving analysis of DNA by GC/MS/SIM (and by the COMET assay discussed below), and analysis of uric acid oxidation products and products of aromatic hydroxylation are currently being evaluated. Measurement of DNA damage by free radicals using the technique of gas chromatography with selected ion monitoring has been discussed in the chapter by Aruoma and Halliwell in this volume.

<u>Establishing a biomarker for DNA damage in lymphocytes</u>

The COMET assay (single cell gel electrophoresis assay) was discussed as a method for measuring DNA damage in isolated cells and as a method for studying genotoxic and antigenotoxic effects in the gastro-intestinal tract *in vivo*. The assay is performed as follows (contributed by Dr Andrew Collins); cells suspended in a low melting point agarose are layered on a microscope slide and the agarose allowed to set. The cells are then lysed by incubating at 4°C with triton X 100 and histones are removed from DNA with 2.5 M NaCl. The slides are transferred to a solution of high pH (0.3M NaOH) and electrophoresed. DNA is attracted to the anode but it is able to move only if there are strand breaks. After neutralisation, DNA is stained with a suitable dye, such as DAPI and the slides are examined by fluorescent microscopy.

In control untreated cells, the fluorescent image resembles a nucleus with little or no DNA extending on to the anode. When cells contain DNA damage, the images are 'COMET' like, as DNA is pulled from the 'nucleus' into a 'tail', and the relative intensity of fluorescence in the tail increases with the amount of DNA damage. As few as 100 DNA breaks per cell can be detected.

The COMET assay is rapid, simple and reproducible. It is readily applied to lymphocytes isolated from a small sample of blood. It can be used to examine *in vivo* effects of treatment with genotoxic agent and/or a particular nutritional regime in terms of DNA breakage. It will also detect variations between individuals without experimental treatment, for example, in comparison of human populations representing different lifestyle, diet or exposure to occupational or environmental mutagens.

The DNA repair assays with *E. coli* K-12 strains

DNA repair assays with *E. coli* K-12 strains are based on the comparison of the survival rates of otherwise isogenic strains which differ in DNA repair capacity (uvrB/recB vs. uvr^+/rec^+). In animal mediated assays, mixtures of the two strains (1-2 x 10^8 cells per animal) are injected iv. into animal hosts (mice) which have been treated with a DNA damaging agent and additionally with various doses of a putative antigenotoxin. Furthermore, positive and negative control groups are included. After 2-3 hrs exposure, the bacteria can be recovered from various organs (liver, spleen, kidneys, blood, testes, stomach, intestine, and colon) and the individual strain survival determined by plating appropriate dilutions of the organ homogenates on Neutral red-Streptomycin agar (three plates per dilution). Longer exposure times in the host animals are not feasible due to intrinsic genotoxicity occurring also in chemically untreated animals which is probably due to phagocytosis. In order to enable precise measurements in stomach, intestine, and colon, the animals have been deprived of feed 24 hrs before exposure of the indicator cells and the remaining contents of the GI tract have to be removed before homogenisation. The strains can be distinguished by their colour morphology: The repair deficient strain is lac^+ and forms red colonies, the repair proficient parental strain is lac^- and forms white colonies; both strains were made streptomycin resistant to prevent contaminations of the selective media plates. Reduction of the viability of the repair deficient counterpart serves as a measure for the induction of repairable DNA damage. The test system is sensitive towards a variety of genotoxins including those contained in foodstuffs such as nitrosamines, cooked food mutagens, mycotoxins, and polycyclic aromatic hydro-carbons. In order to obtain positive results with PAHs, it is necessary to permeabilize the indicator cells by short EDTA treatment. Representatives of various groups of putative interceptor compounds have been tested. It was possible to show that (i) results obtained in long term carcinogenicity experiments are in good agreement with findings obtained in DNA repair assays in *vivo*. For example, the decrease of carcinogenic potency in nitrosamines by isothiocyanates is paralleled by reduction of DNA damage. (ii) several compounds which act as antimutagens *in vitro* were effective or gave only marginal effects at extremely high doses *in vivo*. (iii) In contrast to *in vitro* procedures the system enables one to define the experimental conditions under which a protective compound is effective, e.g. chlorophyll and isothiocyanates were only protective when given simultaneously or shortly before the genotoxins. Discussions reported here were contributed by Dr Knasmuller and his colleague Dr

Schulte-Herman.

Effects of dietary flavonoids on the binding of ^{3}H-aflatoxin B_1 to hepatic DNA

The experiment contributed by Dr LeBon involved feeding rats a purified diet supplemented with 3000 ppm flavonoid for two weeks. The animals were then treated with ^{3}H-AFB1 (intraperitoneal administration) two hours before sacrifice. Hepatic DNA was isolated and the level of specific binding of ^{3}H-aflatoxin B1 to DNA measured. Rats fed non-hydroxylated flavonoids such as flavone, flavonone and tangeretin showed lower AFB1 binding to DNA. In contrast, polyhydroxylated compounds such as quercetin had no effect on the aflatoxin binding to DNA.

Simultaneous determination of variation carotenoids, retinol and tocopherol in serum samples by means of HPLC

Dr Begona Olmedila informed the workshop that the characterization of these reportedly protective compounds both in foods and human serum, is essential for a better interpretation of epidemiological studies. *In vivo*, most of the compounds act synergistically and must not be considered separately with regard to their role in cancer preservation. Carotenoids are normal constituents of human blood and tissues. Carotenoids are introduced into the human body in their natural form through dietary intake, mainly from fruits and vegetables and in the form of food additives. Their presence in greater or lesser proportion in human serum varies according to the origin of the population studied. It is generally accepted, however, that such carotenoid levels and composition is proportional to the amount of carotenoid ingested in the diet, although their destruction in the gastrointestinal tract and the pharmacokinetic profile of the individual can affect the levels *in vivo*. An HPLC method that allows simultaneous determination of carotenoids is now available, and is applicable to human samples and vegetable samples (see the chapter by Olmedilla *et al* in this volume).

Evaluation of a simple, direct technique to assess changes in colonic cell proliferation *in vivo*

The workshop discussions then switched to considerations of colorectal cancer and the techniques for the identification of intermediate biomarkers of neoplasia and to gain an insight into the relationship between dietary factors and colorectal cancer.

Gee and Matthew informed the workshop of technique to assess increased cell proliferation (the full version is described in their paper in this volume). The method involves counting dividing cells in microdissected crypts from human biopsies, and provides information on their distribution within the crypt. The technique was reported to be fast and relatively inexpensive and could be applied to stored tissues. The technique is suited to large scale experimental studies concerned with the relationship between diet and colorectal cancer.

Role of dietary components in the aetiology of colorectal cancer

Dr John Mathers commented that intervention trials provide some of the most convincing evidence about the role of food components in the aetiology of colon cancer. However, such studies are difficult to carry out successfully with volunteers from the general public because the relatively low risk for any one individual means that a large number of people must be studied over a long period of time to have any hope of demonstrating a significant effect. Poor compliance may be an additional problem.

An alternative strategy is to work with individuals who are at enhanced risk and who may be more readily motivated to participate in the necessary experiments. Individuals carrying the gene for Familial Adenomatous Polyposis (FAP) represent an ideal human model of colorectal cancer. Most affected individuals develop multiple colonic polyps in the teenage years, one or more of which will develop into cancer in 10-15 years. In some individuals polyps do not occur until the 20s or 30s and dietary factors may be important in this delay. The adenomas in FAP are identical to those in sporadic cancer. Evidence available to data suggests that the formation of adenomas in FAP can be modified by dietary or pharmalogical means despite the strong genetic influence.

DMH rat model for colon cancer study

The colon carcinogen 1,2-dimethylhydrazine (DMH) is frequently used to study colon carcinogenesis in animal models. DMH induces tumours which are similar to those seen in humans. Alink *et al* in this volume, have discussed their study which examined the modulating effect of heat processing and of vegetable and fruit in human diet and of vegetable and fruit in animal diets on the DMH-induced colon carcinogenesis in rats. Dr Graeme McIntosh observed that the DMH rat model is a convincing model of cancer. Studies take 6-8 months. However, unless users choose a responsive strain of rat and use a well defined diet they will not be able to produce reproducible and comparable results.

Secondly, with DMH given in smaller and fewer doses, one can reduce number of tumours/animal and incidence to a level which maximises the sensitivity of dietary perturbation. We have been able to produce some interesting observational data on differing influence of protein sources and dietary fibre types (fibres are very different in their effects) on incidence, tumour burden and tumour mass index (10g transformed area of all tumours per rat).

I would like to thank Andrew Collins, Siegfried Knasmuller, Anne-Marie LeBon, Begona Olmedilla, Jenny Matthew, John Mathers, Jenny Gee, Graeme McIntosh and Beatrice Pool-Zobel for their contribution to the workshop discussions and hence this report.

WORKSHOP REPORT: IN VITRO METHODOLOGY

G. Williamson

AFRC Institute Of Food Research
Norwich Laboratory
Norwich Research Park
Colney Lane
Norwich
NR4 7UA

The workshop considered the ways of measuring protective or carcinogenic properties of dietary small molecules. The methodology involving macromolecules and the action of, for example, dietary fibre was not discussed.

The use of the Talalay assay using Hepa1c1c7 cells in culture was extensively discussed. The assay detects compounds that induce quinone reductase in mouse hepatoma cells. The effect on the levels of some cytochrome P_{450} enzymes can also be determined in this system by the use of mutants defective in the Ah receptor. It was agreed that this method is an excellent screening method, provided that the limitations were appreciated. Rather than detect all phase II inducers, which includes other enzymes such as UDP-glucuronyltransferase and other glutathione S-transferases, it is specific for compounds which interact via either the Ah receptor/xenobiotic responsive element (including P_{450}1A1 or 1A2) or the antioxidant responsive element (glutathione S-transferase α or quinone reductase). Other assays are therefore required for detection of compounds which do not act via these systems.

The detection of carcinogens was also dealt with. The methodology involved in the Ames Salmonella mutagenicity test was discussed, and it was generally agreed that this assay is a good indication of the potential carcinogenicity of a compound but that the answer tends to be either "yes" or "no" without quantitative information. The use of this test together with the Williams hepatocyte assay, was recommended for the general detection of carcinogens.

PART 9 IMPLICATIONS FOR PUBLIC HEALTH

IMPLICATIONS FOR DIETARY GUIDANCE

W. P. T. James

Rowett Research Institute
Bucksburn
Aberdeen AB2 9SB

1 INTRODUCTION

Other plenary lectures have been concerned with the detailed mechanisms and issues relating to the link between diet and cancer. The question is whether we are now in a position to provide advice on dietary prevention.

Rather than assessing the application of previous contributions I propose to take an unusual tack in order to anticipate problems which those involved in policy-making will meet when they come to advocate dietary change. My assumption is that those who do propose dietary prevention will be exposed to criticisms which range from the cogent to the personal. Only two factors may mitigate the criticism: the recognition that the suggested changes are justified primarily because they will prevent other conditions, e.g. coronary heart disease, and secondly an acceptance that cancer is so unpleasant that preventive measures may be justified even without reasonable evidence for the efficacy of these proposals.

Fat intake in relation to cardiovascular disease has a very strong 40-year-old base of intensive physiological, biochemical and molecular biological research. Serum cholesterol measurements are now considered crude risk factors for those advocating dietary changes for heart disease because any self-respecting physician knows that the array of lipoproteins, each with their metabolic role and physiological control, contribute to this crude index. Physicians, unused to thinking about multiple effects of several dietary components on these lipoproteins, demanded fully controlled intervention trials, the results of which are now intensely disputed[1].

What a contrast then with our understanding of the dietary basis for carcinogenesis! Although saturated fatty acid intake has been linked, as has total fat intake, to colon and breast cancer, these associations are essentially based on cross-cultural human studies and on experimental studies where different types of fat have been added to the diet of animals given carcinogens. In Willett's prospective epidemiological studies the links between fatty acid intakes and breast cancer are negligible or even inversely related[2]. This finding has been criticized on the grounds that the range of fat intakes within the U.S. group is comparatively small[3], but a plan to assess the value of low fat diets in the prevention of breast cancer has been stalled.

Developing a Strategy for Cancer Prevention

Issues which need to be considered are (a) the unusual problems in cancer prevention in terms of development time and individual susceptibility; (b) the current paucity of biomarkers of risk; (c) the multiplicity of inhibitors, blockers, promoters and retarders of carcinogenesis and, finally, in a different domain the retention of scientific credibility by those who advocate preventive measures. If all these problems can be dealt with then we have another series of issues: (i) current concerns relating to energy intake, both in aetiological terms and when translating dietary advice into practice for individual use; (ii) the potential value of identifying high risk groups; (iii) the practical problems of considering the role of prevention in individuals who are middle-aged or elderly; (iv) how to use population goals when advocating individual action; (v) how to effect dietary change in populations with no overriding sense of personal responsibility for health, and (vi) how best to combat the commercial pressures of those whose interests are vested in promoting or at least maintaining current inappropriate diets.

The Long-term Nature of Carcinogenesis

The long-term nature of carcinogenesis presents substantial problems in analysing the role of diet and these are not just confined to dietary monitoring. Carcinogenesis requires a series of different steps each of which may be affected by different dietary factors. Thus, were we to concentrate on the initiation step with nutritional change, then we might need to set up a very different study from that which would be required for assessing the factors which modulate the promotional phase. One example, stomach cancer, should suffice to show some of the contradictions in preventive policies.

Stomach Cancer

Although the rates of stomach cancer are falling throughout the world, it is still the commonest cancer. Evidence suggests that the first phase in the carcinogenic process may involve mucosal changes in the stomach, occurring in early childhood, with metaplastic transformation induced by bacterial infection. Thus the gastric mucosa changes to the intestinal form with a loss in the acid secreting capacity of the stomach. There is then a greater likelihood of sustained bacterial growth in the stomach if bacterially contaminated foods are ingested. Migrants with this form of gastric mucosa retain their high risk of stomach cancer, even if they migrate early from a high risk country such as Colombia to a lower risk country, e.g. the U.S.[4]

The initiation of mutational change may depend not only on nitrosamine ingestion, e.g. from smoked fish, but on nitrosamine formation from gastric nitrite. This formation of N-nitroso compounds may well be inhibited by ascorbic acid but the production is markedly enhanced by gastric bacteria which readily proliferate in a stomach with a reduced capacity to secrete acid. Thus the enhanced risk of gastric carcinoma in pernicious anaemia has been ascribed to the bacterial proliferation in the stomach and the formation of endogenous nitrosamines from nitrite[5]. Nitrite in turn is now recognized to be very dependent on endogenous nitrite formation within the body from ingested nitrate.

Based on this plausible sequence of metabolic transformations, it was proposed that dietary nitrate, nitrite and N-nitroso compounds should be restricted. In the absence of 1% of the evidence needed for regulatory change to prevent cardiovascular disease, extensive monitoring of the nitrosamine content of foods was started and changes in food smoking were introduced. Production systems for beer, fish and meat products changed. The use of nitrite as a food preservative was then re-examined with alternatives being rapidly introduced by the food industry. Now we are confronted by legislation which sets down limits to the nitrate concentrations of drinking water which, on a European scale, is involving society in huge investments on water purification systems and massive changes in fertilizer practice. All these changes, it should be noted, were introduced at great expense on the basis of a suggested metabolic sequence for dietary nitrate involvement in stomach carcinogenesis. Yet there is no real evidence that dietary nitrate intakes determine nitrosamine formation and no formal trials have been made of the value of nitrate intake reduction. Nevertheless the medical profession has, for the most part, quietly accepted the politician's response to popular concern about the supposed risk of stomach cancer.

Stomach Cancer and Salt Intake

It is claimed that the use of highly salted foods helps to maintain an abnormal and rather atrophic gastric mucosa or that the salt damages the mucosal barrier which otherwise resists the penetration and action of N-nitroso compounds[6]. Joosens[7] has confidently linked the worldwide decline in stomach cancer to the concomitant decline in the incidence of strokes. The risk of a stroke is now widely accepted as related to an individual's blood pressure and societal stroke rates show a strong correlation with the population's average blood pressure[8]. Yet it is noticeable that the preventive push for reducing salt intake has come from those involved in trying to combat hypertension.

Given the multiplicity of problems in convincing the medical establishment that salt had anything to do with the development of hypertension, consider how much more difficult it would have been if monitoring of blood pressure had not been introduced and if, without this biological marker of the body responses to sodium and the value of blood pressure monitoring as a risk marker for stroke, we had to contend with attempting to link salt intakes to the incidence of strokes. That, in effect, is the problem we deal with when discussing the role of sodium in the development of stomach cancer.

High Risk Group Strategies

This concept is high on the agenda of those who deal with cardiovascular disease. Physicians, dominated by their clinical view of the idiosyncratic nature of individual susceptibility to disease, feel more comfortable dealing with concepts of genetic susceptibility and high risk groups as do toxicologists and others who advise food industrialists on the latest food/health scare. All three groups are very suspicious of what are seen to be grand proposals for social engineering the population's food intake by those who have a public health perspective. Unfortunately, in cancer prevention, it is much more difficult to identify high risk groups than in cardiovascular disease. Genetic or familial factors do apply but their specificity is modest at best. In a high risk Colombian population it is possible to identify a recessive autosomal gene with variable penetrance depending on age and whether or not the mother has chronic atrophic gastritis (CAG). This determines the risk of developing CAG but this has a low rate of prediction for stomach cancer itself[9]. Similarly there is now clear evidence of a familial propensity to breast cancer. In women with a strong family history of breast cancer, e.g. in a young sister, then the empirical risk of breast cancer by the age of 65 approaches 50%, a risk compatible with a fully penetrant dominant condition[10] but when the population is assessed, genetic susceptibility is identified as applying to only 4% of the families studied[11]. Again in colonic cancer there is the well-recognized familial disease of polyposis coli with an enhanced susceptibility to colon cancer; this is also true of those with specific gene constructs[12] but genetic probes are not yet available to assess how much this could contribute to a high risk approach to cancer prevention.

Smokers as a High Risk Group

We are left with only one high risk group that is readily identifiable and which has been woefully neglected in prevention strategies, i.e. the smokers. Smokers have obviously been targeted to encourage them to give up smoking, but no effort seems to have been made to modify their dietary habits as they give up smoking nor when they continue to smoke despite advice to the contrary. Smoking induces a marked increase in micronuclear formation in bronchial epithelium this being reduced by ß-carotene supplements[13] and smoking accounts for an extra 30 mg/day oxidation of ascorbic acid, now recognized as needed for the stability of DNA, e.g. in the sperm of young men[14]. Given the increasing evidence for the preventive role of ß-carotene in ameliorating the risk of lung cancer in heavy smokers[15] it seems extraordinary that so little emphasis has been put on attempting to reduce the high risks of smoking other than by attempting to persuade people to overcome their addiction. Dietary measures are required to prevent people from gaining weight after stopping smoking[16] but it seems even more important to encourage a plentiful consumption of fruit and vegetables.

Block and her colleagues[17], in reviewing the literature on about 200 trials which have examined the possible link between fruit and vegetable consumption, finds an amazing consistency of evidence with a 2-4 fold benefit in risk for a huge range of cancers if the subjects were eating well above average intakes for that population. With such coherence from so many trials it seems reasonable to identify this issue as the single most convincing dietary relationship in the field. It is also interesting to note that those cancers with the strongest evidence for a link with smoking were those where the greatest benefit was evident when people consumed a plentiful supply of vegetables and fruit.

A special dietary preventive strategy for smokers seems to me overdue and the promotion of vegetables and fruit consumption seems now justified as a cancer preventive measure on a societal basis. This advice is presented in the absence of formal clinical controlled trials which is increasingly being demanded as the only acceptable form of rigorous assessment before public policies are developed. To impose that demand in relation to carcinogenesis seems, however, unreasonable.

Dietary Energy Intake

It has been accepted for over 40 years (e.g. Tannenbaum[18]) that animals which grow more slowly by having their total food intake or their protein intake restricted develop fewer spontaneous tumours and live considerably longer than *ad libitum* fed animals. This has led to the concept that energy intake itself is of crucial importance to carcinogenesis and that we should attempt to persuade people to restrict their food intake as a preventive measure. The pressure to do this was amplified when a number of studies seemed to show that those groups with a higher energy intake also had the highest cancer risk. Some biological plausibility for the argument also developed when Ames showed a cross-species relationship between energy turnover and free radical induced DNA damage[19].

Those of us who are involved in the physiological regulation of energy balance recognize that the total energy need of individuals is heavily influenced by four components: height, which tends therefore to influence weight, weight itself once corrected for height, age and physical activity[20]. Thus a population which is tall, overweight but physically active, e.g. some groups of young Americans, will have much higher energy needs than short, thin and perhaps relatively inactive Indonesians. Thus, cross-cultural studies of energy intake in relation to carcinogenesis are often flawed because in simple terms the human machine is bigger in one society than in another. The metabolic rate per unit active tissue mass is, however, usually identical with very little evidence of energy adaptation to supposedly poor conditions[21]. An individual's metabolic rate is highly consistent and appetite, despite social pressures, is amazingly well-regulated such that attempts to semi-starve demand intense self-discipline to overcome the physiological drive to eat. Advising people to cut down on their food intake as a preventive measure is therefore crude and unscientific advice which is likely to meet with little or no success as many involved in treating overweight and obese patients will agree.

Physical activity, however, is another component of increased energy expenditure which is sometimes associated with a protective role in cancer despite increasing evidence that it does impose a free radical stress on the body presumably because of free electron leakage from the highly active muscle mitochondria. However, local scavenging systems seem to deal with this problem and tumour formation is exceedingly rare in muscle.

This dismissal of the role of energy intake in human carcinogenesis does not mean that Tannenbaum's studies were ill-conceived, nor that the issue of energy requirements is not fundamental to the development of dietary advice (see below). Indeed, Tannenbaum's studies may highlight fundamental issues relating to the altered hepatic metabolism of components, e.g. steroids or carcinogens which modulate carcinogenesis. The programming of oncogene responsiveness, mitochondrial free radical scavenging systems or the efficacy of DNA repair systems may also be affected. Biochemical and molecular biological approaches to these issues are now underway at my Institute: early programming of gene expression has been highlighted recently but similar work now needs to be undertaken on gene stability.

Interpreting Nutrient Goals

In WHO[8] we developed a set of nutrient goals (Table 1) which have led to considerable controversy either because vested interests, e.g. in the sugar industry, chose to misinterpret the proposals, or because some scientists who also earn money from journalism decided to produce a polemic against nutrient goals in general[22]. This was happily backed by some components of the food industry, e.g. the confectionery, soft drinks and butter fat industries, to the embarrassment of the more responsible food industrialists who recognize the importance of responding to long-term consumer requirements rather than short-term marketing needs. One justified criticism of the WHO report, however, was that we failed to spell out for the older scientists and doctors associated with the food industry what the new concepts in public health meant and how to use these nutrient goals.

As the original WHO report on cardiovascular disease made clear[23] a population strategy depends on identifying populations as well as individuals at risk and shifting population distribution rather than extensive consensus in an effort to reduce disease. This concept has been beautifully set out by Rose more recently[24]. Thus a total fat goal of 30% energy is the average for a population. This allows a distribution of intakes around the 30% value and does not mean that a specific intake of 30% is prescribed for everybody. Similarly it does not prescribe any of the many dietary means by which an individual might achieve a nutrient target of say 25-35% fat. The translation of nutrient goals into dietary goals is a society specific and indeed an individual matter which those of us in public health policymaking choose not to tackle. This neglect, however, opens the way for much misinterpretation by dietitians, the public and industrialists. There is therefore a real need to tackle this issue.

The second misunderstanding about the WHO targets was our introduction of a lower set of goals. This stemmed from a sense of global responsibility rather than a parochial U.S. or Northern European approach. Many societies with far greater populations than in the West have very different diets, e.g. China, with a fat intake of about 14-15%. To specify a fat goal of 30-35% would then be grossly irresponsible, particularly since our cancer specialists on the WHO study group perceived that as fat intakes rose beyond 15% proportionately more cancers might occur. We therefore chose to assess whether there was a minimum level of a nutrient which was necessary.

Table 1 Population Nutrient Goals

	Limits for population average intakes	
	Lower	Upper
Total energy	see important footnote[a]	
Total fat (% total energy)	15	30[b]
Saturated fatty acids (% total energy)	0	10
Polyunsaturated fatty acids (% total energy)	3	7
Dietary cholesterol (mg/day)	0	300
Total carbohydrate (% total energy)	55	75
Complex carbohydrate[c] (% total energy)	50	70
Dietary fibre[d] (g/day)		
As non-starch polysaccharides (NSP)	16	24
As total dietary fibre	27	40
Free sugars[e] (% total energy)	0	10
Protein (% total energy)	10	15
Salt (g/day)	–[f]	6

[a] Energy intake needs to be sufficient to allow for normal childhood growth, for the needs of pregnancy and lactation, and for work and desirable physical activities, and to maintain appropriate body reserves of energy in children and adults. Adult populations on average should have a body mass index (BMI) of 20-22 (BMI = body mass in kg/[height in metres]^2).

[b] An interim goal for nations with high fat intakes; further benefits would be expected by reducing fat intake towards 15% of total energy.

[c] A daily minimum intake of 400 g of vegetables and fruits, including at least 30 g of pulses, nuts, and seeds, should contribute to this component.

[d] Dietary fibre includes the non-starch polysaccharides (NSP), the goals for which are based on NSP obtained from mixed food sources. Since the definition and measurement of dietary fibre remain uncertain, the goals for total dietary fibre have been estimated from the NSP values.

[e] These sugars include monosaccharides, disaccharides, and other short-chain sugars produced by refining carbohydrates.

[f] Not defined.

In the case of free refined sugars, dietary cholesterol and saturated fatty acids, there is not a known absolute requirement for these nutrients, so a value of 0% was assigned much to the fury of the industrialists who perceived this, incorrectly, as threatening. Where there was a minimum need, e.g. total fat, sodium or fibre, a judgement had to be made. This involved complex issues including the energy needs of the varying populations around the world. Thus nations with a high birth rate and a disproportionate population of young people have in general a lower food need per head than an aging population where adults predominate[20].

The issue of diet and cancer was considered extensively. It led to a modest upper goal for polyunsaturated fatty acid (PUFA) intake because of increasing concern that too high a PUFA intake might be disadvantageous. The 30% upper value for total fat was also specified as possibly too high, mainly because of the concern about cancer rates worldwide. The innovative piece of advice, however, was to advocate a 400 g goal for daily fruit and vegetable consumption (potato consumption is additional). This goal was derived by reference to the food balance sheets for the Mediterranean countries and stemmed from a wish to recognize the probable protective role of fruit and vegetables.

The fibre goal was expressed primarily in non-starch polysaccharide (NSP) terms but was expressly not related to cancer rates. At that stage we had our original data on the Scandinavian cross-cultural studies on large bowel cancer[25] but this was considered insufficient. It was also thought politic to calculate NSP needs purely on the basis of preventing constipation. By using the then unpublished faecal weight to NSP intake relationship and variances produced by Cummings we were able to back calculate to the likely needs on an energy basis for different populations. We set an upper and a lower limit which took account of varying population energy requirements and the intake needed to minimise the proportion of people who would run the risk of becoming constipated by having a faecal output below 100 g per day. Many a would-be critic, hoping to castigate us for invoking a protective role for fibre in colon cancer, has fallen silent when the method and purpose of the calculation is explained!

Translating Nutrient Goals into Dietary Targets

It is important to appreciate that individuals vary in their energy needs and that the use of nutrient goals in nutrition education is currently nonsensical because it is beyond the wit of anyone to work out rapidly how to achieve an intake of total fat, for example, which is 20% of energy needs. Considerable training and a well-above-average intelligence, combined with computational skills are needed to achieve this target. We therefore developed in the Coronary Prevention Group a new mode of food labelling based on the energy content, not the weight of a food[26]. This is fundamental to consumers because expressing nutrients on a weight basis is only helpful if an absolute intake is required. This applies to non-starch polysaccharide or protein intake, the latter being expressed on a weight basis. Nevertheless, the big issues of the day relate to dietary factors, many of which are given targets proportional to energy needs. There is currently little governmental or international response to these suggested measures for labelling food because insufficient effort has been made by voluntary organisations and there is huge inertia in governmental circles by officers who either do not understand the issues or feel foolish for advocating inappropriate approaches for so long.

A different and practical approach to implementing dietary change is shown in Figures 1A & B, based on simple, energy-related procedures for estimating adults' needs

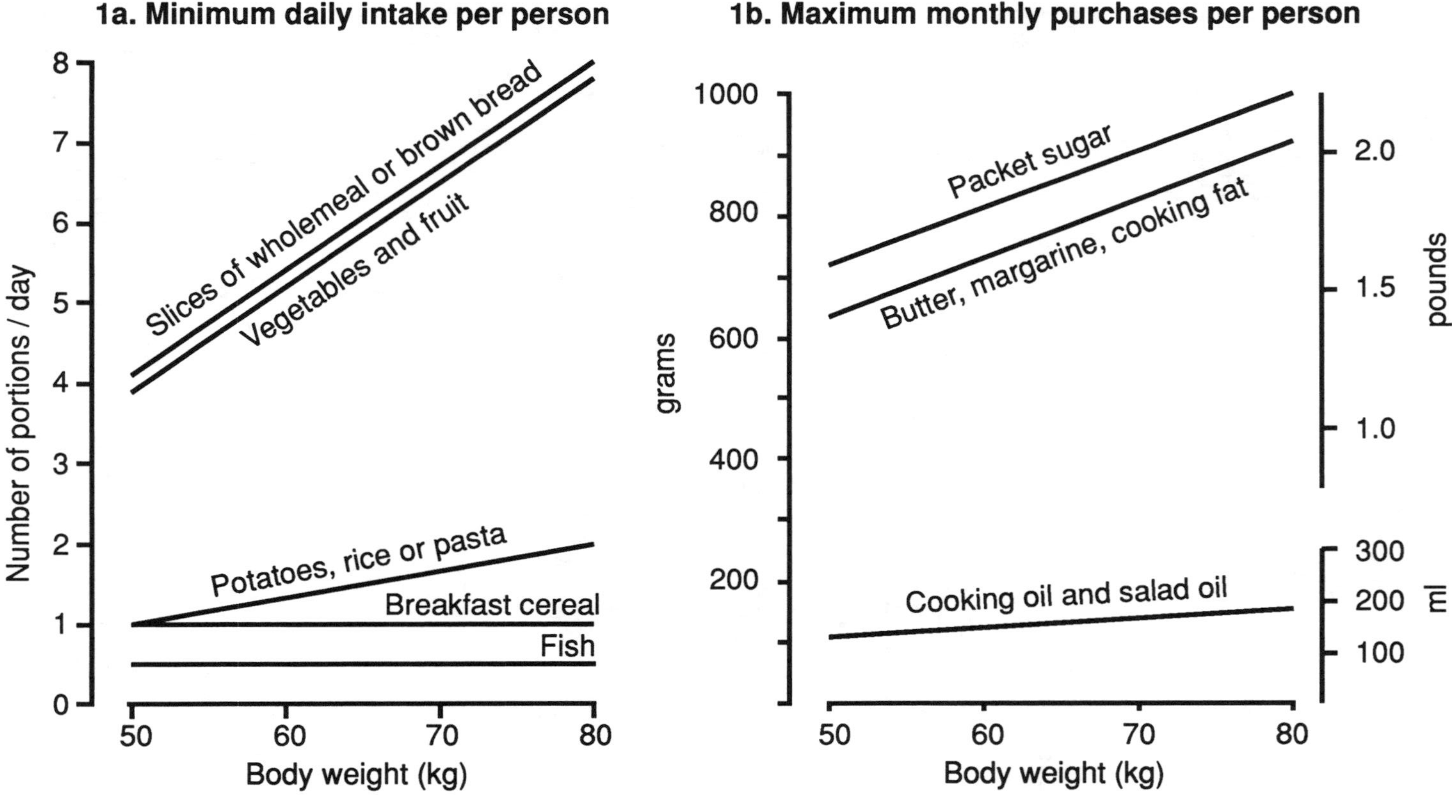
1a. Minimum daily intake per person
Number of portions / day
0
1
2
3
4
5
6
7
8
Slices of wholemeal or brown bread
Vegetables and fruit
Potatoes, rice or pasta
Breakfast cereal
Fish
50
60
70
80
Body weight (kg)
1b. Maximum monthly purchases per person
grams
200
400
600
800
1000
Packet sugar
Butter, margarine, cooking fat
Cooking oil and salad oil
1.0
1.5
2.0
pounds
100
200
300
ml
50
60
70
80
Body weight (kg)

for NSP, total fat and the WHO goals for free sugars, saturated fatty acids and vegetable and fruit intake. Note that NSP intakes will be proportional to body weight thus the population goals (Table 1) should **not** be applied to children who need a proportional goal based on their energy needs when compared with a population reference energy target of 10 MJ. Thus young children should receive only 50% of the 24 g advocated, i.e. 12 g once they are over the age of 2 years and on a full mixed diet. Similarly, salt intake should not be set at 6 g/day for everyone. Very little salt comes from discretionary use[27] so salt intakes tend to be proportional to energy needs also and can be calculated as 3-6 g/10MJ and then related to individual energy needs.

Advice to the Middle-aged and Elderly

The accumulating evidence on stomach, breast, colon and prostate cancer suggests that we need to take a fresh look at the question of whether preventive advice should be developed for the middle-aged and elderly. It seems that the propensity to stomach and breast cancer may be set at an early age. Yet, for stomach cancer, the progressive fall in its incidence, with an arrest in this fall during wartime in Norway, and the preventive role of adult vegetable intake, all point to the opportunity for changing the incidence rates of stomach cancer during adulthood. If the experimental evidence for ß-carotene suppressing the progression of early gastric cancer to infiltrating tumours in rats[28] holds true in current studies on the role of ß-carotene in preventing gastric cancer in heavy smokers then this will amplify the potential importance of dietary change in middle life.

It should also be remembered that our approach to the elderly is undergoing drastic revision since the elderly are physiologically very similar to the middle-aged - at least up to the age of 75 years. For the following decade 85% of elderly live at home so we are coming to recognize that one should consider a life expectancy of 25 years for those retiring at 60 years of age. This 25 year period is a time when profound effects might be achieved by maintaining gene stability by dietary means. This will, however, require a completely different approach to the diet in the elderly since they have usually been targeted simply for food supplements when their real need is to maintain absolute intakes of micronutrients and other protective dietary factors in the face of a progressive fall in energy need as they become more inactive and their lean tissues atrophy.

However, the development of a cancer prevention policy in the elderly is likely to be greeted with scorn because of the lack of proof of the efficacy of such measures and the sense that the elderly should be allowed to eat what they like for their limited lifespan. Nevertheless one can advocate the same practical measures on general health grounds and perhaps achieve the same ends (see below).

Vested Interests

Much of the controversy relating to the NACNE report has been set out in The Food Scandal[29]. This should come as no surprise to those who have studied the role of tobacco companies seeking to prevent new public health policies relating to tobacco use[30]. Cigarette companies are now buying food companies to help them diversify and, it is claimed, to give themselves access to Congressmen in the U.S. who refuse to be lobbied by tobacco interests. The problem arises from single commodity groups, e.g. meat, milk, butter, sugar and confectionery industries, because they have to diversify or adjust to criticism and see their market contract. The meat and milk industries are particularly vulnerable if they fail to respond swiftly and appropriately because there is then a tendency to advocate a reduction in total meat and milk consumption rather than moving rapidly to produce products with a low fat content. The meat industry is currently being handicapped by the high fat content of meat products which is therefore harming the image of the industry. This is a challenge which, unless met, will mean that the current wave of vegetarianism induced by concern for animal welfare, will have strong backing from those advocates of public health who seek to use simple messages to achieve a reduction in saturated fatty acid intakes.

2 CONCLUSIONS

The current obsession with reducing energy or fat intakes to prevent carcinogenesis depends on animal, not human, evidence. If standard criteria for developing public health policies are used then there is no case to be made for implementing these policies except on other health grounds. The single feature of current studies, which is extraordinarily consistent, is the preventive role of fruit and vegetable consumption. The evidence in smokers is particularly persuasive and should be implemented as a special need for this group as well as for the rest of the population. Logically the middle-aged and the elderly should be included in these prevention strategies. The credibility of these preventive campaigns will be enhanced substantially by applying new techniques which provide biomarkers of risk. These will be most readily applied to high risk groups, e.g. those with colonic polyps, specific breast conditions and smokers. Translating nutrient goals or WHO values for population average intakes of fruit and vegetables requires a recognition of the differences in energy needs of different subgroups. European populations know the importance of preventive dietary change but rarely perceive themselves as at risk. Novel legislative and other strategies will be needed if current recommendations are to be implemented effectively.

3 REFERENCES

1. U. Ravnskov, BMJ, 1992, 305, 15.
2. W.C. Willett, M.J. Stampfer, G.A. Colditz, B.A. Rosner, C.H. Hennekens and F.E. Speizer, NEJM, 1987, 316, 22.
3. J.R. Herbert and E.I. Wynder, NEJM, 1987, 317, 165.
4. N. Muñoz, 'Gastric Carcinogenesis', Elsevier Science Publications, Amsterdam, 1988, p. 51.
5. Editorial, Lancet, 1977, 2, 281.
6. H. Ohshima, B. Piguatelli, C. Malaveille, M. Friesen, S. Calundo, D. Shuker, N. Muñoz, and H. Bartsch, 'Gastric carcinogenesis', Elsevier Science Publishers, Amsterdam, 1988, p.175.
7. J.V. Joossens, 'Epidemiology of arterial blood pressure. Developments in cardiovascular medicine', Martinas Nijhoff, The Hague, 1980, p.489.
8. WHO, 'Diet, nutrition, and chronic diseases', WHO, Geneva, 1990, Technical Report Series, No. 797.
9. G.E. Bonney, R.C. Elston, P. Correa, W. Haenszel, D.E. Zavala, G. Zarama, T. Collazo and C. Cuello, Genetic Epidemiol., 1986, 3, 213.
10. A.G. Schwartz, M.D. King, S.H. Belle and V.A. Satariano, J. National Cancer Institute, 1985, 75, 665.
11. J. Higginson, C.S. Muir and N. Muñoz, 'Human cancer: epidemiological and environmental causes', Cambridge University Press, 1992.
12. Editor, Lancet, 1981, 1, 1236.
13. TNO Nutrition and Food Research Annual Report 1991, TNO Toxicology and Nutrition Institute, The Netherlands, 1992
14. C.G. Fraga, P.A. Motchink, M.K. Shigenaga, H.J. Helbock, R.A. Jacob and B.N. Ames, Proc. Natl. Acad. Sci. USA, 1991, 88, 11003.
15. W.C. Willett, Nature, 1989, 338, 389.
16. W.P.T. James, Clinics in Endocrinology and Metabolism, 1984, 13, 635.
17. G. Block, B. Patterson and A. Subar, Int. J. Epid., 1992, in press.
18. A. Tannenbaum, Cancer Res., 1945, 5, 616.
19. B.N. Ames, Free Rad. Res. Comms., 1989, 7, 121.
20. W.P.T. James and E.C. Schofield, 'Human Energy Requirements: A Manual for Planners and Nutritionists', Published by arrangement with the Food and Agriculture Organization of the United Nations by Oxford University Press, 1990.
21. W.P.T. James and P.S. Shetty, Hum. Nutr.:Clin. Nutr., 1982, 36C, 331.
22. P. Skrabanc, M. Gibney and J. LeFanu, 'Who needs WHO?', Social Affairs Unit, 1922.

23. WHO, 'Prevention of Coronary Heart Disease' WHO, Geneva, 1982, Technical Report Series, No. 678.
24. G. Rose, Nutr. Metab. Cardiovasc. Dis., 1991, 1, 37.
25. International Agency for Research on Cancer, Large Bowel Cancer Group, Nutr. Cancer, 1982, 4, 3.
26. The Coronary Prevention Group, 'Nutrition Banding: A scientific system for labelling the nutrient content of foods', CPG, London, 1990.
27. W.P.T. James, A. Ralph and C.P. Sanchez-Castillo, Lancet, 1987, 1, 426.
28. L. Santamaria and A. Bianchi, Preventive Medicine, 1989, 18, 603.
29. C. Walker and G. Cannon, 'The Food Scandal', Century Publishing Co. Ltd., London, 1984.
30. P. Taylor, 'Smoke Ring: The politics of tobacco', The Bodley Head, London, 1984.

Subject Index